Physical Education, Health and Sports: An Integrated Approach

Physical Education, Health and Sports: An Integrated Approach

Editor: Albert Plummer

Callisto Reference
www.callistoreference.com

Callisto Reference,
118-35 Queens Blvd., Suite 400,
Forest Hills, NY 11375, USA

Visit us on the World Wide Web at:
www.callistoreference.com

ISBN: 978-1-64116-293-7 (Hardback)

The publisher's policy is to use permanent paper from mills that operate a sustainable forestry policy. Furthermore, the publisher ensures that the text paper and cover boards used have met acceptable environmental accreditation standards.

Printed in China.

Cataloging-in-Publication Data

Physical education, health and sports : an integrated approach / edited by Albert Plummer.
p. cm.
Includes bibliographical references and index.
ISBN 978-1-64116-293-7
1. Physical education and training. 2. Health. 3. Sports. 4. Athletes--Health and hygiene. I. Plummer, Albert.
GV206 .P49 2020
613.7--dc23

Table of Contents

Preface

Physical education is related to maintaining the human body through physical exercises. It is very important for student's health and overall well-being as it encourages psychomotor learning in a play or movement exploration setting to promote health. The technologies that are used in physical education are video projectors, GPS, games and gaming systems. It focuses on developing good activity habits through team sports such as football, basketball, etc. Yoga is also being included in the modern practice as a stress reduction technique. All of these activities enhance the muscular strength and cardiovascular endurance of individuals. This book is a compilation of chapters that discuss the most vital concepts and emerging trends in the field of physical education. It strives to provide a fair idea about this discipline and to help develop a better understanding of the latest advances within this field. This book will serve as a reference to a broad spectrum of readers.

Various studies have approached the subject by analyzing it with a single perspective, but the present book provides diverse methodologies and techniques to address this field. This book contains theories and applications needed for understanding the subject from different perspectives. The aim is to keep the readers informed about the progresses in the field; therefore, the contributions were carefully examined to compile novel researches by specialists from across the globe.

Indeed, the job of the editor is the most crucial and challenging in compiling all chapters into a single book. In the end, I would extend my sincere thanks to the chapter authors for their profound work. I am also thankful for the support provided by my family and colleagues during the compilation of this book.

Editor

1

Learning Model of Physical Education Locomotor Basic Learning in Grade III Primary School

Eka Nandasari[1], Agus Pujianto[2], Tri Nur Harsono[3]

SD N Larikan, Jl. Ds. Larikan-larikan, Kecamatan Doro Kabupaten Pekalongan, Indonesia, 51191[1]
Jurusan Pendidikan Jasmani Kesehatan dan Rekreasi, Fakultas Ilmu Keolahragaan, Universitas Negeri Semarang, Indonesia[23]

Article History

Keywords:
Game Letter Word; Basic Motion Locomotor; Game

Abstract

The purpose of this study is to produce games letter word in the learning of basic locomotor movements physical education at Elementary School third-grade students in District Gunungpati 2016. This research is the development, product development procedure includes needs analysis, literature review and observation, the initial product manufacturing, design validation by the experts, the trials I, product revision, the second large-scale trials, expert review and the final product. Data is collected using questionnaires obtained from the expert evaluation, field observations and the student questionnaire. A descriptive data analysis techniques percentage. The results of the analysis of the initial product of 91% then declared eligible. The observation and the student questionnaire on a small scale trial gained (81.6%). The test results of large-scale expert (95%) to be eligible and could be used. The observation and questionnaire on large-scale test was (86.6%) are feasible and can be used. On a small scale trials and large-scale increase in the observation and questionnaires to students of (5%). It can be concluded that the game is a good letter word that is feasible and can be used as an alternative to the basic motion locomotor learning materials in elementary school third-grade students in District Gunungpati.

Correspondence address :
Dk. Bamban, Ds. Lemahabang, Kec. Doro, Kab. Pekalongan, 51191
E-mail: e_nandasari@yahoo.com

INTRODUCTION

The progress of a nation can only be achieved through the arrangement of a good education. Efforts to improve the quality of education continually done either conventionally or innovative, so that education must be adaptive to changes of the times in accordance with the demands in the national education goals contained in Act No. 20 National education system in 2003 on chapter II article 3, declared the education function and purpose as follows: National Education serves to develop the ability to form character and the civilization of the peoples dignity in the framework of the intellectual life of the nation, aims to develop the potential of students in order to become a man of faith and taqwa to God Almighty, precious, healthy, have learned, accomplished, creative , independent, and become citizens of a democratic and accoun Table.

In accordance with regulation No. 28 1990, Chapter 3, the function of the elementary school was the first elementary school, through his protégé provided basic capabilities. Second, the primary school is an educational unit which provides basic education to follow on the next level.

One of the subjects that could use a game developed in learning are the subjects of physical education. Physical education is an integral part of an overall education process through a variety of physical activities that aim to develop organically, neuromuscular, intellectually and emotionally. Physical education is a process of education through physical activity designed to improve physical fitness, develop motor skills, knowledge and behaviour of healthy and active living, sportsmanship, and emotional intelligence. Learning environments are carefully arranged to enhance the growth and development of the entire realm of physical, cognitive, psychomotor and affective each student (Samsudin, 2008).

Physical education Health Sports are compulsory subjects taught range from basic to secondary or vocational secondary education through activity, with physical activity is expected to learners have a good physical fitness in flower growing age students become subjects in the learning process (Setiadi, 2013).

Physical education has a very important role because it gives the opportunity to students to engage directly in a variety of learning experiences through physical activity, play and exercise that is done in a systematic. A supply of that learning experience geared to fostering, as well as to form a healthy and active lifestyle throughout life.

Physical education is the media to encourage the development of motor skills, physical abilities, knowledge, reasoning value awareness (attitude-mental-emotional-spiritual-social), and conditioning pattern of healthy living that rises to stimulate growth as well as a balanced development. With physical education students will acquire a range of expression that is closely related to the impression of a pleasant and personal expression that are creative, innovative, skilled, have physical fitness, healthy lifestyle habits and have knowledge and understanding of human motion (Sasminta, 2012).

In the national standards of education (SNP article 1, paragraph 15) expressed that the Curriculum unit level education (KTSP) is the operational curriculum are organized and carried out by the respective educational units. The arrangement was done by KTSP with attention to the education unit and based on the standard of the competition as well as the basic competencies developed by the national standards bodies of education (BSNP). (Mulyasa, 2007).

In the process of learning of physical education teachers are expected to teach various skills and basic motion sports and strategy games with respecting sport values (honesty, sportsmanship, cooperation, tolerance, etc.) so that the implementation of teaching not just solely to provide the material, but to build the character of students (Pujianto, 2015). One of the basic competencies in the curriculum KTSP class III to be achieved, namely the standard competition: 6. Practice range of motion of the basics in simple games and values contained therein. The basic competency: Practice a combination of the basic motion path, run and jump with a good coordination in a simple game, as well as the value of cooperation, tolerance, honesty, responsibility and respect for the opponent or yourself. Where the basic locomotor motion should be taught in school.

Motor ability stage owned at the age of 9-10 years (class III) include: (1) learning to relax when you feel tired, (2) studying the problems of nutritional barriers, (3) can use a good mechanics, (4) Overcoming shortcomings as good as possible, (5) trying to master his skills as best as possible, (6) reproduce the activities to enhance physical capabilities with basic exercises, (7) develop muscular strength, muscular endurance, and flexibility (Sukintaka, 1992).

Physical education in elementary school it's very appropriate for the growth of flower children because at that time the children have a lot to get the motion variations are many, with wide variations are many, the child is able to add his knowledge in motion (Rumini, 2014).

Based on explanation above that physical education, basic competence and character at age level (9-10) it can be concluded that learning requires students in terms of movements with lots of free motion of the students become active. Students are given the knowledge of a wide range of motion according to the level of its development, so that students can develop motion capabilities and confident in doing the activities of motion in everyday life. Seen in terms of the development of learning basic locomotor motion then is very instrumental in everyday life by moving students could do something fun. The base is the locomotor motion is the most basic and important is taught to students. For basic locomotor motion from it should be taught as attractive as possible so that the learning of physical education more fun by giving modifications. These modifications raised the values contained in the game. As well as the modification of the game can be make as a medium for reaching the goal of physical education. Based on the background, then route the researchers ' observations to find out how the physical education learning process in particular the basic locomotor motion in elementary school.

Based on the preliminary studies that have been carried out by the researchers ' observations directly and did the interview against the physical education teachers about learning the basic locomotor motion on 7 March to 8 april 2016 in three elementary schools: Kalisegoro State Elementary School, Ngijo 1 2 State Elementary School in Ngijo District, Gunungpati Semarang State Elementary School obtain information that in learning basic locomotor motion class III yet done learning using a modification of the game. Students tend to be passive and less enthusiastic in learning. Concerning the existing infrastructure belongs to quite good, consisting of the school yard, appliances, plastic ball hitter kasti, kasti ball, ball, volleyball, Table tennis equipment, tennis balls and bed. Empirically in the implementation of the basic locomotor motion study found several things, among them: (1) the lack of variation in learning (2) yet the existence of a modification to the game. With game modifications there yet for basic locomotor motion material, thus causing the lack of active participation of students in learning.

From some of these observations the learning process in particular basic locomotor motion material it can be concluded that the need for variation in learning basic locomotor motion through a modification of the game. Based on the background of researchers wanted to give science and innovation regarding new learning basic locomotor motion by using a modification to the process of physical education learning activities that are fun. For it researchers provide material about the basic locomotor motion combined with the games contain elements of locomotor motion learning of physical education with the goal of keeping the learning of physical education became a thing of fun and in accordance with the PAIKEM GEMBROT (Active, innovative Education, creative, effective, fun, joyous and weighing).

Letter Word is a series of game modification of locomotor circuit motion or track, in the game the students doing the game carrying a letter, in the letter there are words that are related to the basic motion of locomotor and students practice what is contained in those words.

Tools used in this sport are in fact very simple, and easy to come by because the instrument used is using some of the unused material namely as: cardboard, bottles, rubber bands, balloons, and pipe. This letter word game can be played in various types of field i.e. rough field, field, and the field of sand.

Based on explanation above, the authors held a study with the title "Physical Education Locomotor Basic Learning Model on Grade III elementary school in Gunungpati district 2016". Based on the above background, the issues examined in this study is: "How Physical Education Locomotor Basic Learning Model on Grade III elementary school in Gunungpati district 2016?". This research aims to produce a model letter word that is effective and in accordance with the characteristics of the students so that they can cope with the problems that occur in learning.

The research of relevant reference literature review was made in this study is associated with the issue of the development of the basic locomotor motion. Researchers did a study of some of the results in the form of theses and journals over the internet.

METHOD

The method used in this research is a method of research and development or Research and Development. According to Sugiyono (2015) methods of research and development or in English language Research and Development is a research method that is used to produce a particular product, and test the effectiveness of these products.

The model that will be developed is the

game letter word basic locomotor motion material on grade III elemntary school in Gunungpati district Semarang

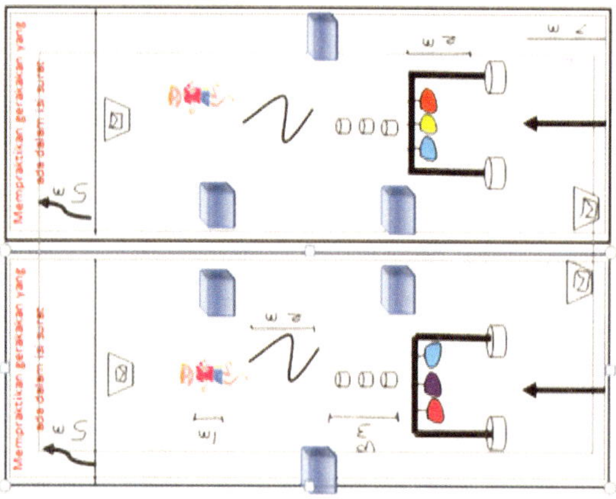

Figure 1. Design

The type of the data obtained in this research is quantitative and qualitative data. Quantitative data are obtained from the results of a questionnaire assessment of elementary school students in Gunungpati district, Semarang city on game letter word. While qualitative data obtained from the results of the evaluation of physical education experts and experts in the form of learning, criticism and suggestions, as well as observations on aspects of psychomotor and affective student. So the data will be retrieved in the form of a descriptive percentage.

The instruments used in this research is a form of evaluation sheets, questionnaires, interviews, observation, and documentation. Data analysis methods used by researchers to study this development is using the technique of descriptive analysis of shaped percentage. In data processing, the percentage is obtained by the formula of Muhammad Ali (1987).

$$NP = n/N \times 100$$

NP = Value in %
N = obtained value
N =the total number of values/sum of all data

Percentage criteria based on (Source Ali, 1987)

Table 1. Percentage Classification

Percentage	Classification	Meaning
0-20%	Not Good	Doesn't Worth
20,1%-40%	Less Good	Less Worth
40,1%-70%	Good Enough	Worth Enough
70,1%-90%	Good	Worth
90,1%-100%	Very Good	Very Decent

RESULTS AND DISCUSSION

Table 2. First Product Validation Design by Physica Education Expert

Physical Education Expert	Number of Scoring
Sum	68
Average	4,5
Percentage	91%
Clasdification	Very good / Very decent

Based on the evaluation of physical education experts after the pre research conducted trials, then the product of the game letter word is expressed very well, so it is feasible to use in subsequent trials, namely test I.

Table 3. The Results Of The Quality Model Of Small-scale Trials Game

	The amount of the assessment score	
	PE Experts	Learning Experts
Sum	72	61
Average	4,8	4,1
Percentage	96%	81%
Percentage Average	88,5%	

Source: trials (2016)

Based on **Table 3** the results of model tests on small scale games obtained on average 88.5% so well stated and worthy of use. In addition to assessment by an physical education expert and learning, do also use assessment questionnaire students and direct observation. Following are the results of the assessment through the student questionnaires and observation.

Table 4. The results of the Questionnaires and Observations students in Test I (small scale)

Assessed Aspect	Average %	Criteria	Meaning
Psychomotor Aspect	75.3%	Good	Worth
Affective Aspect	82,8%	Good	Worth
Cognitive Aspect	86,9%	Good	Worth
Percentage Average	81,6%	Good	Layak

Source: trials (2016)

Based on **Table 4** observations and student questionnaires in small-scale trials seen that psychomotor aspect, recap of the results obtained average percentage is good i.e. 75.3%. Recap of the affective aspects of the obtained average good 82.8%. While the cognitive aspects of the obtained average good i.e. 86.9%. The third aspect of the obtained average percentage 81.6% said that good so worth used in research trials on a large scale.

Large scale trials conducted in three primary schools namely Ngijo 2 State Elementary School, Ngijo 1 State Elementary School, and Kalisegoro State Elementary School. This trial aims to expand the scope of products used in the study of material motion basic locomotor.

Table 5. The results of the quality assessment Model of large-scale Trials Game

Quality Assessment Model In The Game Of Large-scale Trials By Experts				
	A	B	B1	B2
Score Summary	69	70	71	73
Percentage	92%	93%	95%	97%
Avergae Percentage	94,2%			

Source: researchers (2016)

Description
A = Physical Education Experts
B = Learning Experts 1
B1 = Learning Experts 2
B2 = Learning Experts 3

Based on the results of the quality assessment **Table 5** model test on a large scale game, then the implementation of large scale trials are conducted in 3 elementary school, where a third elementary school, Ngijo 2 State Elementary School, Ngijo 1 State Elementary School, and Kalisegoro State Elementary School. The results of the quality assessment model of the game letter word by penjas 92%, earn a percentage to expert learning 1 gain percentage 93%, to expert learning 2 obtain a percentage of 95%, and 3 learning experts to obtain the percentage of 97%. So the results of the quality assessment model of the game letter word by physical education learning experts and earn a percentage of the average 94.2% then it can be said to be very good and very worthy of use. The assessment was also done using cognitive aspects of learning, i.e., affective, and psychomotor through questionnaires and observations of students directly. Following are the results of the assessment of these three aspects of learning.

Table 6. The results of the Questionnaires and Observations students in large scale Trials In Ngijo 2 State Elementary School

Assessed Aspects	Average %	Criteria	Meaning
Psychomotor Aspect	89,8%	Good	Proper
Affective Aspect	85,8%	Good	Proper
Cognitive Aspect	90%	Good	Proper
Average Percentage	88,5%	Good	Proper

Source : trials (2016)

Based on **Table 6** the observations and student questionnaires in large scale trials in Ngijo 2 State Elementary School held on Monday 10 October 2016. The results have been obtained from these three aspects, where aspects of psychomotor 89.8% average with good results then so decent, average affective aspects 85.8% then with the result that it deserves, and cognitive aspect with an average 90% then good results and declared viable. So the retrieved results from these three aspects with average 88.5% percentage of declared good and proper use.

Table 7. The results of the Questionnaires and Observations students in large scale Trials In Kalisegoro State Elementary School

Assessed Aspects	Average %	Criteria	Meaning
Psychomotor Aspect	85,8%	Good	Proper
Affective Aspect	83,6%	Good	Proper
Cognitive Aspect	85,7%	Good	Proper
Average Percentage	85,0%	Good	Proper

Source : trials (2016)

Based on **Table 7** observations and student questionnaires in large scale trials in Kalisegoro State Elementary School held on Tuesday 18 October 2016. The results have been obtained from these three aspects of psychomotor aspect, where an average of 85.8% good results then so decent, average affective aspects of 83.6% then by the results that it deserves, and cognitive aspect with an average of 85.7% then good results and declared viable. So the retrieved results from all three aspects of the good and decent use. the infrastructure, the entire exercise program that is planned can be implemented optimally and can get the results as expected.

Table 8. The results of the Questionnaires and Observations students in large scale Trials In Ngijo 1 State Elementary School

Assessed Aspects	Average %	Criteria	Meaning
Psychomotor Aspect	90,4%	Good	Proper
Affective Aspect	85,2%	Good	Proper
Cognitive Aspect	84%	Good	Proper
Average Percentage	86,5%	Good	Proper

Source: trials (2016)

Based on **Table 8** observations and student questionnaires in large scale trials in SDN Ngijo 1 took place on Wednesday 19 October 2016. The results have been obtained from these three aspects of psychomotor aspect, where an average of 90.4% of good results with so so worthy, affective aspect of an average of 85.2% then with the result that it deserves, and cognitive aspect with an average of 84% of good results and then declared it deserves. So the retrieved results from these three aspects with the average percentage of 86.5% declared good and proper use.

Based on the results of large-scale trials that have been conducted in three elementary schools in Gunungpati district, Semarang i.e. Ngijo 2 State Elementary School, Ngijo 1 State Elementary School, and Kalisegoro State Elementary School. Then the retrieved data from the recap of the third school in a large scale test with comparison results average assessment aspects of cognitive, affective and psychomotor aspects of aspects as follows.

Table 9. Recapitulation of data from all three schools in large scale trials

Aspect	School Name		
	Ngijo 2 State Elementary School	Kalisegoro State Elementary School	Ngijo 1 State Elementary School
Cognitive	90%	85,7%	84%
Affective	85,8%	83,6%	85,2%
Psychomotor	89,8%	85,8%	90,4%
Average	88,5%	85%	86,5%
Total	86,6%		

Source: researchers (2016)

From **Table 9** recapitulation of data results from large-scale trials in the three elemntary school Gunungpati district, Semarang then obtained an average percentage of aspects of cognitive, affective and psychomotor aspect aspect. For the average cognitive aspects of the obtained of 86.5%, to aspects of affective obtained an average of 85%, to aspects of psychomotor obtained an average of 88.4%. Of the overall aspect can be dirata-rata the amount acquired for 86.6% therefore it can be concluded that the overall aspects of the three primary schools with game model letter word can be said that it is worth to use.

Letter Word is a set of game modification of locomotor circuit motion or track, in the game the students doing the game carrying a letter, in the letter there are words that are related to the basic motion of the locomotor and students practice what is contained in those words.

Game rules

1) This game is divided into 2 teams, each team matched with the number of students that were in the school
2) this game is not bound by time, because the aim of the game is the student able to do basic locomotor movements in the game letter word and can mendemontrasikan a word that exists in the letter,
3) order of the players performed based on mobile number sort students because for ease in his judgement.
4) Before the game starts students are given an explanation of game rules letter word
5) The game starts when there is a whistle from the steady starting line
6) Then the students perform game letter word to finish
7 finish line) when the students read the words in the letter then practice those words.
8) When the words in the letter that's not true in practice it, then friends in one group can be put into practice those words. By way of bringing the letter and given to friends.
9) Students must play to completion

How to play

1) students are divided into two groups, the number of groups adapted to the amount that is in the class
2) students marched according with the group his team
3) then when the steady whistles-students took the letter and ran
4) then the students perform a jump with one hand touching the balloon over bergelantung dipralon, students must touch the balloon a balloon without it regardless
5) students passed the hurdles bottles with spring
6) after which students follow the line, the line here meant that students practice walking follow the line, then the students perform the movement skipping 5 times, after the completion of new students open the mail and putting into practice the word disurat to the finish line.
7) when the words in the wrong students practice letter then the letter given to another friend in the group so that it can help put into practice the existing words in the letter.
8) after completion of the movement in accordance with the practice of the letter then the students ran back to the starting line waiting for their turn letter word games do.
9) do the game until one group has done all and turns to other groups.

CONCLUSION

The end result of this is the development of research activities in the form of product model game letter word according to data based on a test I (N = 23) at grade III Ngijo 2 State Elementary School, and II trials (N = 23) at grade III Ngijo 2 State Elementary School, (N = 26) Kalisegoro State Elementary School, (N = 22) at grade III Ngijo 1 State Elementary School.

Based on the results of observation and analysis of the questionnaire is very influential in the aspect of cognitive, affective and psychomotor. The presence of repetition of motion and repair weaknesses then gained greater psychomotor outcomes compared with cognitive and affective aspects.

Based on the results of the evaluation of expert penjas, expert teaching and students point of view it can be concluded that the game letter word meets the criteria of the product well then the game letter word is worth to be used for the grade III elementary school in Gunungpati district Semarang.

Based on the percentage of the results that can be analyzed for expert evaluation trials I obtained an average of 88.5% so well stated and feasibility, to the observations and questionnaire student trials I obtained an average of 81.6% so well stated and worthy of use. Percentage results for expert evaluation trials II obtained an average of 94.2% so declared is excellent and is well worth the use, for the observations and questionnaire student test II obtained an average of 86.6% then declared good and worth to be used. So the trial results of the analysis I and II an increase in trial observations and questionnaires students by 5%.

REFERENCES

Ali, M. (1987). Penelitian Kependidikan Prosedur dan Strategis. Bandung: Angkasa.

Mulyasa, E. (2007). Kurikulum tingkat satuan pendidikan sebuah panduan praktis. Bandung: PT Remaja Rosdakarya.

Peraturan Pemerintah. (1990). Pendidikan Dasar

Pujianto, A. (2015). Pengembangan Model Pembelajaran Gerak Dasar Lari Melalui Permainan Throw And Run Pada Siswa Berkebutuhan Khusus (Tunarungu) di SDLB Negeri Semarang Tahun 2015. *ACTIVE: Journal of Physical Education, Sport, Health and Recreation*, 4(7).

Rumini. (2014). Pembelajaran Permainan Kids atlhletics Sebagai Wujud Pengembangan Gerak Dasar Atletik Pada Anak-Anak. *Journal of Physical Education Health and Sport*, 1(2), 98-107.

Samsudin. (2008). Pembelajaran pendidikan jasmani Olahraga dan Kesehatan SMP/MTS. Jakarta: Litera

Sasminta. (2012). Permainan Kecil. Malang: Wineka Media

Setiadi, A. F., & Widyasari, H. (2013). Model Pembelajaran Gerak Dasar Melompat Dalam Penjasorkes Melalui Permainan Lompat Bergandeng Pada Siswa Kelas IV Sekolah Dasar. *ACTIVE: Journal of Physical Education, Sport, Health and Recreation*, 2(3).

Sugiyono. (2015). Metode Penelitian Pendidikan Pendekatan Kualitatif, Kualitatif, dan R&D. Bandung: Alfabeta.

Sukintaka, T. R., & Soeprijo, B. (1992). Teori Bermain Untiik D2 PG5D Penjaskes.

Undang-undang. (2003). Sistem Pendidikan Nasional. Nomor 20.

2

Development of A Sensor For Measuring Endurance Athletes While Doing A Kick in Tae Kwon Do

Muhamad Faozan[1], Imam Santosa[2], Mohamad Annas[3]

Department of Health Physical Education and Recreation, Sport Science Faculty, Universitas Negeri Semarang, Indonesia[123]

Article History

Keywords:
Endurance; Tae Kwon Do; Sensor; Development

Abstract

The purpose of this research is to design and know the effectiveness of tools developed to measure endurance athletes when kicking in Taekwondo. The approach used in this research is Research and Development (R & D) method. Research subjects were athletes and coach. The subjects of the study were athletes and experts. Taekwondo expert validation results are good with a total score above 83, Expert validation Electro one is good with a total score of 86, For the two Electro experts stated both with a total score of 85. And also from the results of small-scale trials I obtained data that the product has not been effectively used. In large-scale trials the product is declared effective and can be used to measure the endurance of the athlete when kicking. The conclusions of this study resulted in an athlete endurance sensor product during a kick in Taekwondo, And also this product can be used for measuring endurance athletes when kicking. For trainers and athletes it is recommended to try the product as a tool to measure the endurance of the athlete while kicking in Taekwondo.

Correspondence address :
Dk. Cilincing Rt 13/Rw 04 Ds. Datara Kec. Warungpring, Pemalang District, 52354
Central Java
E-mail: muhamad.faozan161@gmail.com

INTRODUCTION

Tae Kwon Do is a Korean national martial artist. Taekwondo is also the most popular Korean Martial Sports and is also our National Sports. This is the most widely played martial art in the world and also in the Olympic games.

In the 70s, Taekwondo in Korea split into two (2) streams, namely the International Taekwondo Federation (ITF) that existed at the time led by General Chong Hi, who was then headquartered in Toronto Canada. The World Taekwondo Federation (WTF) at that time was led by Dr. Un Yong Kim, based in Kukkiwon, Seoul, South Korea. Un Yong Kim, based in Kukkiwon, Seoul, South Korea.

The Indonesian National Organization for Taekwondo is Taekwondo Indonesia. There are two major international organizations that embrace the Taekwondo belt in the world, the International Taekwondo Federation (ITF) and the World Taekwondo Federation (WTF). WTF was established after the ITF. At present, the organization recognized by the international Olympic committee is WTF. At present, the organization recognized by the international Olympic committee is WTF. The WTF makes the official rule of Taekwondo's match at the Olympics. Taekwondo Indonesia also refers to WTF (Gugun Arief Gunawan (Periyadi, 2007)

The match in Taekwondo is twofold, namely kyorugi (free fight) and poomsae (stance show). Poomsae is not contested in the Olympics. The match takes place in an arena measuring 12x12 meters. In this arena there is another 8x8 meter box for the battleground of two Taekwondoin, the fight must still take place within this boundary, beyond the line it is safe. Both Taekwondoin wear Taekwondo standard uniforms along with body armor, head, groin, calf, hand and gum shields (dental rubber). Both types of matches aim to achieve an achievement.

Inside Taekwondo, the use of kicks is very dominant. There are various variations of Taekwondo kicks, all to do with speed and high precision. Taekwondo prefers kick attack, because the kick power is greater than the power hit. Although there are many different doctrines and techniques among Taekwondo organizations, this art generally emphasizes kicks made from a movable attitude, using greater range and leg strength to paralyze the opposite from a distance. Taekwondo has a lot of very effective and deadly kick types to knock your opponent on during the game.

In a match, the 45 degree, forward, ax, and side kicks are the most widely used, the kicks include a jumping, spinning, skip and drop kick, often in the form of a combination of multiple kicks. Kick in the front, with the target of the stomach or the head using the front end of the foot, kick hoeing toward the front using the heel with the target head, lifting the legs as high. The kick toward the back, lifting the knee and then jerking the legs behind the target toward the stomach or toward the head, the kick done by turning the body toward the rear 360 degrees dolke chagi also often called a tornado kick.

The ability of an athlete's kick is one of the important things in Taekwondo, because at the time of one of the biggest points contributor got from the kick. To get a good kicking ability an athlete must continue to improve quality both in terms of speed, endurance and strength.

One way to improve the quality of the kick in Taekwondo is that athlete endurance kicks in, a trainer should monitor the development of athlete ability from day to day but this can not work well if a coach does not have primary data about his athlete's condition, one of which is how the endurance condition of an athlete in a kick in a long time. To achieve maximum achievement there are several things that must be integrated into a form of integrated program of sports achievement. No less than medical science, physiology or physiology, psychology, nutrition and coaching. Hosted by their respective experts, in its integrity to handle athletes at both local and national levels. (Sajoto, 1988)

However, the current problem is there is no tool or technology that can to measure or record the endurance of athletes in a kick with a cheap price and easily obtainable in the wider community. During this time to train endurance only with continuous training and without being able to get data or record that the athlete has increased or decreased in practice Taekwondo kick.

With the obstacles that are in the effort to improve the performance of athletes, in this case the endurance when Taekwondo kick about the absence of data or recordings of the results kick karna training because there is no tool that can to record the endurance of kicks from athletes. So in an effort to increase endurance while doing taekwondo kick and also increased athlete performance is still less than the maximum because there is no data on the results of exercise that shows increased or decreased endurance which later used as a comparison of previous exercises and subsequent exercises.

With the problem so that researchers feel interested and challenged to create and develop the required tools, a tool that is cheap and can easily get in the wider community. Athletic endurance gauge when kicking In Taekwondo is a new innovation tool for measuring the endurance of the athlete when kicking, the purpose of this tool is made one of them to find out how far the endurance of the athlete itself when kicks, the athlete kicks in the pyongyo has attached a vibrating sensor.

Once the vibrating sensor receives vibration, the sensor emits voltage and is received by the next Arduino in the process of extracting binary code which is then emitted by bluetooth for subsequently received by the laptop to be displayed in the form of a display graph.

The harder the athlete's kick will be on the highest scale, and vice versa if the athlete's kick has decreased, the graph will show a decrease on the scale. And the results of the graph can be stored or recorded in the laptop and can also be printed to be able to compare with the previous exercises and the next exercise.

After the preliminary research that the researchers conducted on 9, 11, 13, 14 and 16 February 2017 at dojang taekwondo Semarang City, including Best Gunungpati, PPLP, Mandala, New Star, SSP Thunder, GTC, Sandi Baru, Manunggal Jati, HTC, BSB City.

Obtained a data showing that during this time to monitor the development of endurance athletes when kicking has not been monitored optimally, due to lack of supporting data from the results of kick exercises conducted. And also the trainers need a tool to record the results of the exercises done for comparison of previous exercises and subsequent exercises.

The problem formulation is (1) how is the design of the athlete endurance sensor development product when kicking in Taekwondo? (2) Is an effective development product used for measuring endurance athletes when kicking?

The purpose of this development study (1) to produce a product in the form of development of the athlete's endurance sensor during kicks. (2) Knowing the effectiveness of the developed product.

METHODS

The research design used is a research-based development model (Research and Development). According Sugiyono (2010) research and development model (research and Development) is a study used to produce a specific product and test the effectiveness of the product.

The data collection techniques in this study are by: Observation, Interview, Documentation, Expert Validation.

The subjects of the trial classify the subjects of the trial into two are as (1) Taekwondo expert is referred to is the coach of Taekwondo Central Java who plays a role to determine whether the product of this development is appropriate material and truth. (2) electro expert, electro expert in this research is lecturer / expert who usually handle in electro. Validation is done by using a questionnaire about the design of Electro circuit tools and the effectiveness of the tool. In the experimental product test subjects were 5 athletes in Dojang TC Kota Semarang, while the trial use of this research was 15 athletes in Dojang Taekwondo PPLOP Central Java.

The design of an athlete endurance sensor development product when kicking in the Taekwondo is a new innovation tool for measuring endurance athletes when kicking, the purpose of this tool is to one of them to find out how far the endurance of the athlete is when kicks, athletes kick on a pyongyo that has attached a vibrating sensor.

Once the vibrating sensor receives vibration, the sensor emits voltage and is received by the next Arduino in the process of removing binary code which is then emitted by bluetooth for subsequently received by the laptop to be displayed in the form of a graph display.

The harder the athlete's kick will be on the highest scale, and vice versa if the athlete's kick has decreased, the graph will show a decrease on the scale.

And the results of the graph can be stored or recorded in the laptop and can also be printed to be able to compare with the previous exercises and the next exercise

Way of data analysis This research uses qualitative approach and model development method.

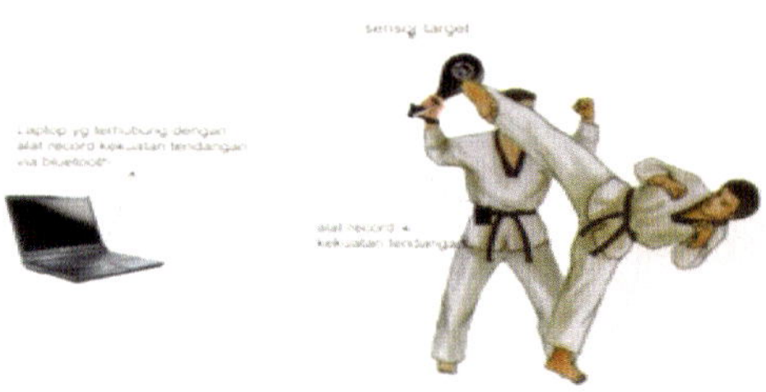

Picture 1. Design plan

Product design drawings:

Development of the athlete's endurance sensors during a kick on the pyongyo that has been installed a vibrating sensor. Once the vibrating sensor receives vibration, the sensor emits voltage and is received by the next Arduino in the process of extracting binary code which is then emitted by bluetooth for subsequently received by the laptop to be displayed in the form of display graphics.

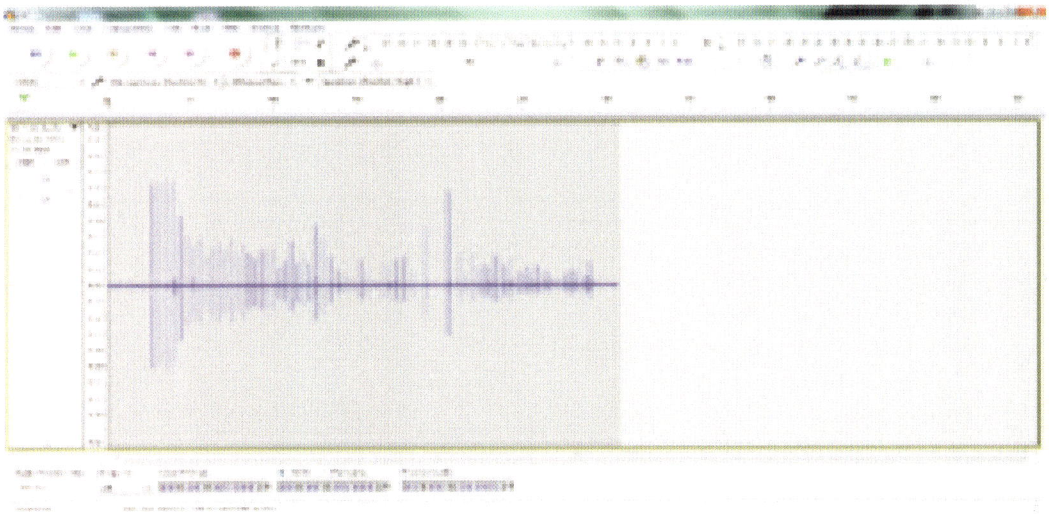

Picture 2. Graphics display

How to read the resulting graph **(Picture 2)**:

Athletes kick at the target with a fast intensity and in a long time, the graph generated after the measurement will show whether endurance athletes when the kick down, fixed or even increased. Because basically the harder the kick done by the athlete then the graph will show on the highest scale, so also vice versa if the kick done by the athlete decreased then the graph will show the decrease on the scale and the results of the graph can be stored or in record in laptops and can also be printed with previous exercises and subsequent exercises.

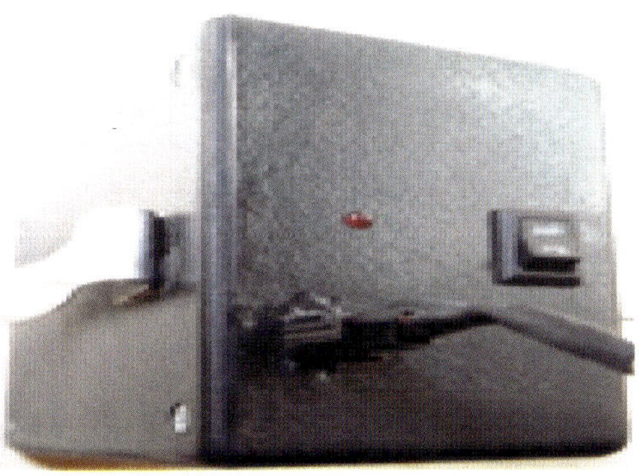

Picture 3. Model boks mikrokontro

In this microcontrol box there are several components as a support for the measurement, the first is the on-off switch to activate the microcontrol box, the second is the indicator light that serves as a marker that the tool is active.

This microcontrol box that receives, processes and sends data generated by kicks on target-mounted sensors and displayed on a graphic laptop.

To be able to open the graph there is an application that must be installed on the laptop, this application can be installed to all types of laptops.

To be able to connect the microcontrol box to the laptop using a Bluetooth connection, but in the validation results of electro experts to connect using Bluetooth is still less stable and it will affect the accuracy of the resultingIn the microcontrol box there are several components as a support for measuring, the first is the on-off switch to activate the microcontrol box, the second is the indicator light that serves as a marker that the tool is active.

This microcontrol box that receives, processes and sends data generated by kicks on target-mounted sensors and displayed on a graphic laptop.

To be able to open the graph there is an application that must be installed on the laptop, this application can be installed to all types of laptops.

To be able to connect the microcontrol box to the laptop using a Bluetooth connection, but in the validation results of electro experts to connect using Bluetooth is still less stable and will affect the resulting accuracy

RESULTS AND DISCUSSION

This small-scale trial was conducted at Dojang TC Kota Seamarang with respondents 5 athletes and aimed to identify and identify various problems such as weakness, deficiency, or product effectiveness when used for measuring. The data obtained from the interviews conducted by the researcher to the respondent or the trial subjects were used to evaluate the product before it was used in a large-scale trial.

The results obtained by researchers in small-scale trials I are as follows. A total of 5 athletes stated:

1. It is safe to use for endurance measurements when kicking
2. Products useful to help athletes to know how good the power tahanya.
3. Four athletes say the product is comfortable to use for endurance measurement when kicking
4. The product can be used for the next exercise, to help improve the quality of the kick by looking at the recording of the exercise.
5. Product has the advantage of innovation, which is in the form of primary data that can be used as a reference for increased endurance in kicks.
6. Three athletes claimed to have never seen a similar product in the Sports world especially Taekwondo.

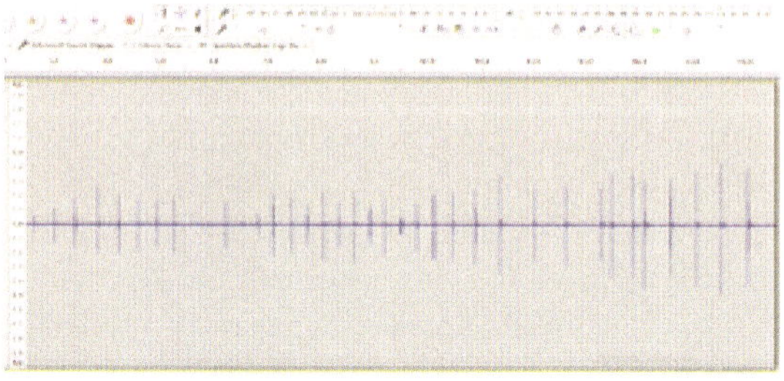

Picture 4. Graph of measurement results on small-scale trials I

Based on the above graph it can be concluded that the endurance of the athlete when the kick is not stable but has increased in the last moment.

Small-scale trials II were conducted with the same respondents and the same number of 5 athletes. The results obtained by researchers in small-scaltrials II are as follows. A total of 5 athletes stated:

1. It is safe to use for endurance measurements when kicking
2. Products useful to help athletes to know how good the power tahanya.
3. Four athletes say the product is comfortable to use for endurance measurement when kicking
4. The product can be used for the next exercise, to help improve the quality of the kick by looking at the recording of the exercise.
5. Product has the advantage of innovation, which is in the form of primary data that can be used as a reference for increased endurance in kicks.
6. Three athletes claimed to have never seen a similar product in the Sports world especially Taekwondo.

A large-scale trial was conducted at Dojang Taekwondo PPLOP Central Java on June 19, 2017 with a total of 15 athletes, along with detailed interview results on a large-scale trial. The results obtained by researchers in the Larger scale trial are as follows. A total of 15 athletes stated:

1. It is safe to use for endurance measurement when kicking
2. The product is comfortable to use for the measurement of endurance when doing kicks
3. The product can be used for the next exercise, to help improve the quality of the kick by looking at the recording of the exercise.
4. Product has the advantage of innovation, which is in the form of primary data that can be used as a reference for increased endurance in kicking.
5. Seven athletes claim to have never seen a similar product in the Sports world especially Taekwondo.

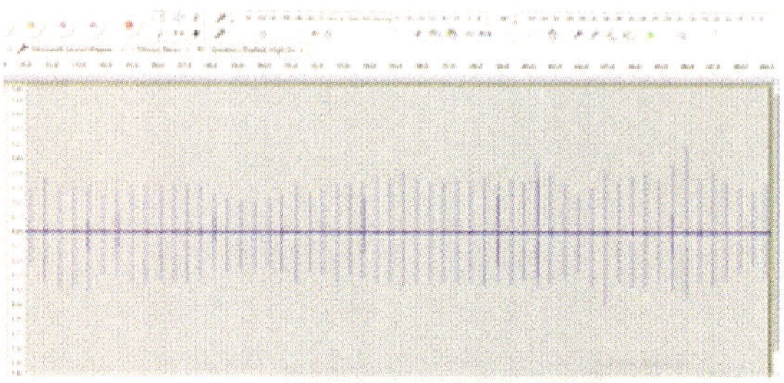

Picture 5. Graph of measurement results on a large-scale trial

From the graph above can be concluded that the endurance of one athlete while doing the kick is still fixed from the beginning to kick until the finish of the chart remains stable.

Based on the analysis of research results and discussion in this thesis, then made some revisions include:

1. Use also a standard pyongyo type, because it relates to comfort and quality.
2. Cables used from pyongyo to microcontrol

box should not be too long can be disturbing for exercise or measurement.

The result of the research is based on the analysis of data description of trial, implementation in Semarang City. for the weariness of the tool how far this tool can be used for measuring endurance athletes when kicking, experimenting effectiveness, observation techniques, interviews, documentation and discussion. Researchers made a new innovation in the form of development of the athlete's endurance sensors during a kick in Taekwondo. In the initial draft description, in the initial design, the researcher focused on aspects of criteria that have been used by Kemenpora in selection and research for innovative sports technology competition participants in 2011.

Prior to the small-scale test, the development of the athlete's endurance sensor when kicking in Taekwondo first need to be validated by expert experts in accordance with this field of research. To validate the resulting product, the researcher involves a material expert consisting of 1 trainer of Central Java taekwondo Dereck Afsa and Electrical experts from academics and practitioners from the Faculty of Engineering, Semarang State University. I Made Sudana, M.Pd. and Tatyantoro Andrasto, S.T., M.T

Validation is done by a team of experts by observing the development product of the athlete's endurance sensor during a kick accompanied by an evaluation sheet along with a suggestion and input sheet. Evaluation sheet is a questionnaire that contains aspects of product quality. The suggestion sheet is used as a revision as well as input given to the researcher regarding the developed tool.

The evaluation result is the value of product quality aspect of development of athlete endurance sensor during kick in Taekwondo by using 100 (1-10 scale) scoring range. The questionnaire evaluation sheet for the quality of the development of the athlete's endurance sensor for kicks in Taekwondo.

The data obtained from the evaluation sheet or questionnaire by expert experts is the determination of the next step whether the development of the athlete endurance endurance sensor during a kick in Taekwondo can be used for small-scale trials and field trials (large-scale trials) the results of filling the evaluation sheet of expert Taekwondo and expert electro experts.

Revise the initial draft of the product, based on the advice of an expert on the development of the athlete's endurance sensor when kicking, the product revision is made with the following details:

The effectiveness of this product is based on the results of large-scale trials. The effectiveness of the product includes effectiveness for the measurement and effectiveness of automated products.

During the discussion to implement the development of biometric sensors for the net of volleyball that was considered final, the researchers presented expert experts. This activity aims to deliver the development outcomes (process procedures and products) to users and professionals through discussions to find out the extent to which research success is achieved.

This development product can be used for measuring the power of an athlete when doing a kick equipped with a graphical data as a reference for the next exercise.

The indicator of success of this product is in the form of analysis from observation result, interview, documentation and discussion with expert expert team that is Taekwondo and Electro expert. According to the product test, it was found that the development of kicker strength sensor in Taekwondo can be effectively used for measuring the endurance of the athlete during a kick. The results of large-scale trials show that the product has functioned properly, athletes and trainers can also see the results of measurements made.

CONCLUSION

Based on the results of the analysis and discussion, the conclusions can be drawn from this research is mengahsilkan product sensors measuring endurance athletes when doing kicks that are suitable for measurement. For athletes and coaches may recommend to try as an athlete's endurance gauge when kicking. See the limitations of this product, to further develop the endurance gauge product of the athlete while doing this kick to fit as expected.

REFERENCES

Periyadi, A. (2017). Hubungan Motivasi, Agresivitas, Dan Mental Terhadap Prestasi Olahraga Beladiri Taekwondo Pada Atlet Kyoreugi. Jurnal Dosen Universitas PGRI Palembang.

Soegiyono. 2010. Metode Penelitian Pendidikan, Pendekatan Kualitatif dan R&D. Alfabeta; Bandung

Sajoto, M. 1988. Pembinaan KondisiFisik Dalam Olahraga. Jakarta

3

Influence of Difference Exercise Anaerobic Interval Methods Against The Results of The Shooting Ratio of Underbasket Height and Long Limbs

Agni Herarta Anindya Satria[1] ✉, Sugiyanto[2], Agus Kristiyanto [3]

Prodi Ilmu Keolahragaan Program Pascasarjana,Universitas Sebelas Maret Surakarta, Indonesia[123]

Article History

Keywords:
Anaerobic Interval Exercise Method; The Ratio of Height and Long Limbs; Shooting Underbasket

Abstract

The purpose of this research is to know (1) the difference between the influence of the ratio of anaerobic interval exercise 1:3 exercise, anaerobic interval and the ratio of 1:5 against shooting underbasket results, (2) the difference between the ratio shooting results underbasket height: long legs and high ratio of height: long limbs are low, (3) the influence of the interaction between exercise anaerobic interval ratio and the ratio of height: the length of the limbs results shooting underbasket. This research uses experimental methods with a 2 x 2 factorial design. Based on the results of the analysis of the data shows that: (1) there is a significant influence on the differences between the ratio of anaerobic interval exercise 1:3 exercise anaerobic interval and the ratio of 1:5 against results shooting underbasket, pvalue < 0, 05. Influence of exercise anaerobic interval with the ratio of 1:5 has better results than an anaerobic interval workout with a 1:3 ratio with average results respectively 9 and 8, 43, 43. (2) no difference shooting results significant underbasket between height ratio: the ratio of height and limb length height: long limbs, pvalue < 0.05. Results of shooting underbasket earned by the sample with a ratio of height: the length of the limb with a low category better than the sample with a ratio of height: long limbs with high category with average results each 19.14 and 16.67. (3) there is the influence of the interaction between exercise anaerobic interval ratio and the ratio of height: the length of the limbs results shooting underbasket, pvalue < 0, 10.

✉ **Correspondence address:**
Jl. Rifle 1 No. 13 09/18 kadipiro village sub district of banjarsari, solo, 57136
E-mail: Pkojaya100@gmail.com

INTRODUCTION

Was a complex game included his movement that is made up of the combined elements of a coordinated motion neatly so it takes quite a long time to master the basic techniques of the game was right. Priest Sodikun (1992:18) "was the basic techniques can be distinguished into: techniques of throw and catch, dribble, shoot or shooting technique, technique pivots or pivot engineering and lay up shot". Of some of the basic techniques of the game was on top of the most dominant in the game was is throwing a catch (passing & cyc-catching), dribble (dribbling) and shoot the ball (shooting).

According to Danny Kosasih (2008:50-52) shot is divided into five kinds, i.e. a lay up shot, set and jump shots, free throw shot, three point shot, and the hook shot.

The goal was in the game is to create the right shots and got a number on every occasion, which is a requirement of that squad was declared the winner. According to Machfud Irsyada (1999:14) that in accordance with the primary purpose of the games was itself i.e. inserting the ball as much as possible to your opponent's basket with a sportive manner in accordance with the agreed rules. The success rate of a person entering the ball into the basket can be affected by habits and a good shooting technique mastery.

Required proportion of proper exercise to improve shooting underbasket. In practice, application of the principles of compulsory exercises note, namely sustainable, overload, the load increases, individual and reversibilitas.

In shooting exercises, problems encountered underbasket teachers is determining the magnitude of the ratio used. Fox and Matthew (1981:262) said the ratio between work and rest in practice speed was 1:3. However, the employment ratio and the rest 1:3 and 1:5 for short intervals is an exercise to develop the endurance (Rushall and Pyke, 1992:210). Shooting is shooting techniques underbasket done quickly and repeatedly recurring, so obviously the element of speed and endurance is dominant in its implementation. Based on this theory, need to research experiments aim to know the increase results from the exercise ratio underbasket shooting interval anaerobic 1:3 and 1:5.

Shooting underbasket divided into 3 stages: prefix, repulsion, while in the air, and landing are performed to the maximum and repetitive. The series of movements that are affected by the performance of the muscles, joints, and bones in the limbs as pengungkitnya. The long limb, in Biomechanics was able to do the leap over and over again quickly, but still efficient in energy use so that the suspected individual is very helpful in doing the shooting underbasket. The individual must be able to maximize the length of tungkainya to produce a high leap closer to the basket, and efficient in energy use so that it is able to improve the results of shooting underbasketnya.

The students at the University of Surakarta Development Shoots can not achieve maximum results in the lecture Was theory and practice of stage 2, this is demonstrated with at least students who pass the test of shooting underbasket. Addressing this, it is necessary to consider the approaches and methods of the exercise of the right to produce a better underbasket shooting, then the authors conducted a study entitled "the influence of Difference Exercise Anaerobic Interval Methods against the results of the Shooting Ratio of Underbasket Height length of limbs".Based on the background of the problem, identification of the problems and limitations of problem then the problem can be formulated as follows:

1. Is there any difference between the ratio of influence of anaerobic interval exercise 1:3 exercise anaerobic interval and the ratio of 1:5 against shooting underbasket results?
2. Is there a difference between shooting results underbasket height ratio: the ratio of height and limb length height: length of low limbs?
3. Does the influence of the interaction between exercise anaerobic interval ratio and the ratio of height: the length of the limbs results shooting underbasket?

Based on the above problems then the purpose of this research is to find out:

1. the difference between the ratio of influence of anaerobic interval exercise 1:3 exercise anaerobic interval and the ratio of 1:5 against shooting underbasket results?
2. The difference in results between underbasket shooting height ratio: the ratio of height and limb length height: length of low limbs?
3. The influence of the interaction between exercise anaerobic interval ratio and the ratio of height: the length of the limbs results shooting underbasket?

The Study Of Theory

The game Was the game's team is a game was played by two good squads of both men and women who each team consists of five players. Played on a rectangular field with a certain size aimed at inserting the ball towards the opponent's basket and holding opponents to not enter the ball. The victory of a team is determined by the number of balls that are put into the opponent's basket (Perbasi, 1990:2).

Basic techniques of Basketball Sodikun Priest (1992:47) elaborated on the elements contained in the basic skills of the game was composed of: the technique of throwing and catching the (passing), dribble Technique (heel), shoot (shoting), motion Technique pivots (pivot), lay up shoot, Merayah.

Shooting Underbasket

Shooting underbasket is a very important shot (fundamental) was in the game. The basic technique is underbasket shooting in the game that was easy to do because it is close to the basket, but difficult to learn, more so for students who have not skilled.

An effective method of exercise to improve the results of the shooting interval exercise method is underbasket anaerobic, because according to the characteristics of the underbasket shooting done quickly and requires great endurance in order to minimize the fatigue which can reduce results. About interval exercise, there are two basic elements must be taken into account, i.e. the ratio between working time and rest periods.

In General, the sport was using 60% of ATP-PC + LA, LA-20% oxygen and 20% oxygen. As for shooting underbasket, work activities with high intensity within 30 seconds, the energy used is the ATP-PC + DINING table according to Fox, Bowers, and Foss (1993:290; 306). So a test shooting underbasket includes activities that use the energy of ATP-PC system + DINING. Fox, Bowers, and Foss (1993:33) say that thinning the number of PCs and resintesa process of ATP occurs in less than 3 minutes. Of that, taken to the conclusion that the ATP-PC system + LA take place within a maximum of 3 minutes. To provide break time, exercise can be stopped or continued with intensity or lower the load. Therefore, the main purpose of exercises to improve shooting achievements underbasket aimed at the development of the energy system of ATP-PC and plus the development of LA.

Exercise

According to Bompa (1990:3), training is a systematic activity in a long time is increased progressively and that leads to the individual traits of human physiological and psychological functions needed to achieve the objectives that have been determined. According to Fox, Bowers, and Foss (1998:288) principles in the exercise program is knowing the main energy system that is used to perform an activity and through the principle of overload (overload) for putting together a workout program that will develop an energy system that is specialized in sports.

According to Bompa (1990:34) there are two things that perl note in principle of specificity, namely; (1) conduct training exercises in accordance with the specific characteristics of sport, (2) perform exercises to develop special biomotorik ability in sports. Soekarman (1987:60) suggested that the exercise had to be specifically to increase the strength or the energy systems that are used in sport is required. According to Pyke, Robert, Woodman, Telford, and Jarver (1991:119) the exercises should be directed specifically towards the energy system or muscle fibers are used, also associated with special motor skills improvement. Exercise program undertaken must be specific, tailored to the goals to be achieved in the sport.

An increase in the granting of the load should be done progressively and gradually. Progressive load exercise means always increases, from beginning to the end of the exercise. The quantitative nature of the exercise load is, the burden of training can be a heavy burden that must be lifted, the number of repetitions set, long a break per set, speed, frequency per week, and so on. For other sport athletes, certainly bahanlatihannya also will be different, for the purpose of training any different. Sprinter 100 meter athlete practicing in order to run the soonest possible. High jumper athlete training goal is to jump as high as-in height. While the athletes pelempat Javelin train with hopes to throw a lembig as far as possible. With the demikin it can be understandable that why athlete sprinter 100 meters the main exercise does not load erupa lifting weights (dumbbell) seberat-beratnya, but speed, mileage or duration of practice run in a day. The burden of the exercise can be an approximate percentage of intesitas exercises, what percentage of the load be taken at the beginning of exercise exercise and what percentage of its increase.

In principle, each individual is different one by the other. Similarly, in practice, each individual also has a different kemampuanyang. The benefits of exercise will be more meaningful and useful when training programs are planned and implemented on the basis of the characteristics and conditions of the individual athlete. Therefore, the individual characteristics of the atet should participate in drawing up the latihanyang program is considered to be executed. Related to this, according to Harsono (1998, 112-113) suggests that factor-faktorseperti age, gender, body benuk, maturity, educational background, length of practice, the level of physical freshness, psychological traits, and others all must come into consideration in drawing up an exercise program.

Physical ability that is owned by a person not settled, it can be changed according to the activity carried out. The liveliness of a person doing exercise or physical exercise can improve physical ability, rather inactivity or without exercise will menibulkan one's physical abilities decline. According to Soekarman (1987:60) said that, every workout results if not kept then it will be back as before. Based on this principle, physical exercise must be done regularly and continuously.

A coach should consider aspects that a component of the exercise. As mentioned by Bompa (1990:75) "efficiency of an exercise is a result of; time is used; distance traveled and number of repetitions (volume); load and its velocity (intensity); as well as the frequency of appearance (density).

Energy Systems

Principal source of energy in meeting the needs of the everyday muscle activity is ATP. ATP stored in muscle glycogen and in limited quantities, are able to be generated through the process of resintesa ATP through the materials that are available in the body. The main source of energy is carbohydrates, then fats and proteins. In a State of low carb eksersi fat burning, play an important role. ATP can be used as muscular activity energy in three ways, two of which are anaerobic, i.e. energy system ATP-PC system and energy ATP-PC + DINING.

The energy of ATP-PC system + LA is anaerobic energy system which is a continuation of the ATP-PC system. The difference is the resintesa of ATP occurs through the process of Glycolysis in blood, glycogen is broken down into ATP and pyruvate. Pyruvic acid lactic acid would be in the absence of oksgen. This is the end result of anaerobic energy system. The lactic acid that builds up in the muscle will cause fatigue in the muscles.

Interval Workouts

Interval workout is a series of repeated physical exercise system and punctuated the break. Due to anaerobic interval workout consists of activity (anaerobic) and rest (aerobic), then the speed will increase.

An effective exercise program is an exercise program tailored to the energy system. While the energy system identified from time and intensitasnya.

The ratio between working time and rest in practice participate determine the outcome of practice. Determination of the ratio can change the purpose of the exercise.

Anaerobic interval workout with a 1:3 ratio is the ratio of 1 to 3 to work time and rest periods. For example, do the shooting underbasket for 30 seconds, then istirahatnya 3 times 30 seconds that is 90 seconds. In practice shooting underbasket, per Deuteronomy was done with submaksimal up to a maximum effort. When you are finished directly calculated istirahatnya until break time is running out, the sample immediately prepared to do Reps next.

Exercise Anaerobic Interval Ratio

1) ratio of Anaerobic Interval Workout 1:3

Anaerobic interval workout with a 1:3 ratio is the ratio of 1 to 3 to work time and rest periods. For example, do the shooting underbasket for 30 seconds, then istirahatnya 3 times 30 seconds that is 90 seconds. In practice shooting underbasket, per Deuteronomy was done with submaksimal up to a maximum effort. When you are finished directly calculated istirahatnya until break time is running out.

The ratio of anaerobic interval workout 1:3 interval is an exercise with rest periods are not enough to restore the ATP-PC, so fatigue began to arise due to the buildup of lactic acid in the blood and muscles. If this is done continuously, then exercise anaerobic interval with the ratio of 1:3 have turned into a exercise endurance.

2. Anaerobic Interval Exercise Ratio) 1:5

Anaerobic interval workout with a 1:5 ratio is the ratio of 1 to 5 for work time and rest periods. For example, do the shooting underbasket for 30 seconds, then istirahatnya 5 times 30 seconds that is 150 seconds. In practice shooting underbasket, per Deuteronomy was done with submaksimal up to a maximum effort. When you are finished directly calculated istirahatnya until break time is running out, the sample immediately prepared to do Reps next.

Height: Ratio Length Of Limbs

Height and long limbs is one of the areas of study of physical anthropology. The role of physical anthropology or anthropobiologis in sports is not new. According To T. Jacob (1991:1) since the Olympic Games of 1928, and on almost every Olympics thereafter always carried out research anthropobiologis on athletes from various sports.

The ideal body shape in accordance with sport learned is one of the terms in sports achievement. Sajoto (1988:11) States one of the aspects in order to achieve progress in the biological aspects of sports is covering the structure and posture, namely: 1) size height and long limbs, 2) large size, width and weight, 3) form the body. Human limbs are divided into upper and lower limb limbs, so the ratio of height and long limbs are biomekanika allegedly can improve results shooting underbasket.

The role of the ratio of the Height: the length of Limbs in Shooting Underbasket

On shooting underbasket, size height and long limbs, as well as the type of stature becomes very important and can contribute to the achievement. Height was instrumental in the sport was, so the higher bodies, the ease in entering the ball to the basket. The long limb size gives a lot of advantages in doing shooting underbasket. Unequal length will give you a better system of levers rather than shorter limbs. A system of levers by the long limb will result in a stronger repulsion, can bring the body higher and closer to the basket. His long limbs produces a larger cross-sectional area, so as to narrow the space motion of doing shooting underbasket, so as to save time. Thus, it has the size of a long limb and supported by regular exercise will then be retrieved results shooting underbasket.

METHOD

The research method used was experimental research method with a 2 x 2 factorial design. This research is to know the interactions between exercise anaerobic interval ratio is the ratio of height: length limbs to increased results shooting underbasket.

Population and sample the study's son is a student semester V Department of Education University of health and Sports Development 2014/2015 year Surakarta Shoots. The technique used is the sample random sampling to select samples that add up to 60 students. The overall student population numbers Son semester V Department of Education University of health and Sports Development 2014/2015 year Surakarta Shoots is approximately 240 students.

RESULTS AND DISCUSSION

The first hypothesis in this study stated that "there is a difference between the ratio of influence of anaerobic interval exercise 1:3 exercise anaerobic interval and the ratio of 1:5 against shooting underbasket results".The results of the analysis of variance for Anaerobic Interval Exercise Ratio obtained Fhitung of 10.715 with significance of 0.002. Because of the significance of price Fhitung for Anaerobic Interval Exercise Ratio smaller than 0.05, then alternative hypothesis was accepted and the zero hypothesis was rejected. Score average Shooting exercise anaerobic interval ratio underbasketkelompok 1:3 (10.7) larger than average score Shooting exercise anaerobic interval ratio underbasketkelompok 1:5 (9.10). Thus, the first hypothesis in this study can be accepted.

The second hypothesis in this study stated that "there is a significant difference between shooting results underbasket ratio height: long legs and high ratio of height: length of low limbs". The results of the analysis of variance for height ratio: long limbs obtained Fhitung of 6.094 with significance of 0.017. Because the price of the significance of Fhitung to height Ratio: long leg smaller than 0.05, then alternative hypothesis was accepted and the zero hypothesis was rejected.

The third hypothesis in this study stated that "there are differences of Shooting underbasketsiswa of antaraRasio interaction Anaerobl Interval Workouts: 3 and 1:5 with height ratio: long limbs categories high and low". The results of the analysis of variance for the interaction of Anaerobic Interval Exercise Ratio and the ratio of height: length limbs obtained Fhitung of 4, 320dengan the significance of 0.042. Because the price of the significance of Fhitung for Anaerobdan Interval Exercise Ratio interaction ratio height: long leg smaller than 0.05, then alternative hypothesis was accepted and the zero hypothesis was rejected.

CONCLUSIONS

Based on the results of the research and the results of data analysis that has been done, the conclusion can be obtained as follows:

1. There is a difference significant influence between the methods of anaerobic interval exercise ratio and 1:3 ratio 1:5 anaerobic intervals against the ability of shooting underbasket. The method of interval anaerobic exercise 1:5 influence ratio better than anaerobic interval workout 1:3 method against the ability of shooting underbasket.
2. There's a difference between shooting underbasket ability student who has a high ratio of body: long limbs "high" and "low". Students with a high ratio of body: long limbs, the category "low" has the capability of shooting better than underbasket student with height ratio: long limbs category "high".

3. There was a significant interaction between influences the method of interval anaerobic exercise and the ratio of height: the length of the legs against the ability of shooting under-basket.
    a. Students who have a high ratio of body: long limbs category "high" is more suitable if using the method of interval anaerobic exercise ratio 1:5.
    b. the student who has a high ratio of body: long limbs category "low" is more suitable if using the method of interval anaerobic exercise ratio 1:3.

REFERENCES

Abdullah, A. 1981. Olahraga untuk Perguruan Tinggi. Yogyakarta: P.T. Sastra Hudayat.

Adnyana, I. K. S. 2011. Perbedaan Pengaruh Metode Latihan Continous Circuit dan Football Circuit terhadap Peningkatan VO2 Max Pemain Sepakbola Mahasiswa ditinjau dari Rasio Istirahat 1:2 dan 1:3. Tesis.

Ambler, V. 1990. Petunjuk untuk Pelatih dan Pemain Bolabasket. Bandung: Tarsito.

Biyakto, M. 1993. Pembinaan Kondisi Fisik. Surakarta: UNS Press

Bompa, T. O. 1990. Theory and Methodology of Training. The Key to Athletic Performance. Dubuque Iowa: Kendall Hunt.

Fox, E. L., Richard B Bowers. et all. 1988. The Psysiological Basis of Physical Education and Athletics. Philadelphia: WB. Sounders Company.

Harsono. 1988. Coaching dan Aspek-Aspek Psikologis dalam Coaching. Jakarta: Ditjen Dikti.

Harre, D. 1982. Principles of Sport Training. FPOK IKIP Bandung.

Hidayat, I. 1997. Biomekanika. FPOK IKIP Bandung.

Herywansyah. 2010. Perbedaan Pengaruh Pendekatan Pembelajaran dan Persepsi Kinestetik terhadap Hasil Tembakan Lay Up Bolabasket. Tesis.

Imam, S. 1992. Olahraga Pilihan Bolabasket. Jakarta: Depdikbud Dirjendikti Proyek Tenaga Pendidikan.

Johnson, B. L. and Nelson J. K. 1986. Practical Measurement for Evaluation in Physycal Education. New York: Macmillan Publishing Company.

Kirkendall, R.D. 1980. Motor Learning Concept and Application. Iowa. WE. Brown Company.

Kosasih, D. 2008. Fundamental Basketball. Semarang: Karmedia.

Machfud, I. 1999. Bola Basket. Jakarta: Depdikbud.

Munir, M. (2013). Meningkatkan Pembelajaran Passing Bolavoli Dengan Media Keranjang Target. ACTIVE: Journal of Physical Education, Sport, Health and Recreation, 2(8).

Pate, R., Clenaghan, M.B., and Rotella, R. 1993. Dasar-dasar Ilmiah Kepelatihan. Alih Bahasa Dwijawinoto. Semarang: IKIP Semarang Press.

Perbasi. 1990. Pedoman Pelatih Bolabasket Modern. Jakarta: Perbasi

Sarumpaet, A. Zulfar Djazet, et all. 1992. Permainan Besar. Jakarta: Departemen Pendidikan dan Kebudayaan, Direktorat Jendral Pendidikan Tinggi Proyek Pembinaan Tenaga Kependidikan.

Snell, R S. 2006. Anatomi Klinik untuk Mahasiswa Kedokteran Edisi 6. Jakarta: Penerbit Buku Kedokteran.

Sucipto. 2010. Permainan Bola Basket. Jakarta: FPOK Universitas Pendidikan Indonesia.

Sugiyanto. 1993. Pertumbuhan dan Perkembangan. KONI Pusat: Ditjen Diklusepora. PB PBSI. Bahan Penataran Pelatih Bulu Tangkis Seluruh Indonesia.

Suharno. 1985. Kepelatihan Olahraga. Yogyakarta. FPOK.

Triaksama, I. N. A. 2014. Pengaruh Metode Latihan Interval Anaerob terhadap Peningkatan Kecepatan Lari 100 Meter Ditinjau dari Rasio Panjang Telapak Kaki dan Tinggi Badan. Tesis

Welkowits, Ewen and Cohen. 1982. Introduction Statistics for Behavior Sciences. Orlando: HBJ Inc.

Wissel, H. 1996. Bolabasket Dilengkapi dengan Program Pemahiran dan Tehnik. Alih Bahasa. Bagus Pribadi. Jakarta: PT. Raja Grafindo Persada.

Yusmawati, Y. (2014). Upaya Peningkatan Hasil Belajar Lay-Up Bola Basket. Journal of Physical Education Health and Sport, 1(2), 77-85.

2004. Peraturan Bola Basket Resmi. Jakarta: Perbasi.

1993. Ilmu Coaching Umum. Yogyakarta: IKIP Yogyakarta.

4

Mapping The Sports Club Students in Bali

Suratmin[1], Gede Eka Budi Darmawan[2], I Putu Darmayasa[3]

Department of Sport Coaching Education, FOK UNDIKSHA, Indonesia[123]

Article History

Keywords:
Statement of a sports club; Elementary school students in Bali

Abstract

The aims of this research are (1) mapping of student sports clubs in Bali province based on sports achievement at elementary school student sports school, and (2) designing elementary school student sport concept in Bali province. The research method used survey method. Research approach with quantitative and qualitative combination approach. The results of the study were (1) mapping of students' sporting achievements at Bali provincial / municipal elementary schools of various sports competed, (2) establishment of elementary school sports clubs to be undertaken by youth and sports education offices of Bali provincial / 3) the concept of a student sports club district / city in the province of Bali. The conclusions obtained were (1) the profile of the students' sport achievement achieved by the elementary school students in the province of Bali, (2) the elementary school sports club was formed in accordance with the youth and sports education policy of the istrict / city in Bali province, (3) a student sports club district / city in the province of Bali.

Correspondence address :
Kampus FOK Undiksha, Jinangdalem Singaraja Bali
E-mail: ratmin-sgrbali@yahoo.co.id

INTRODUCTION

Achievement sports are done by everyone who has the talent, ability, and potential to achieve achievement. Achievement sports are conducted through the process of coaching and developing sportsmanship in a planned, tiered, and sustainable through the competition to achieve achievement with the support of science and technology of sports (Act No. 3 on the National Sport System in 2005). Field facts show that sporting achievements in Indonesia are still fluctuating, requiring the attention of the government, sports actors, and stakeholders in sports. Various sports organizations in Indonesia recognize that the guidance of sports at the basic level as the foundation of the sports building achievement has weak conditions, so it has not been able to face the challenges ahead (Lumintuarso, 2011).

Table 1. Results of Bali Student Sports Week

MEDALITY REQUIREMENTS									
Kabupaten/ Kota	2014			2015			2016		
	Gold	Silver	Bronze	Gold	Silver	Bronze	Gold	Silver	Bronze
Denpasar	42	34	19	44	34	24	36	46	42
Badung	27	18	24	19	37	30	48	37	31
Buleleng	13	19	34	13	5	15	8	9	25
Gianyar	4	10	26	6	16	25	13	11	23
Bangli	8	4	17	5	6	18	9	7	10
Klungkung	4	14	21	3	6	20	6	11	21
Jembrana	15	12	6	23	9	10	9	8	11
Karangasem	6	4	11	8	13	17	6	11	21
	2	7	14	6	3	16	4	4	24

Source: Report of Student Week Sports Week (PORJAR) Bali Province 2014-2016

Based on the results of PORJAR Bali province above shows that the sports coaching achievement is still dominated by districts and big cities, which are more advanced both from aspects of human resources, facilities, management and sports coaching patterns. Sports training has always been linked to efforts to; (1) improving achievement, (2) maintaining achievement, and (3) achievement retreat. Ability achievement is a manifestation of the overall personality of a person. Achievement ability is the resultant of the many capabilities that determine achievement, which is built in the process of training that lasts for years. (Grosser, et.al. in Paulus L.P, 2012).

A solemn commitment to improving the quality of long-term sports coaching certainly requires good management. Efforts that need to be done are (1) Increase the quantity and quality of sports clubs both at the level of pemasalan, breeding and peak performance. (2) Improving the management, (3) Improving the quality of builders, trainers and athletes, (4) Improving the quality of results (Sudono, 2008). Denpasar City in conducting student sports coaching; (1) coaching is centered on sports clubs, in addition to extracurricular activities, (2) the recruitment system is conducted by scientific selection, in addition to natural selection so that the number of athletes possesses large, (3) training programs are carried out continuously through existing sports clubs and , (4) the qualification of the trainers owned by Denpasar City is very high, in which the trainers who have the certificate of regional or national trainers are relatively many.

Student's sport coaching conducted by Buleleng is (1) the training of the students is concentrated extracurricular in school, because they have not been able to optimize the sports club, (2) the recruitment system is mostly done by natural selection, besides scientific selection so the number of athletes is relatively small) training programs have not been carried out continuously, but are still abrupt or approaching competitions and matches and, (4) the qualifications of trainers belonging to Buleleng are moderate, with trainers with local or national coach certificates limited.

Student sporting achievement obtained by Denpasar is very high, always proven to win the general champion. Student sport achievement of Denpasar always experience improvement in some superior sport, even there is record-breaking, whereas student achievement of student achievement of Buleleng is fluctuate, meaning that achievement is still up and down. Students' sporting achievements of Buleleng often experience a decrease in sporting achievements in several leading sports (Suratmin, I Wayan Artanayasa, and I Made Budiawan, 2009).

The steps in the monitoring of talented athletes (James Tangkudung, 2006) are: (1) Observation of students' attitudes in sports, either at school or outside school or in other places, (2) Observation of student characteristics, (4) Selection, screening, or general or special selection by means of instruments to measure the branches of the sport concerned, and (5) Conducting selection based on anthropometric characteristics, ability and physical development. Characteristics of athletes to be a superior athlete athlete include: (1) Quality innate, (2) Good body shape, according to the sport of interest, (3) Physical and mental health, (4) State of good organs , such as lung, heart, (5) Good basic motion capabilities, such as speed, endurance, (6) Rapid and precise adjustments, both physical and mental to new experiences and new environmental adjustments, (7) since birth that can support the achievement of prime, among others, resilient, brave, confident, and (8) Craze to exercise.

Various efforts to improve the selection process of quality admissions by performing several types of tests to select prospective students and have the ability to type certain sports (Kemenpora, 2006). Some important considerations for attracting talented athletes are: (1) having a healthy physical, no disability, expected posture in accordance with the sport of interest, (2) having the function of body organs, strength, speed, elasticity, endurance , (3) have good basic motion, (4) have good intelligence and emotional, (5) have high integrity, and (6) have innate characteristics that can support achievement of prime achievement, among others; competitive character, strong will, courage, and high spirits.

This study focused on mapping student sports clubs in the province of Bali. The objectives to be achieved in this research are (1) to mapping the student sports club in Bali province, and (2) to design student sport club concept in Bali province.

METHODS

The research method used survey. This study uses a combination approach (quantitative and qualitative). Data obtained through interviews with heads of sports or heads of youth and sports education offices, questionnaires, and archives / documents of Student Sports Week in Bali province. Data and information needed in the research in the form of policy of Education Office of Youth and Sports in the form of; objectives, targets, needs for education and training of students, competent institutions / organizations, club names, sports, sports clubs, sports talent recruitment systems, training facilities, trainers, facilities, management, funding, learning and training systems , try out / championships, and sports achievements. The data obtained are the results of sports achievements, sports club concepts, students, sports coaching system, recruitment system, number of sports clubs, trainers, training facilities and infrastructure as well as competent institutions.

The subject of this research is Head of Sports Department of Education of Youth and Sports district / city in Bali. Data analysis used is triangulation of data. Triangulation is a method used in qualitative research, often also done in quantitative methods. The triangulation approach not only compares data from multiple sources, but also uses various techniques and methods to research and capture data or information from the same phenomenon. This study uses triangulation data of various data sources or information. In data triangulation techniques or information by grouping the program stakeholders and using as a source of data or information.

RESULTS AND DISCUSSION

Mapping of Student Sports Club of Denpasar City Based on Sport Achievement

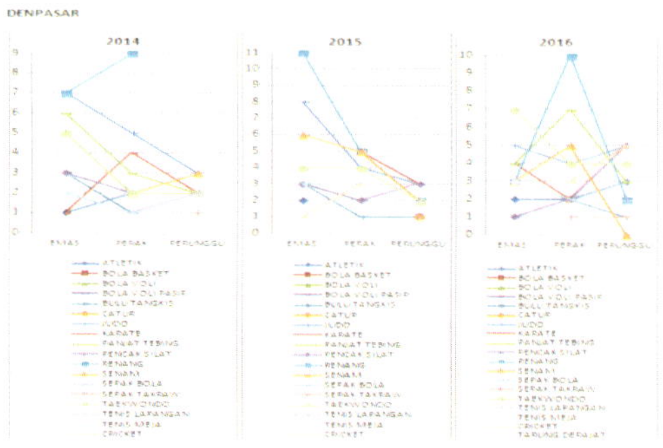

Based on the results of sports achievements in the implementation of the Student Sports Week in the province of Bali 2014-2016 for the city of Denpasar shows achievements as follows: 1) Athletics, 2) Badminton, 3) Chess, 4) Judo, 5) Karate, 6) Rock Climbing, 7) Pencak Silat, 8) Swimming, 9) Gymnastics, 10) Sepak Takraw, 11) Taekwondo, 12) Tennis Court, 13) Table Tennis, and 14) Cricket. The city of Denpasar is a barometer of sports coaching in the province of Bali, so that almost all sports competed or contested medals get continuously. Denpasar city is the defending champion in every organization of PORJAR Bali province.

Mapping of Student Sports Club of Badung Regency Based on Sport Achievement

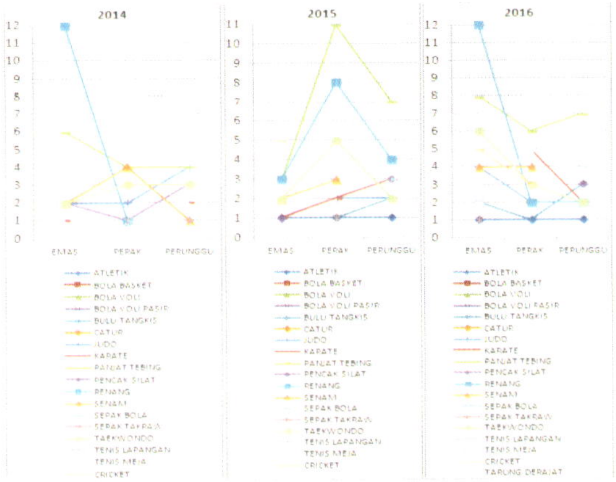

Based on the results of sports achievements in the implementation of the Student Sports Week in the province of Bali 2014-2016 year for Badung Regency shows achievement as follows: 1) Athletics, 2) Badminton, 3) Chess, 4) Judo, 5) Karate, 6) Rock Climbing, 7) Pencak Silat, 8) Swimming, 9) Gymnastics, 10) Sepak Takraw, 11) Taekwondo, 12) Tennis Court, 13) Table Tennis, and 14) Cricket. Badung regency is also a barometer of students' sports coaching in the province of Bali, so that almost all sports competed or competed for medals continuously.

Mapping of Student Sports Club of Buleleng Regency Based on Sports Achievement

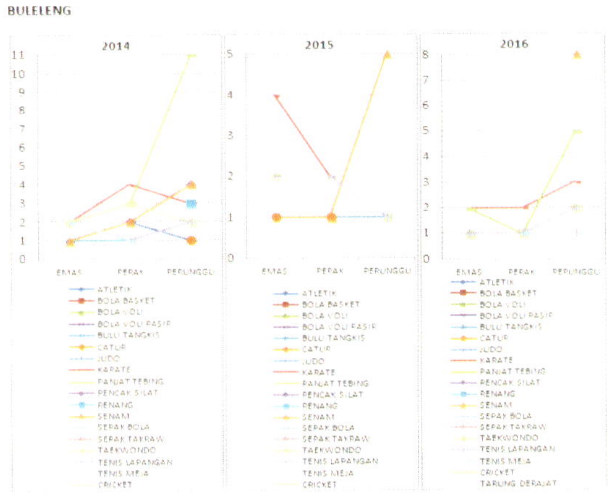

Mapping of Student Sports Club of Buleleng Regency Based on the results of sports achievements in the implementation of Student Sports Week in the province of Bali 2014-2016 for Buleleng Regency shows achievements as follows: 1) Athletics, 2) Badminton, 3) Chess, 4) Karate, 5) Rock Climbing, 6) Gymnastics , 7) Sepak Takraw, 8) Taekwondo, 9) Tennis Court and 10) Table Tennis. Buleleng regency can develop sports 10 sports, so that 60% of sports competed or competed to obtain medals continuously. Sports Achievement

Mapping of Student Sports Club of Gianyar Regency Based on Sports Achievement

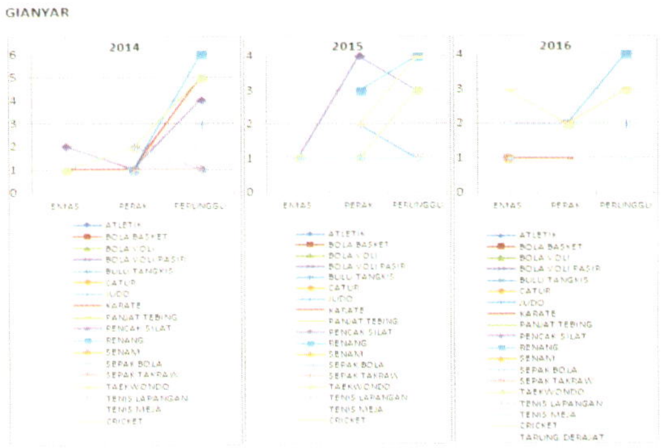

Based on the results of sports achievements in the implementation of the Student Sports Week in the province of Bali 2014-2016 for Gianyar Regency shows achievement as follows: 1) Athletics, 2) Badminton, 3) Judo, 4) Karate, 5) Pencak Silat, 6) Swimming, 7) Sepak Takraw, 8) Taekwondo, 9) Tennis Court, 10) Table Tennis, and 11) Cricket. Gianyar regency can develop sport coaching 11 branches of sports, so 60% of sports competed or competed gain medals continuously.

Mapping of Student Sports Club of Bangli Regency Based on Sports Achievement

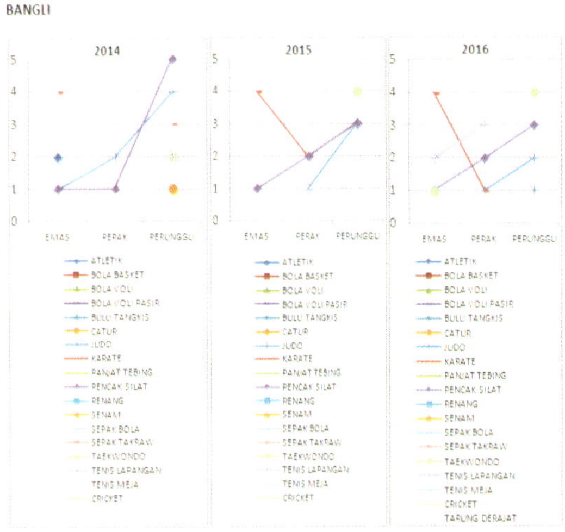

Based on the results of the sports achievements in the implementation of the Student Sports Week in the province of Bali 2014-2016

for Bangli Regency showed achievement as follows: 1) Athletics, 2) Judo, 3) Karate, 4) Pencak Silat, 5) Taekwondo, and 6) Tennis Field. Bangli regency needs to develop the development of students' sports branch, proved that only 6 sports are able to obtain medals continuously.

Mapping of Student Sports Club of Jembrana Regency Based on Sports Achievement

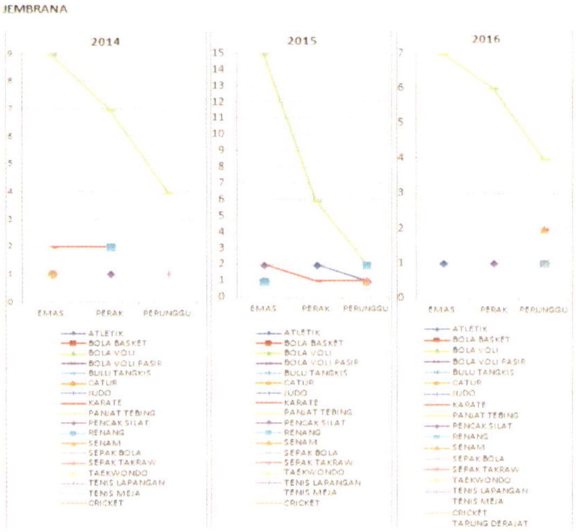

Based on the results of sports achievements in the implementation of the Student Sports Week in the province of Bali 2014-2016 for Jembrana Regency shows achievement as follows: 1) Athletics, 2) Chess, 3) Judo, 4) Karate, 5) Rock Climbing, 6) Pencak Silat , 7) Swimming, 8) Foot Takraw, and 9) Tennis Court. Jembrana regency needs to develop the development of students' sports branch, proved only 9 sports that are able to obtain medals continuously.

Mapping of Student Sports Club of Karangasem Regency Based on Sports Achievement

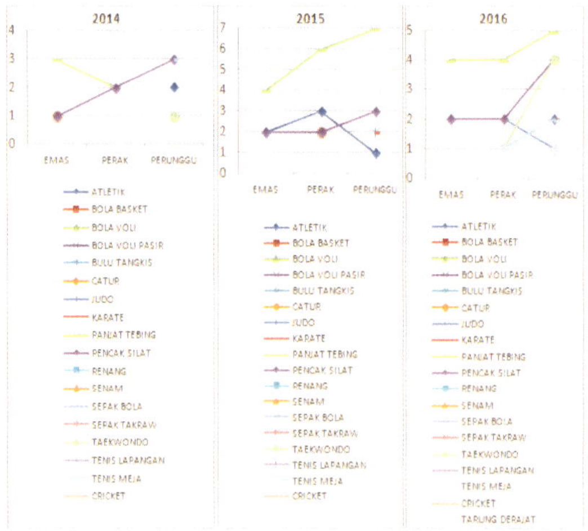

Based on the results of sports achievements in the implementation of Student Sports Week in Bali province 2014-2016 for Karangasem Regency showed achievement as follows: 1) Athletics, 2) Chess, 3) Judo, 4) Karate, 5) Rock Climbing, 6) Pencak Silat , 7) Taekwondo, and 8) Table Tennis. Karangasem regency needs to develop the development of students' sports branch, proved only 8 sports that are able to obtain medals continuously.

Mapping of Student Sports Club of Klungkung Regency Based on Sport Achievement

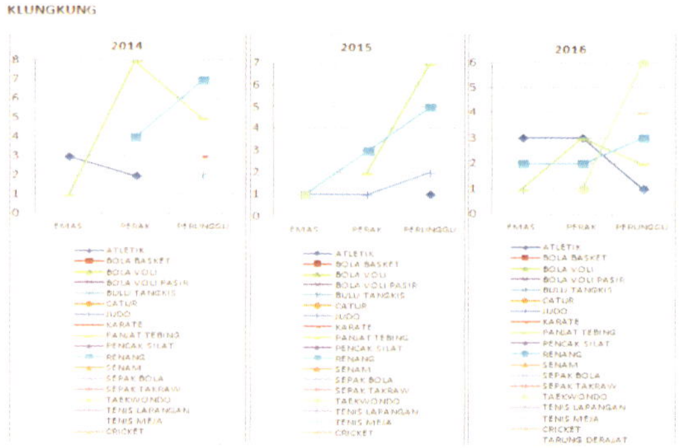

Based on the results of sports achievements in the implementation of the Student Sports Week in the province of Bali in 2014-2016 for Klungkung Regency shows achievements as follows: 1) Athletics, 2) Badminton, 3) Judo, 4) Karate, 5) Rock Climbing, 6) Swimming, and 7) Taekwondo. Klungkung regency needs to develop the development of students' sports branch, proved to be only 7 sports that are able to obtain medals continuously.

Mapping of Student Sports Club of Tabanan Regency Based on Sports Performance

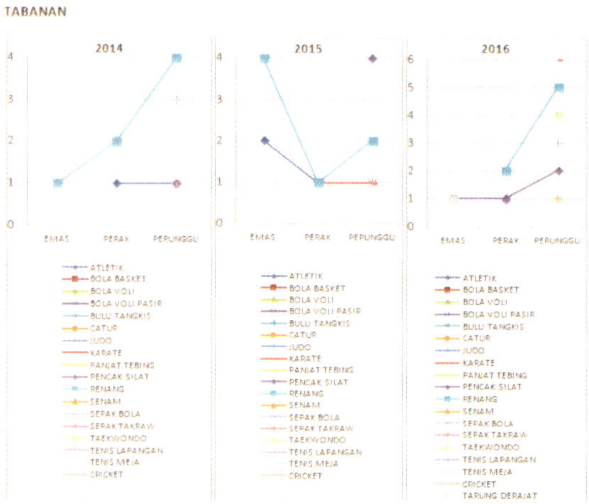

Based on the results of sports achievements in the implementation of the Student Sports

Week in the province of Bali 2014-2016 year for Tabanan Regency shows achievement as follows: 1) Athletics, 2) Chess, 3) Judo, 4) Karate, 5) Rock Climbing, 6) Pencak Silat , 7) Sepak Takraw, and 8) Taekwondo. Tabanan regency needs to develop the development of students' sports branch, proved to be only 8 sports that are able to obtain medals continuously.

Grafik 1. Percentage of Sports Club Policy

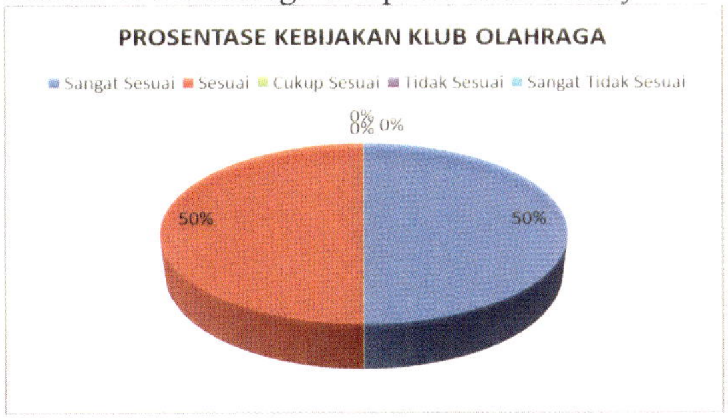

Based on the sample (N = 6) indicated that the perception of Head of Midwife of Sport of Education Office of Youth and Sports of regency / city in Bali province to input of sport club student of elementary school, that is very suitable = 3 people (50%), appropriate = 3 people (50%) .

Grafik 3. Prosentage of Sports Club Input

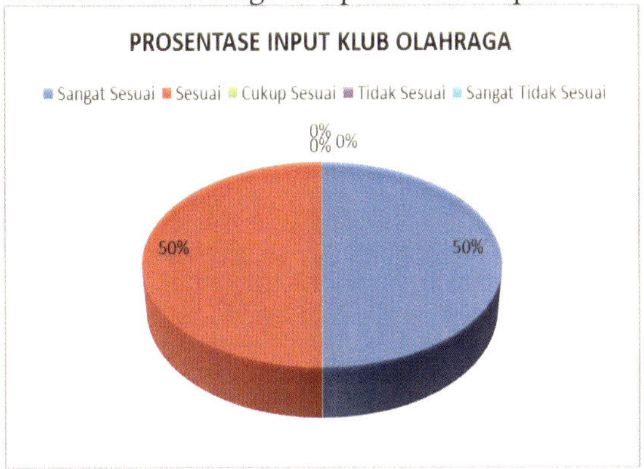

Based on the sample (N = 6) indicated that the perception of Head of Sports Department of Education of Youth and Sports of regency / municipality in Bali province to the policy of establishment of sports club of elementary school student, that is very suitable = 3 people (50%), appropriate = 3 people (50%).

Viewed from the results of sport achievements obtained in PORJAR 2014-2016, the achievement of students / athletes is still dominated by the city of Denpasar and Badung regency, while other areas are still left behind in sports coaching, namely Klungkung, Karangasem, Tabanan and Jembrana districts. Based on the performance achievement, then for the regions that still tend to decrease the achievement, it is necessary to coaching container through the student sports club at the elementary level.

Achievement of achievement is a combination of athlete effort and hard work of trainer, so that both those responsible for the implementation of training program to produce high achievement (Djoko Pekik Irianto, 2009: 7). The sports development of student achievement in Bali province is influenced by the system of training in stages, supported by various facilities, and the target of sport achievement at regional, national, and international level. The coaching of sporting achievements at student sports clubs in the province of Bali refers to the pattern of local and national scale sports coaching, including the involvement of the sports coaches. The training system of students' sporting achievement in the tiered and sustainable Bali provinces needs to be supported by professional sportsman stakeholders and the utilization of sport science and technology.

Development of gold age athletes (golden age), should be able to meet the balance between academic aspects and sports skills. The coaching system considers three aspects of a system, namely: (1) student admissions system, (2) academic development and sports skills process, and (3) evaluation process (Setiono, 2006). Student sports club coaches should be at least a bachelor's degree in sport coaching education, sports education or sports science. Thus the trainer understands the factors of the stages of student development so as to have no difficulty in approaching the students and able to make training planning, make training programs and carry out the training well and programmed in accordance with the plans that have been made with science and technology approach.

A professional trainer is created with authority, educational qualifications, and competence, so that the head coach in his or her job is assisted by a physical assistant trainer, technical assistant coach, assistant strategy or physical trainer, and mental assistant coach. To improve coaching requires a pattern of coach improvement. Qualifications and abilities should be improved. Some of the minimal skills that the trainer must master are; appreciation of professional ethics, the understanding and application of sports science, the mastery of skills in a sport, the mastery of teaching and learning strategies or training, social skills include the ability to socialize, communicate, lead, make humor, influence others, and mastery of training programs.

CONCLUSION

The conclusions obtained were (1) the profile of the students' sport achievement achieved by the elementary school students in the province of Bali, (2) the elementary school sports club was formed in accordance with the youth education and sports regency / city policy in Bali province, (3) a student sports club district / city in the province of Bali.

REFERENCES

AUSSIE Sport. The Search is Over. Australian Sport Commission. 1993.

Djaali. 2013. Psikologi Pendidikan. Jakarta: Penerbit Bumi Aksara.

Grosser, et.al. 2012. Latihan Fisik Olahraga (Conditionstraining) diterjemahkan oleh Paulus L.P. Satuan Pelaksana Prima Pratama (Jakarta: Prima Pratama.

Tangkudun, J. 2006. Kepelatihan Olahraga Pembinaan Prestasi Olahraga. Jakarta: Penerbit Cerdas Jaya

Laporan Hasil Pekan Olahraga Pelajar (PORJAR) Provinsi Bali 2014-2016

Lubis, J dan Heryanty Evalina, 2007. Latihan Dalam Olahraga Profesional. Jakarta : Badan Pengembangan dan Pengawasan Olahraga Profesional Indonesia

Lumintuarso, R. 2011. "Pembinaan Multilateral Dalam Pendidikan Jasmani dan Olahraga Prestasi." Disertasi, Universitas Negeri Jakarta.

M. Furqon H. Teknik Pemanduan Bakat Olahraga (Surakarta: Program Studi Ilmu Keolahragaan Program Pascasarjana Universitas Sebelas Maret, 2003).

Munandar, U. 2009. Pengembangan Kreatif Anak Berbakat. Jakarta: PT Rineka Cipta.

Setiono, H. 2006. Model Sistemik Pembinaan Atlet Berprestasi. Jurnal IPTEK Olahraga, Volume, 8, No. 1

Sudono, S, S. 2000 "Klub Sebagai Ujung Tombak Pencapaian Prestasi Olahraga Indonesia". Seminar Ilmiah Keolahragaan PON XV Tahun 2000. Surabaya : Pantia Seminar Ilmiah PON XV

Sugiyono. 2010. Metode Penelitian Pendidikan: Pendekatan Kuantitatif, Kualitatif, dan R & D, Bandung: Penerbit Alfabet.

Undang-Undang No. 3 tahun 2005 tentang Sistem Keolahragaan Nasional.

5

Development of Stick and Ball Sports on Gateball

Indriyanti[1✉]**, Tri Nur Harsono**[2]**, Rumini**[3]

Department of Health Physical Education and Recreation, Sport Science Faculty, Universitas Negeri Semarang, Indonesia[123]

Article History

Keywords:
Gateball; Stick and Ball; Research and Development

Abstract

The purpose of this research is to make product design development of stick and ball sports in gateball. The approach used in this study is a method of Research and Development. The subject of this research is the Central Java on gateball club event gateball in Semarang and Yogyakarta. Experts and expert expert gateball expert in mechanical engineering. The data analysis phase the work field, and the data analysis stage include observation, observation, interviews, and documentation of the test kefektifan products, expert judgment expert expert gateball and expert mechanical engineering expert. The results of this research are stick and ball exercise for beginner players gateball gateball. The result of the validator 3 expert expert from the expert gateball and expert mechanical engineering product validation data beginning the first phase obtained a score above 73 definitions of the criteria of "good", on the second stage of the product validation data obtained a score above the 81 criteria for "excellent". The results of the interviews to the development of gateball players 19 stick and ball gateball can not be used to play in a match and can be used for subsequent exercises but for beginners a product development tool model stick and ball gateball " INC. "can be used to enhance the ability of basic techniques in motion game for players, gateball.

✉ **Correspondence address :**
Jl. Tangkil-tengah Rt.08 Rw.04 Kec. Kedungwuni, Pekalongan District, 51173 Central Java
E-mail: indripramita10@gmail.com

INTRODUCTION

The sport is any systematic activities to encourage, foster and develop the potential for physical, spiritual and social (Act No. 3 of the year 2005). The scope of the exercise according to the system of National Keolahargaan Indonesia consists of sports education, sports, recreation and sports achievements. Recreational sport is a sport which is performed with a penchant for community and ability to grow and develop in accordance with the conditions and cultural values of the local community for health, fitness, and fun. Recreation of the latin "re-creare", which literally means "reset", is an activity that is performed to return physical and spiritual refreshment. This is an activity that is done the sport whilst working. Activities are generally done for recreation is tourism, sports, games, and hobbies. Recreational sports can also be used as a vehicle of leisure education can provide experience for the child and can shape personality in order to build confidence and improve our ability to know yourself and others.

According to Col gateball is a kind of sport that is unique, as it is played simultaneously between recreational purposes while grabbing feat. Gateball players do not distinguish gender, age (old-young, male, female), this sport is a sport safe, does not require excessive power, no physical contact, as well as a rolling ball above ground level. Gateball is a sport that uses the beater (stick), played by two teams face each other. Each team consists of 5 players, with 5 balls. The first team with a red ball, each ball is numbered 1, 3, 5, 7, and 9. While the second team with white balls numbered 2, 4, 6, 8, and 10. Each player each have 1 ball. Gateball is played in the open field or grassy field was covered with artificial turf, there are no obstacles (trash, stones, etc.), flat square length with size 15 x 20 m or 20 x 25 m (commonly used 15 x 20 m). The uniqueness of sport Gateball is unnecessary physical toughness biasauntuk become players. Age factor is also not snag create playing gateball on national and international events. Thus, gateball is often referred to as a sport without limits.

Gateball sports entered in Semarang areas beginning in 2012 that was introduced to employees of Large Hall area of the river Pemali. Until now in the Hall of the River Pemali Juana has two clubs. Once introduced in a large Hall area of the river Pemali Juana recently spread in Dinasservice area of Semarang, gateball Club which has around the Office of the province of Central Java.

Preliminary results of a study it conducted on February 12, 2017 at the service of the Central Java province PSDA, Mina Clan in Central Java, the Balai Besar area of the river Pemali Juana, PLN Central Java province, Copyright works of Central Java province, Department of youth and Sports Central Java, Bina Marga (Teak Coral Equipment Units), SD N Wells Banyumanik Boto. Obtained results that according to the opinions of the various clubs, Gateball can not develop to its full potential, one of the reasons is the high stick, produced by Japan gateball and balls, the difficulty of getting the gear stick and ball gateball, even though the stick and the ball is the main equipment in the game of gateball. Stick, produced by Japan's existing excess with a stick made by machinery manufacturers so that the result is nice but there are drawbacks, namely the price is expensive and difficult in Indonesia because it had to Import directly from Japan. On the basis of the background mentioned above, then the researchers intend to develop a form of tool stick and ball gateball with title of research in the form of "development of stick and ball sports on gateball".

Development of gateball constraints experienced in Semarang, so have not been able to develop in the society to the maximum, as well as other sports such as soccer, basketball, volleyball, badminton, and others. Whereas gateball already applied to the international arena. (Attaqi, 2016) Indonesia has great potential to become a Hockey stick manufacturer. Indonesia has abundant wood and good quality and skilled human resources, sophisticated and modern wood processing machines are also owned by timber companies in Indonesia. But in reality Indonesia is still dependent on Hockey import stick. If Indonesia continues to rely on other countries' products, it is clear that the achievements and sports industry in Indonesia will not be able to move forward. Problems that can be identified is an expensive tool, tools that are difficult to get, a long bureaucracy to get tools, a new sport, a sport that has not been popular.

A research certainly has problems that need to be researched, analyzed, and kept to a possible solution. In this research the problems that need to be formulated is how product design development of stick and ball sports in gateball. Aiming to make product design development of stick and ball sports on gateball produced by Japan.

METHODS

The research design used in this research is research development (research and development). According to (Sugiyono, 2010) research methods development research is a method used to produce a particular product, and to assess the effectiveness of these products. Another case, to produce a specific product is required and needs analysis to test the effectiveness of these products.

In research and development is focused to produce a tool of stick and ball gateball for athletes beginner. Measures development in the study of appropriate measures of research development of Research and Development (R&D) in **picture 1**.

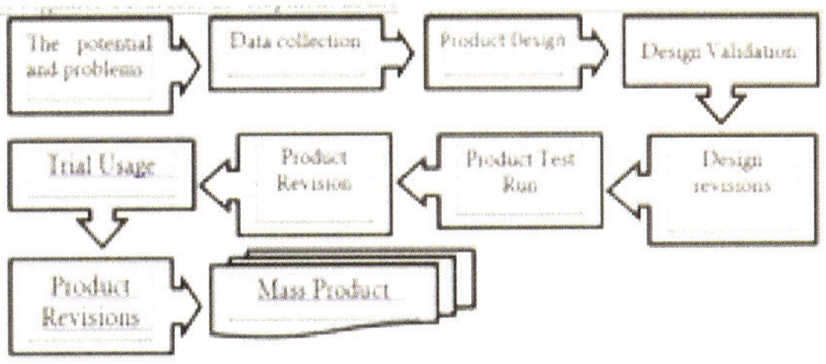

Picture 1. Measures the use of methods of Research and Development (R&D).Source: (Borg and Gall in sogiyono's book)

The subject of small-scale trials I & II implemented in Semarang city with 8 players gateball. And large scale trials in the city of Yogyakarta, with 19 players gateball.

This development in the study, researchers used the experts expert review the material and mechanical experts to observe and measure the quality of products (kevalidan, practicality, and effectiveness) products are made.

Design of products made in the development of stick and ball gateball are as follows:

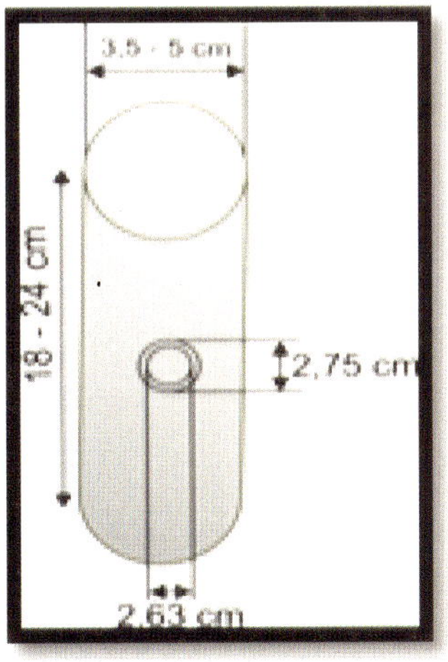

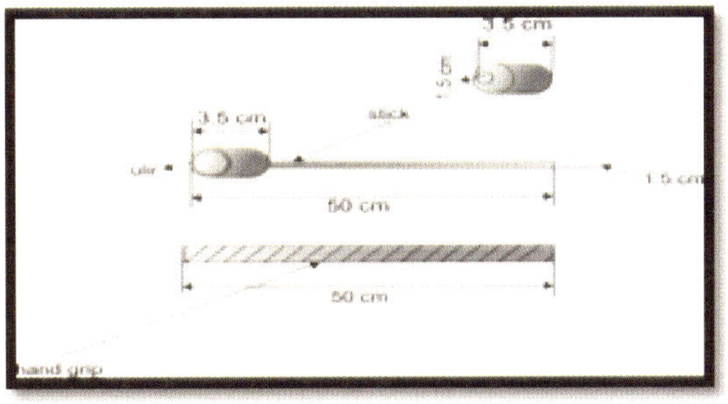

Picture 2. head and body stick
Source : (documenting the researcher, 2017)

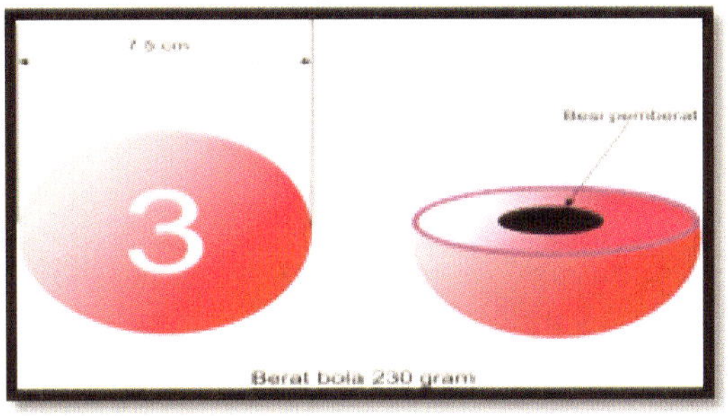

Picture 3. gateball ball
Source: (documenting the researcher, 2017)

Engineering data collection done in research development, as follows: observation, interview and documentation of data analysis techniques used are descriptive use percentage to know the validity of product experts and response receivable expert/experts and players against products stick and ball gateball through question form provided by researchers. While the data in the form of advice and reason of choosing the answers are analyzed using qualitative analysis techniques. The formula used in the percentage of data processing are as follows:

$$P = \frac{\sum Xi}{\sum Xi} \times 100\%$$

Description
P = Presentage
$\sum Xi$ = The amount of Score study by coach or Athlete
$\sum Xj$ = The Amount Of The Maximum Score
100 % = Konstanta

From the results of the percentage obtained is then classified to derive the conclusion of data, in table 1 will be presented the classification of percentage

Table 1. The Classification Of The Percentage

Percentage	Classification	Meaning
75 – 100 %	Very Good	Very Decent Used

50 – 75 %	Good	Feasibility
25 – 50 %	Less Good	Fixed
0 – 25 %	Not Good	Not Worth To Use

Source : (Sugiyono, 2016)

RESULTS AND DISCUSSION

Small-scale Trials I & II

After the product development of stick and ball gateball treated small-scale trials I & II and revised and discussed with experts and expert engineers gateball product development model stick and ball gateball ready to do a test scale small II in gateball players.

The following is a breakdown of the number of players gateball (respondent) used in small-scale trials II:

Table 2. List Of Small Scale Trials Of Gateball

Name	Age	Team
Apriyandi Idris	28	Pen
Purbo rokhman	31	Pen
Sugeng priyono	45	Pen
Mada ikrar S	35	Pen
Bayu Edhi C. S.	30	Pen
Budhi Santoso	41	Pen
Yoyok Haryo	50	Pen
Sri Wahyuningsih	49	Pen

This test aims to find out and identify the various weaknesses, deficiencies, excess, and the effectiveness of the product when used by players of gateball. The photo attached to the attachment.

Data obtained from the results of interviews conducted by researchers to the respondents or subjects of a test used to evaluate a product before it is used in a tested wide scale usage. The **table 3** details the results of the interviews have been done researchers in small-scale trials II against gateball players is as follows.

By looking at the **table 3**, then the results obtained by researchers in a small scale test II is as follows:

1. The product is safe to use for gateball players exercise
2. Products already comfortably used for gateball players exercise
3. The product is in compliance with the physical size of gateball players
4. The product still used for gateball players exercise
5. The product can not be used to play
6. The product can not be used for the next exercise

For complete data and as part of a triangulation carried out discussions with experts experts gateball. After the test run finishes placing experts discussion experts to assess whether the development of the product stick and ball and gateball are effective when used by players of gateball.

After the inspection data with through discussion with 3 people and 1 gateball expert expert expert expert mechanical engineering, then obtained the results that the product development model stick and ball and gateball are effective when used for players gateball in small trials I headed to small scale II and can proceed to test your usage (broad-scale trials). After small-scale trials I towards small-scale II and prior to the implementation of the broad-scale trials, much needed feedback, suggestions and comments on the development model of stick and ball gateball.

Table 3. The results of the interview against the players in gateball small-scale trials

Substance	The results of the interviews the cast of gateball								Result
	1	2	3	4	5	6	7	9	
Security	√	√	√	√	√	√	√	√	Secure products
comfort	√	√	√	√	√	√	√	√	Cozy products
Size	√	√	√	√	√	√	√	√	The size corresponds to the size of the physical
A load of stick and ball	_	_	_	_	_	_	_	_	The weight of unresolved
Uses to play	_	_	_	_	_	_	_	_	The product can not be used to play
Uses for the next exercise	_	√	_	_	√	_	_	_	The product can not be used in the next exercise

Product Revision After Tests Small Scale II

Based on advice from experts of the expert on the development model of tool stick and ball of gateball which has tested cobakan in scale, then the focus of researchers to prepare product development to prepare to test the use (test wide scale).

Wide scale Trials

Wide scale trials conducted in the field of Shiva of Prambanan, Yogyakarta. The number of athletes that used in a trial of a wide scale is 3 club. (Picture attached documcntation) thc following is a breakdown of the number of players gateball (respondent) used in wide scale test:

Table 4. List of gateball wide scale trials

Athlete Name	Age	Team
Apriyandi Idris	28	Pen
Purbo rokhman	31	Pen
Sugeng priyono	45	Pen
Mada ikrar S	35	Pen
Bayu Edhi C. S.	30	Pen
Sugeng Santoso	48	Pen
Ali Sodiqin	21	Retto
Astriana Yasika Maida	22	Retto
Dandy Prastyanto	24	Bengawan Solo
Deni Purwani	24	Retto
Muhsin Catur	24	Retto
Fathurahman	38	Borobudur
Sukar	40	Borobudur
Aryanto	41	Borobudur
Masrufan F	38	Borobudur
Anton S	40	Borobudur
Adi Panuwun	37	Borobudur
Rafael Warsidi	39	Borobudur
Bayu Kristiaji	45	Borobudur

At this stage of the analysis of the trial data, this wide scale data observations, interviews and documentation analyzed in analytical diskriptif by doing pencermatan and in-depth examination of the information and or feedback that can be dijaring from the test subjects try. To selengkapi data and as part of a triangulation carried out discussions with experts experts gateball. Indicator to determine whether the results of the development of the product stick and ball gateball is in compliance with the purpose of the research was to the way athletes do short punches and blows away with using the product development of stick and ball gateball the observer (researcher and expert scholars) doing observations and pencermatan. As well as collecting the results of the interview against the respondents (subject tests). The table details the results of the interview that has channeled researcher in wide scale trials against players gateball.

From **table 4.** then results obtained by researchers in the wide scale trials are as follows:

1. The product is safe to use for gateball playcrs cxercise
2. Products already comfortably used for gateball players exercise
3. The product is in compliance with the physical size of gateball players
4. The product still heavy when used for gateball players exercise
5. The product can be used to play
6. The product can not be used for the next exercise

After completing the data and as part of a triangulation carried out discussions with experts/expert team validator and a gateball players also be respondents at large scale trials/area. Discussions do give some questions that aims to see the extent of the feasibility of the development that has been done. Summary of trial results testing/usage wide scale i.e. products in both the criteria and the product is said to be worthy of use for beginner players.

Comparison of initial and final products can be seen in the following **table 5**:

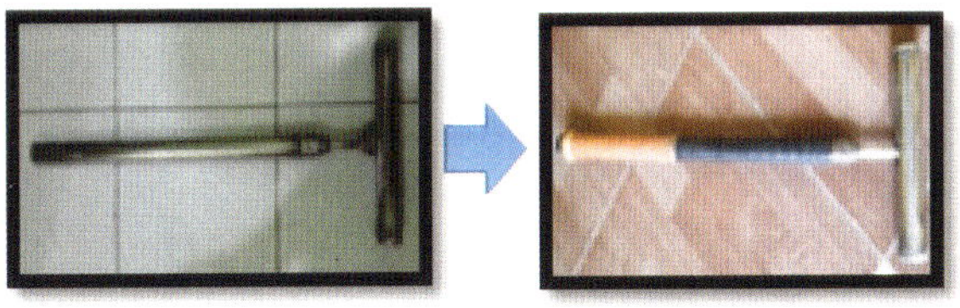

Picture 5. Initial products and end products

Table 5. product comparisons early and final product

Early product	The end product
Grip stick still in a State of open without a grip that wraps.	Grip stick already bundled in with a neat denghan grip using the basic rackets.

The end of the handle still open without any cap on the handle grip dipunggung.	The end of the handle of the stick already covered by using a pedestal table that is made of rubber.
The color stick still naturan with metal scrap welding	The color stick is already diamplas and already cleared from the former las.
The length of the stick 50 cm	same
Diameter of stick 4.47 cm	3.9 cm in diameter
The weight of the head of the stick 600 grams	Weight 400 grams
The weight of the ball 300 grams	Same

Product specifications development of Stick and Ball Gateball. Development of gateball ball and stick model has specifications:

1. The head of the Stick gateball has a length of 20 cm
2. The Diameter of the head stick 3.9 cm
3. The length of the rod stick 50 cm
4. Material stick stainless
5. natural Color stick
6. The weight of the ball 300 grams
7. ball Diamater 7.4 cm
8. The color of the ball that is already a patent that is red and white.

By looking at the comparison chart between the stick and the local stick then import can be drawn the following conclusions:

Aspects of Orisinilitas

Product development model stick and ball gateball is a result of researchers with distinguishing features compared to existing sports technology, so it is the tangible results of ideas, thoughts, concepts of invalid constructs which belonged to researchers with intent and purpose is as a business as well as its efforts in helping to increase achievement and develop the sport of gateball.

Aspects of Innovation Excellence

Product development model stick and ball have in the work of innovative gateball, materials, use and maintenance. By looking at the ingredients used in the manufacture of using only local ingredients.

Economic Aspects

Product development of stick and ball gateball have economical and affordable and have a high effectiveness for a broad audience in favor of sports coaching gateball. By looking at the price that must be removed if we see a product stick import costs Rp. 700,000.00 USD 1,000,000.00 >-and the price of imported ball costing Rp > 600,000.00. Product development with a stick and a ball of gateball for Rp. 400,000.00 to stick and IDR 250,000.00 for the ball. It also could provide jobs and empower local communities in making product development of stick and ball gateball.

The aspect of comfort and security

Product development of stick and ball gateball have safety and comfort level is good for players gateball. Evidenced by the stick adjustable short length according to the size of the physical Jock gateball stick without feeling and mind.

To facilitate us in looking at the effectiveness, advantages or weaknesses between the product stick gateball import compared to product development stick gateball. You can see the **table 6** as follows:

Table 6. table product development effectiveness of stick and ball gateball

Product import	Local Product	Result
Stick and ball made of gateball import	The ingredients stick and balls made local gateball dri local ingredients	The product has the edge on the orisinilitas
Price from Rp import gateball stick. 700,000.00 USD 1,000,000.00 >-and priced the ball imports reached Rp. 700,000.00.	The price of the local Rp gateball stick 400,000.00 and local Rp 250,000.00 ball.	The product stick and ball have the advantage of local Economical gateball.
Making use of machine technology	The manufacturing process by means of empowering communities (the welder)	Product development of stick and ball Orisinilitas aspects have the advantage of gateball and Economics

The weight of the head of the stick: 500 g	The weight of the balls stick: 400 g	The product has an innovative excellence aspect
Long head stick: 18-24 cm	Long head stick: 20 cm	
The surface of the stick: 3.5-5 cm	The surface of the stick: 4.47 cm	
Length: 50 cm stick rods	Length: 50 cm stick rods	
Ball weight: 230 g	Ball weight: 300 g	
Ball diameter: 7.5 cm	Ball diameter: 7.4 cm	
Color in accordance with the terms of the factories	Colors can be customized with a desire	The product has the advantage of innovative

CONCLUSION

After going through the process of model development tools through a stage which is a modification of the Brog and Gall then researchers produce a product development tool models are stick and ball gateball named "Inc. (Indri Colection)". Based on the results of the discussion in this research it can be concluded that: 1). product development model stick and ball gateball "INC." can be used as a means of practicing the blow for the player, 2 gateball). product model development tool stick and ball gateball "INC." can be used to enhance the ability of basic techniques in motion game for the players of gateball, 3).Product development model stick and ball gateball "Inc." can be used to play a game of gateball players.

REFERENCES

Attaqi, I., et all. (2016). Pengembangan Model Alat Stick Hockey Untuk Latihan Pemain Pemula Hockey. ACTIVE: Journal Of Physical Education, Sport, Health And Recreation, 5(3), 151-157.

Kotler, P. & Garry, A. 2001. Prinsip-prinsip Pemasaran. Alih Bahasa Imam Nurmawan. Jakarta:Erlangga. (dalam Tommy Soenyoto, 2013)

Kotler, P. 2002 Manajemen Pemasaran, Jilid I, Ed. Milenium. Jakarta: PT. Prebalindo. (dalam Tommy Soenyoto, 2013)

PB PERGATSI. 2015. Peraturan Gateball dan Pedoman Wasit WGU 2015. Jakarta

Purnomo, E. 1997. "Peranan Iptek Dalam Olahraga". Jurnal Cakrawala Pendidikan (XVI), 3: 63-69

Sugiyono. 2010. Metode Penelitia Pendidikan, Pendekatan Kuantitatif, Kualitatif, dan R&D. Bandung: Alfabeta

Undang-Undang Republik Inonesia Nomor 3 Tahun 2005 tentang Sistem Keolahragaan Nasional. 2007. Jakarta: Kementrian Negara Pemuda dan Olahraga Republik Indonesia.

6

Study of Extracurricular Karate Evaluation Towards Achievement of Students Karate

Gestiawan Candra Pramulyarso[1], Imam Santosa CWW[2]

Jurusan Pendidikan Jasmani Kesehatan dan Rekreasi, Fakultas Ilmu Keolahragaan, Universitas Negeri Semarang, Indonesia[12].

Article History

Keywords:
Evaluation Study; Development; Extracurricular; Karate

Abstract

The purpose of this research is to figure out the development of karate extracurricular in SMA N 1 Slawi, SMA N 2 Slawi and SMA N 1 Bojong. This is a qualitative research with percentage descriptive approach. The result shows that there are some disadvantages in the development of karate exracuriccular so that the student's karate achievement in Tegal Regency is not maximum. First, there is no selection for athletes. Second, the programs for training have not been implemented well. Also the coaches do not have legal certificate. Third, the infrastructures for karate have not supported the athlete's achievement yet. Fourth, the management of karate organization does not run well. The last, karate extraxurricular does not get enough funds to support their activities. Based on the data obtained from the research, it can be concluded that there are some constraints which hamper the efforts to get higher achievement in karate.

Correspondence address: :
Desa Bumijawa, Rt 06-Rw02 Kecamatan Bumijawa, Kabupaten Tegal, 52466
E-mail : candragestiawan@gmail.com

INTRODUCTION

Sport karate martial art that originated in Japan spread to all corners of the world and well known in the vicinity of the 1950s, but at that time not yet visible entry into Indonesia. Then in 1964, a number of Indonesia founded PORKI karateka (Persatuan Olahraga Karate Indonesia).

In the early 1960s, the Government of Indonesia managed to claim the Japan war appropriation to pay as compensation for past events when Japan never invades the nation Indonesia 1942-1945 years. One of the compensations was awarded scholarships on student Indonesia to study in Japan.

In addition to general studies in various disciplines in the College, the youth also have the chance studied Japanese martial arts, namely Karate. They practice karate like Shotokan from various schools, Gojukai, Wadokai and others. The flow of the most widely followed karate is the flow of Shotokan. The youth brought in karate to Indonesia.

After entering in Indonesia, Karate is thriving and appears many colleges in addition to Shotokan. Therefore, PORKI later renamed FORKI (Federasi Karatedo Indonesia). FORKI be the parent of the whole College karate in Indonesia. FORKI later recognized by KONI (Komite Olahraga Nasional Indonesia) the Centre, and the program for the first time in PON 1973. However, the regulation of their games continues to use regulations PORKI.

Pay attention to the development of karate in Indonesia grew rampant, then in 1972 by as much as 24 College karate in Indonesia agreeing to join entry in the shadow of one of the national mentoring organization container FORKI. The names of 24 College karate which States, joined the FORKI, yaitu: AMURA, BKC, BLACK PANTHER, FUNAKOSHI, GABDIKA SHITORYU, GOJUKAI, GOJU RYU ASS, GOKASHI, INKADO, INKAI, KALA HITAM, KANDAGA PRANA, KEI SHIN KAN, KKNSI, KKI, LEMKARI, MKC, PERKAINDO, PORBIKAWA, PORDIBYA, SHINDOKA, SHI ROI TE, TAKO INDONESIA, WADOKAI.

FORKI later acknowledged his existence by KONI. FORKI become a representative WKF (World Karate Federation) for Indonesia. Under construction FORKI, the karateka Indonesia can compete in international fora is mainly sponsored by the WKF.

In some areas in the province of Central Java is still a little extracurricular performing karate school. Extracurricular is one form of coaching achievements and print speeds of athletes. Tegal Regency, of 11 high school, there are only 3 schools that hold extracurricular karate.

The author chose karate as an object of study because only extracurricular karate including members FORKI who can follow such a the karate Championship O2SN and POPDA. Of the three schools that hold extracurricular karate above, yet showed significant achievements.

In POPDA, karate has never been overachievers at the provincial level. Even though every year following the karate O2SN, Tegal Regency have not though obtain the champion.

Yet the achievement of a maximum achievement is inseparable from a number of factors, among others: athletes, coaches, availability of infrastructure, organization, and funding activities. That is where all of these factors are part of the activities of coaching achievements.

Coaching achievements in Tegal, in practice directly charged to the school. Through extracurricular activities at each karate school. Own office party impressed off the hands of subject construction in Tegal Regency karate achievements. This is evident by the lack of information that can be excavated from the DINPORA and FORKI Regency.

The construction of a particular sport cannot be separated from the principles of the construction of the sport in General. To develop the required integrated coaching achievements, directional, continuous and from a young age. From the author of reason to feel interested in researching the karate Coaching in some school through extracurricular activities. The research goal is the high school level because in the age of high school health conditions, physical ability, mental aspects, social aspects and more prepared than the junior high school age children. Thus researchers interested in drawing up scientific papers entitled "evaluation studies Extracurricular Coaching Karate Karate Student Achievement Against"

Having known and understood the background of the title selection reasons, then the question in this study is:

1. What is coaching karate in extracurricular high school 1 Slawi, 2 public High Schools of the province and the high school 1 Bojong seen from athletes and Talent Scouting system?
2. What is coaching karate in extracurricular high school 1 Slawi, 2 public High Schools of the province and the high school 1 Bojong seen from extracurricular coach owned?

3. What is coaching karate in extracurricular high school 1 Slawi, 2 public High Schools of the province and the high school 1 Bojong views of facilities and infrastructure support?
4. How the extracurricular coaching karate in high school 1 Slawi, 2 public High Schools of the province and the high school 1 Bojong views from organisations that run?
5. How the extracurricular coaching karate in high school 1 Slawi, 2 public High Schools of the province and the high school 1 Bojong seen from the funding source used?

The purpose of the research is the primary means to know everything that is in the research, according to the title that the author pointed out, then the purpose of the research

1. To know karate athletes in high school 1 Slawi, 2 public High Schools of the province and the high school 1 Bojong.
2. To know the coach extracurricular karate high school-owned Land 1 Slawi, 2 public High Schools of the province and the high school 1 Bojong.
3. To know the facilities and infrastructure support in the construction of karate in extracurricular high school 1 Slawi, 2 public High Schools of the province and the high school 1 Bojong.
4. To know the structure of the organization that is run in the extracurricular activities of karate in high school 1 Slawi, 2 public High Schools of the province and the high school 1 Bojong.
5. To find out the sources of funding used in the construction of karate in extracurricular high school 1 Slawi, 2 public High Schools of the province and the high school 1 Bojong.

METHOD

The research approach used in this study is a qualitative approach. The research process is based on the theory that are relevant to the matter is examined to find the solution of these problems. This research using survey method, which means the process of data collection was done specifically and precisely or rigorously in an actual situation.

The selection of the approach is based on the consideration that the data sought is about coaching in karate extracurricular high school 1 Slawi, 2 public High Schools of the province and the high school 1 Bojong

The subject of research

The source of the informant this research as many as 55 people consisting of the vice principal, extracurricular Builder karate, physical education teachers, coaches, and athletes.

Object Of Research

The object of this research is the athletes, coaches, facilities and prasrana, organizational structures, and funding.

Location Research Research is a place intended to execute all the processes of research, the selected location to conduct research in high school 1 Slawi, 2 public High Schools of the province and the high school 1 Bojong Tegal Regency, Central Java. The research was carried out in all three of the school because the school is the school that held the extracurricular activities of karate.

Data Collection Instruments

The instruments used in this research is the observation: in this case with regard to the implementation of extracurricular karate Coaching in high school 1 Slawi, 2 public High Schools of the province, and high school 1 Bojong, interviews: interview conducted in this study was carried out by way of the submission of the question which was made before, the speaker is concerned, documentation: documents relating to the implementation of cxtracurricular karate Coaching in high school 1 Slawi , High school 2 Slawi, and high school 1 Bojong, retrieved from data that already exists, the achievements have been achieved, implementation activities photos and other documents and questionnaire: this questionnaire is addressed to the respondent, the respondent lived choose the answers already prepared. This data is used as supporting data in search of information about the implementation of extracurricular karate Coaching in high school 1 Slawi, 2 public High Schools of the province, and high school 1 Bojong.

Data Analysis Techniques

A descriptive analysis of the percentage of a way or method used to analyze the researcher or mendeskripikan answers of the respondents from each variable, so that research in the writing of the discussion will become easier and can be better understood.

The percentage of the results obtained is then classified for obtaining data conclusions.

Table 1. percentages of the Interval score

Interval The Percentage Score	Criteria
> 84 % - 100 %	Very Good
> 68 % - 84 %	Good
> 52 % - 68 %	Enough
> 36 % - 52 %	Less Good
≥ 20 % - 36 %	Not Good

Reduction of data means to encapsulate, choosing things, focus on the things that are important, look for themes and pattern. Researchers will be guided by the objectives that will be achieved in the reduction of data. Data reduction is the process of thinking that requires sensitive intelligence, collusion, and depth of insight that high.

Presentation of data can be done in the form of tables and descriptions. Through the presentation of the data, then the data are organized, arranged in the pattern of the relationship, so it will be easy to understand.

RESULTS AND DISCUSSION

Public high school athletes 1 Slawi A karate athlete recruitment process in high school 1 slawi is done at the beginning of the year lessons began with the promotion of extracurricular activities GMB (Gladi Manggala Bhakti). The extracurricular activities on karate was given the opportunity to present an appearance to attract new students. After these activities, schools provide time for three days to all extracurricular activities include karate to open extracurricular stand where new students can dig up more information on extracurricular activities of interest. The last stage of the recruitment process the athlete is student memillih extracurricular interest via the question form provided by vice principal field of studentship.

After the process of recruitment, extracurricular karate members following the construction of the memorial programs, exercise routine which was held twice in one week, namely, on Tuesdays and Fridays. The exercises done during the 90 minutes from 15.30 till 17.00 West Indonesia Time. An exercise program is divided into three sessions, namely, core, warming and cooling. In a session of heating and cooling all the members get the same portion of extracurricular activities. There is no difference between male students and female or color belt worn. A new exercise portion of the difference can be that on the core training session. Member with white belt underwent an exercise separate from the Member with a belt that is already colored or higher degree from a white belt.

Outside the exercise routine, members get an extra physical exercise for a month before the game. Physical exercise was carried out on Sunday in a week for 120 seconds, which is housed in the building of sports Trisanja. A given physical exercise program include: 2.4 km run, 100 m sprint running, push ups, sit ups, and concludes with a sparing session partner.

High school 2 Slawi

Karate athlete recruitment process at high school 2 Slawi beginning at the time of the year at the new lesson activities MOS (Masa Orientasi Sekolah). In the event the senior doing extracurricular demonstration before new students with the aim to attract new students against certain extracurricular activities. Students indirectly decided to become a member of one of the extracurricular activities in high school 2 Slawi. They are given the opportunity to think about the choice of extracurricular activities of interest. Extracurricular Member registration is done on the first week of teaching and learning activities running through the extracurricular question form provided by vice principal field of studentship.

After the process of recruitment, extracurricular karate members following the construction of the memorial programs, exercise routine which was held twice in one week, namely, on Wednesdays and Saturdays. The exercises done during 120 minutes starting from 15.00 until 17.00 West Indonesia Time. An exercise program is divided into three sessions, namely, core, warming and cooling. In a session of heating and cooling throughout the extracurricular exercise portion gets members the same. There is no difference between male students and female or color belt worn. The difference can exercise portion of that on core training session where members with white belt underwent an exercise separate from the Member with a belt that is already colored or higher degree from a white belt. This is done because a member with white belts need to be conditioned to practice basic karate movements in advance.

The portion of the exercise will be members of the extracurricular karate about one month ahead of the karate match. After a routine training session is completed, the members perform sparing partner or trainer to deal with fellow members of the extracurricular activities in accordance with the class match that followed. Additional exercises are usually performed for 30 minutes menjelas workout routine ends. Special physical training outside the regular workout schedule is not granted to members of karate in extracurricular high school 2 Slawi.

High school 1 Bojong

A karate athlete recruitment process in high school 1 Bojong made at the time of the year at the new lesson activities MOS (Masa Orientasi Sekolah). In the activities of the students were given the now-playing in a vice principal student field that contains a list of extracurricular activities in high school 1 Bojong. Senior Superintendent extracurricular or not doing demonstrations or special dishes for new students.

After the process of recruitment, extracurricular karate members following the construction of the memorial programs, exercise routine which was held twice in one week, namely, on Wednesdays and Saturdays. The exercises done during 120 minutes starting from 15.00 until 17.00 West Indonesia Time. An exercise program is divided into three sessions, namely, core, warming and cooling. In a session of heating and cooling throughout the extracurricular exercise portion gets members the same. There is no difference between male students and female or color belt worn. The difference can exercise portion of that on core training session where members with white belt underwent an exercise separate from the Member with a belt that is already colored or higher degree from a white belt. This is done because a member with white belts need to be conditioned to practice karate basic movements first.

Karate in extracurricular high school 1 Bojong undergo additional exercise or special exercises to prepare the athletes who will compete. The entire exercise program is executed at the moment an exercise routine only.

High school coach 1 Slawi Karate in extracurricular high school 1 Slawi has a coach who is chosen by the school through recommendations from previous coaches. The coach holds a black belt Dan 2 Karate and has been a coach for about 12 years. Although it has been trained in a long time, the coach does not yet have a formal coaching certificate. In organizations FORKI Tegal Regency coaches occupy positions as Secretary FORKI Regency. Coaches get the knowledge to train karate when still an athlete. The highest achievement earned by athletes is his third place Kumite at kejurnas 2005.

The target given by the school to coach among others produces athletes who have superior performance and can donate the Medal for schools of karate Championships at least some on the district level. The target has yet to be fulfilled to the maximum because of the resistance of his own coach. Barriers experienced by caused by factors of time because of work to train karate is not a major job coach. The coach also has a responsibility in its main job which causes the time taken to train.

Coaches make exercise programs, namely exercise routine twice a week and an extra workout on Sunday and physical exercise if the approaching matches. If approaching the event increases the belt, then the exercise is only emphasized on basic techniques and the words that will be examined at the time of the event increases the belt. The program has not been implemented fully due to the constraints mentioned above. The trainers sometimes do his, precisely after the workout. Discuss the existing problems and find solutions together.

High school 2 Slawi

Karate in extracurricular high school 2 Slawi has a coach who is chosen by the school through a recommendation by a FORKI. The coach holds a black belt and karate and has been a coach for a little over 2 years. Coach already has a certificate of the official level of training in Central Java, and routinely follow penataran coach every once a year in the province. Up to this point the coach is also still an active practice as an athlete, and the most recent achievements earned as an athlete was the bronze medal at the Championship DULONGMAS. While his latest achievement as a coach was managed to bring his athletes won 2 Kumite champion and 2 kata in POPDA.

The target given by the school to coach among others produces athletes who have superior performance and can donate the Medal for schools of karate Championships at least some on the district level. The target can be met by the coach because of the magnitude of the support from the school, parents, and athletes themselves.

The program that made coach is fighting techniques that directed breeding for the provincial level, arranged schedule between the physical techniques that gradually that later will be higher. The program has been already able to walk, but still has some constraints as mentioned above. Coaches don't do direct evaluation of students, the evaluation is only a report to Pembina extracurricular karate.

High school 1 Bojong

Karate in extracurricular high school 1 Bojong has one coach who was elected by a INKANAS upon request of the school. The coach holds a black belt Dan 3 Karate. The coach has been the coach of the karate for about 20 years. The coach has had a certificate to train karate officially issued by the INKANAS, but the coach has never followed the upgrading of coaches because upgrading INKANAS always held in Jakarta. Coaches get the knowledge to train karate Kumite athletes when it becomes. The highest achievement ever won by the athlete is his third place national level at the Open Championship SBY CUP in 2009.

The target given by the school to coach among others produces athletes who have superior performance and can donate the Medal for schools of karate Championships at least some on the district level. The target can be met, but haven't been fullest. It is caused by the existence of several barriers. In addition, because of weather factors, obstacles also come from the coach himself. The coach house location away from the school and a long commute time cause the workout schedule does not run as expected. In addition, the number of trainers karate INKANAS district bordering with the numbers is still a little bit, so that the school can not choose the coach of his more affordable locations from the school.

An exercise program that applied to coach at the high school karate 1 Bojong is an exercise routine twice a week without an additional workout schedule. The first one that is preferred basic motion and shape, after that goes into engineering and physics. So far the program has already run. But still there are constraints that make the exercise program yet. The coach is simply not doing evaluation exercise on athletes. Sarana dan Prasarana Sekolah menengah atas Negeri 1 Slawi

Karate extracurricular facilities and infrastructure owned by public High Schools of the province are presented in table 2 below.

Table 2. List means Karate in Extracurricular high school 1 Slawi

Type	Total
Hand protector	4 pairs
Body protector	4 pairs
Leg protector	4 pairs
Face mask	4 pairs

High school 2 Slawi

Karate extracurricular facilities and infrastructure owned by public High Schools 2 Slawi is presented in the table below.

Table 3. Lists mean of Karate in Extracurricular high school 2 Slawi

Type	Total
Hand protector	3 pairs
Body protector	2 pairs
Leg protector	3 pairs
Kaca	1 pairs

High school 1 Bojong Karate extracurricular facilities and infrastructure owned by public High Schools 1 Bojong is presented in the table below.

Table 4. Lists the means the Karate in Extracurricular high school 1 Bojong.

Type	Total
Hand protector	2 pairs
Body protector	2 pairs
Leg protector	2 pairs
Face mask	2 pairs

Organization of high school 1 Slawi Extracurricular organizations karate high school located in 1 in the province under the auspices of the OSIS. Extracurricular organization at the INKAI karate high school 1 Slawi is a branch of the Organization of the Tegal Regency of the INKAI. The organization is managed by students who are members of the extracurricular activities of karate. The organization is in charge of extracurricular karate constructor also acts as a bridge between the organizations with the school.

High school 2 Slawi High school 2 Slawi has no special organization for extracurricular karate. Extracurricular karate under the auspices of OSIS. Administrators field VII about physical freshness and creations. Due to not having a special organization than any extracurricular activities are organized less karate maximal, and yet can run management functions in it. Despite having no organization specifically, extracurricular high school karate 2 Slawi has a builder who oversees the operations of the entire karate extracurricular activities in high school 2 Slawi.

High school 1 Bojong Extracurricular organization of karate in high school 1 Bojong under the auspices OSIS. Extracurricular organizations karate INKANAS in high school 1 is from the Organization branch Bojong INKANAS Tegal Regency. The organization is managed by students who are members of the extracurricular activities of karate. The organization is in charge of extracurricular Builder karate is also the vice principal field of student in high school 1 Bojong.

Funding public high school 1 Slawi Sources of funding at the extra-curricular activities karate high school 1 of the province derives from a school party, twig INKAI Tegal Regency, branch and cash from members of the public High School karate 1 Slawi. From the school the funds budgeted for the coach and Championship events such as POPDA and O2SN. The school awarded school students earn achievements in the form of tuition fee waivers, to champion the free school fees 1 3 months, champion 2 cost-free school 2 months, and third place free of cost schools 1 month. Apart from the school, the coach also gave awards to athletes can earn achievements. From twig branches INKAI URANIUM funds allocated for public competitions Championships and a minimum level of resident students. And cash funds from members for activities budgeted increase belt exams and treatment means of karate in high school 1 Slawi. To date the construction of karate in extracurricular high school 1 Slawi hasn't been getting financial support from sponsors.

High school 2 Slawi Sources of funding at the extra-curricular activities, karate high school 2 Slawi derives from a school party, twig INKAI Tegal Regency, branch and cash from members of the public High School karate 2 Slawi. From the school the funds budgeted for coaches, promotional activities and the recruitment of new members, and Championship events such as POPDA and O2SN. The school awarded school students earn achievements in the form of waivers of school costs money, Free 1st champion For school fees 3 months, champion 2 cost-free school 2 months, and third place free of cost schools 1 month. The school also provides transport for cars complete with money every time a driver and petrol following a Championship. From twig branches INKAI funds allocated for public competitions Championships and a minimum level of resident students. And cash funds from members for activities budgeted increase belt exams and treatment means karate high school 2 Slawi. To date the construction of the extracurricular high school karate 2 Slawi haven't been getting financial support from sponsors.

High school 1 Bojong Sources of funding at the extra-curricular activities, karate high school 1 Bojong comes from the school and from cash Member karate high school 1 Bojong. From the school the funds budgeted for transportation trainer, coach, and events such as Championship POPDA and O2SN. The school awarded school students earn achievements in the form of funding or relief money school fees, to champion free school fees 1 3 months, champion 2 cost-free school 2 months, and third place free of cost schools 1 month. And cash funds from members for activities budgeted increase belt exams and treatment means of karate in high school 1 Bojong. To date the construction of karate in extracurricular high school 1 Bojong hasn't been getting financial support from sponsors.

DISCUSSION

Athletes

Based on the results of the findings in the field note that management coaching athletes in the school's three research not yet running to its full potential, as yet refers to the theory advanced by (Djoko Pekik 2002;27) stating that the achievements need to be systematic planning, implemented gradually and continuously, starting from pemasalan, nurseries and coaching until you reach the pinnacle of achievement. The fact that there has not been such as to the stage of recruitment in the schools rely solely on three prekrutan at the time of initial receipt of the new learners in the absence of the selection process, students follow the extracurricular karate based solely on the interest and not views of potential, talents, background and student achievement. Students who get into extracurricular karate still many who have not known and mastering skills in martial arts, karate. To stage a coaching in schools is simply lasts for 3 years only, so if you only rely on the selection of learners who have entered into the high school is not enough, because there is a good idea to stage the selection as early as possible as it gives socialize in the first high school has extracurricular karate, karate match monitor at the level of junior high school Tegal Regency to trawl the talented students and further given the opportunity entry into high school. This was done so that activities in the implementation of the coaching program may be running optimally.

In general the process of recruitment of athletes at the three schools who became the object of the research belongs to the natural selection process, where students follow an extracurricular karate as a result of environmental influences, wish parents and peer influence. Development and advancement of the athletes are very slow, because of selection of sport and ideal for him nothing, less or not right.

The recruitment process and identifying talent in order to achieve high achievements can be done more quickly when using the selection in accordance with scientific theory Bompa (1990) the cited KONI in the project Garuda Emas. This method selects the Fellowship considers, among other factors: height and weight, speed, reaction time, coordination and strength.

Breeding process and coaching athletes who performed only distinguished from the color or level of the belt. There should be some indicators that need to be noted as criteria for identifying and selecting talented athletes seeds objectively according to Cholik (1994:234) cited by Djoko Pekik Irianto. Such as: health (medical examination, especially the kardiorespiorasi system and the muscular, nervous system), antopometri (height and weight, the size of the body fat, body parts, etc.), physical ability (speed, power, coordination, Vo2 max), psychological abilities (attitudes, motivation, power tolerance), the offspring, long exercise that has followed previous and is there a chance to thrive, and maturasi. The system is applied to schools in the process of recruitment and Scouting talent result in less maximum achievement athlete karate students.

Coach

The next aspect is the coach. The coach is a professional whose job helping sportsmen and teams in improving the appearance of the sport. Because the coach is a profession, then should the coach should be able to provide the services in accordance with the professional standards or size. Whereas in accordance with the profession is the coach should be able to provide training services in accordance with the development of cutting-edge scientific knowledge in the field who pursued according to Pate Rotella in the book (Sanusi Hasibuan Dkk, 2009:8). Just coach high school 2 Slawi and high school 1 Bojong who already have a certificate coach and has expertise in the compliance field. While the high school coach 1 Slawi does not yet have certificates of trainers. A coach in its field of competence is required to have in order to become the Foundation of a trainer early in the running training program, the competence of a must-have sports karate know about techniques chat, know the rules of the game, able to improve the athletes ' capability. Although recently a small part of the task that is already running certainly persists in natural increase. The coach's third most already have expertise in their field but in happen coach not yet fully run the program, exercise, not to become a teacher and motivator for athletes, and it could not discipline him because at the time of exercise often arrive late not even present other work due to investments.

In general the selection of trainers karate school in the three objects is done through the selection of coaches who are members of a Member FORKI. The third coach had been already able to exercise its role as a coach, that's been able to improve the fitness of athletes. Seen in terms of educational background the third coach of the meet because it already holds a black belt karate. If ditijau according to theory Rubianto Hadi (2007:27) in terms of experience in exercising the third coach is pretty good because the third coach has experience as a karate athlete. A trainer who has experience as an athlete will be more skilled in fostering athletes. In terms of additional education just coach high school 2 Slawi routine follows penetration-upgrading a coach. Additional education is very necessary for improving the quality of training because a coach can discuss and exchange ideas, experiences, and methods of the latest best practice with fellow coaches as well as with trainers from other branches as well as other scientific experts are closely related to the profession of coaching.

From the above theory there are still some who have not been executed by the coach, one of which is to be a motivator and teacher for athletes dibinanya, task coach is not only a skill honed athletes alone but should be able to guide the athlete in order to have a good personality and has a high confidence. For the current coach is expected to further maximize the exercise program was assigned in order to additionally be maximum achievement.

Facilities and infrastructure After the coach, the next aspect is infrastructure. Infrastructure and facilities in sports coaching is one of the important factors to improve achievement and determine the quality of coaching accomplishments. Facilities and infrastructure, there is also a need to meet the national standards even to international to support the achievement of the accomplishments of the athletes. The number of existing infrastructure must be in accordance with the number of athletes that exist, such as the availability of a sufficient hand protector, leg protector, body protector, tatami (mats) and the target for practice, besides karate facilities and infrastructure should have a place in indoor or indoor exercise so if erratic weather activity exercise can still walk. From the results of the findings in the field in the General and infrastructure used in the construction of the three karate school extracurricular which becomes the object of research is not yet supporting coaching for maximum achievement. It can be seen from the facilities and infrastructure amount was minimal and yet meet the standards given the number of members more than many existing tools. The available means and conditions already need to be updated due to lack of maintenance. This is because there are no officers specifically for the care of the equipment and lack of funds for the procurement of equipment. In addition to these three schools still do not have tatami (mats) and target punch or kick for target practice. These three schools where research has an exercise that its use in conjunction with other extracurricular activities, thus reducing the focus and concentration of athletes in practice. In high school 1 Bojong still do not have an indoor exercise so if rain does not exercise activities can take place. Moreover, the geographical condition of layout of high school 1 Bojong residing in the mountains, the weather is often erratic so exercise program can not run optimally. The school is expected to be more concerned with extracurricular karate so that achievements can be more optimally and can bring the name of the school.

Organization The next aspect is organization. Data from the results of research conducted at the three schools who became the object of research, just an extracurricular high school karate 1 Slawi and high school 1 Bojong who have the organization. Though in high school has extracurricular organization slawi 1 karate organization's function, but that there was insufficient due to the number of members which is very little. While the organization of karate in extracurricular high school 1 Bojong has been running quite well because it has many members that allows more easily the Division of duties in the running throughout the extracurricular activities of karate. With the pretty much the function of organizing and pengkoordinasian can run.

In high school 2 Slawi no particular organizational structure created. The arrangement of its administrator is still not complete as the absence, Secretary, Treasurer, and sections required in an organization. For the Organization of extracurricular activities in high school 2 Slawi shaded by the field of the student and the school principal as the person in charge, Coach Builder karate and extracurricular activities. Based on the findings of the field and data analysis the school just give target achievement who wish to attain and provide facilities in the form of facilities and infrastructure as well as the funds needed, besides the school appoint a teacher to become a Builder to monitor the course of extra-curricular activities karate 1 week once, patrons rarely hold periodic evaluation in extracurricular activities. For coaching and training program is fully given to the coach. Walking or whether a coaching is highly determined by the Organization in implementing, and if there is no full support, cooperation and coordination of the school a coaching program will not run to its full potential.

The above findings are not yet in compliance with the principles of organization that is diungkapan by (Harsuki 2012:118) that the Organization must be a clear purpose, organizations must be accepted by everyone in the Organization, the Organization must be understood by everyone in the Organization, there is a unity of direction, there is a unity of command, there is a balance between the authority and the responsibility of a person, the existence of a duty, the organizational structure must be composed as simple as possible, the basic pattern of organization should be relatively permanent.

The influence of the existence of the Organization against karate athletes can be seen in terms of Scouting talent and communication with the school. Organizations can facilitate the distribution of information about training programs. In addition, the existence of a special organization, the athlete can establish better communication with the school.

Funding Last aspect was funding. In general the sources of funding of the extracurricular activities of karate in the third school that became the object of research derives from a school and cash members. Help from twig branches only to a minimal level of activity in the County Championship. The funds budgeted for the extracurricular activities of karate schools budgeted for such Championship and coach POPDA and O2SN, at public school Championships do not issue funds, the school does not issue funds for the procurement and maintenance of the equipment. It is less in accordance with the opinion of the Said Junaidi (2003:64) To extracurricular activities needed funding to finance include: honor coaches, purchase tools and sports equipment, rent/field matches and competitions. Kas members used to increase activity levels of belt. The existing funds should be used to the maximum possible because the schools themselves could not issue the funds origin, there should be special details arranged for proposing budgeting funds. Funds that there is still not enough in the improvement of coaching achievements, such as funds for the activities of the test match, the school itself only spends the funds for activities of bullfights held each year, funds for the procurement of infrastructure still hasn't quite like the absence of mattresses and the target, the lack of number of guardians of the existing bodies for practice. With the limited funds that there is the school required to organize the system of allocating funds for extracurricular activities, the school must provide appropriate facilities and infrastructure standards and needs in order to meet the needs of achievement.

Fund management in public High School 2 Slawi is insufficient as there is no special organization that manages the extracurricular activities of karate. Finances should be managed properly for smooth and the achievement of business objectives of the organization. In the absence of such an organization, then funds will be paralyzed. The efficiency of the use of funds will fertilize the activity of the organization. Good management in the management of the Fund brings the real activity of the Organization in.

A third school had never gotten relief funds from sponsors. Existing funding sources have not been able to meet the needs of karate in particular funds for extracurricular procurement means. It has yet to be resolved because the communication between the school with extracurricular members running less well.

CONCLUSION

Based on the results of research conducted in public High Schools 1 Slawi, public High Schools of the province, and 2 public High Schools 1 Bojong extracurricular about coaching against his karate and karate student achievement in Tegal, then it can be inferred that the extracurricular coaching karate in high school 1 Slawi, 2 public High Schools of the province, and a public high school in the category of Bojong 1 less. This occurs because there are still some obstacles in five aspects that becomes a factor in restricting the following maximum achievement:

1. In the aspect of the recruiting system, athletes and coaching program being run has not been fullest because the achievements already won only as the present District and County have yet to ketingkat the province of Central Java. The exercise program applied has not been fully executed according to the existing theory.
2. On the coaches, there is still a coach who can be said to be professional yet because it has no official coach certificate. The designated coach sued for more can lead athletes in order to have a good personality.
3. Facilities and infrastructure, there is still yet to be said well, there is still need for procurement, replenishment, and quality improvement tools.
4. Organizations that there are still less well because in the management of the organization still has not been fullest, there is even a school that does not yet have a special karate organization.
5. The last aspect of funding, the funding comes from the school are still not sufficient in an effort of coaching achievements so that the school is required to find ways in the fulfillment of the budget coaching. In particular funds for procurement of facilities and infrastructure.

REFERENCES

Harsuki. 2012. Pengantar Manajemen Olahraga. Jakarta: PT. Raja Grafindo Persada.

Hasibuan, S., Akhmad, I., Hariyanto, E. 2009. Evaluasi Program Pembinaan Pusat Pendidikan dan Latihan Olahraga Pelajar di Kalimantan Timur, Riau, dan Sumatra Barat.Jakarta:Asisten Deputi IPTEK Olahraga.

Pratiwi, P. (2015). PEMANDUAN BAKAT DAN MINAT CABANG OLAHRAGA MELALUI METODE SPORT SEARCH PADA SISWA SMP NEGERI SE KECAMATAN KARANGANYAR KABUPATEN DEMAK TAHUN 2013/2014. ACTIVE: Journal of Physical Education, Sport, Health and Recreation, 4(3).

Rubianto, H. 2007. Ilmu Kepelatihan dasar. Semarang: Cipta Prima Nusantara.

Rumini, R. (2015). MANAJEMEN PEMBINAAN CABANG OLAHRAGA ATLETIK DI PUSAT PENDIDIKAN DAN LATIHAN PELAJAR (PPLP) PROVINSI JAWA TENGAH. Journal of Physical Education Health and Sport, 2(1), 20-27.

Android-Learned Media Learning Media With Health Material For Students of Class X

Pandora Wahyu Herjanata[1],

Department of Health physical education and recreation, Sport Science Faculty, Universitas Negeri Semarang, Indonesia

Article History

Keywords:
Development; Health; Media; Education; Android

Abstract

Seeing the potential of untapped learning media. Creativity of teachers to create learning media not only for solving problems, but also exploit the potential that exists. Therefore the author tries to design an Android-based program to improve learning experience of Physical Education, Sport and Health to be more interesting. Using Pre test and Post test method in trial scale. The results showed that, (1) the results of media expert and health expert validation showed 80.475% in the "excellent" category and small-scale trials showed an average of 54.114 results in pre test and 79.2 in the post test. (2) The results of data analysis on large-scale trials in 3 schools showed 52,867 results in the test and increased to 75.2754 in the post test. (3) The students' assessment on the product was 77.091% or in the "good" category and the assessment of the learning expert was 89, 5% in the category of "very good." Learning media product of Physical Education, Health and Sport in Android-based named APPJOK with focused on subject types of foods and beverages that are beneficial to the health of growth and development can be practiced to the subject of the trial.

Correspondence address :
Kupang Tanjung Sari RT 06, RW 11, Kupang, Ambarawa, Semarang District, 50612 Central Java
E-mail: pwherjanata@gmail.com

INTRODUCTION

The development of technology today makes the human work easier, in recent years technology is growing in various aspects of human life. One of the most rapid technological advances in the development of communication technology.

Information and Communication Technology is part of Science and Technology (IPTEK) in general all technologies related to the collection, collection (acquisition), processing, storage, dissemination, presentation of information (Darmawan, 2011). In various fields, the development of various technologies creates constraints in the space of time and place can also be bypassed by the existence of ICT, the emergence of various jargon e, ranging from e-book, e-learning, e-laboratory, e-education, e-library where e interpreted electronics aka digital electronic technology.

People now almost all have mobile phones, the distance that used to be a barrier for someone to communicate now is not something that is difficult, this long distance communication tool is very helpful to the community communication process is not limited in space, time and place to the technology in a phone grasp progressively. Mobile phones are no longer just a means to communicate remotely or send messages, in the mobile phone there are various features or applications that can make a mobile phone like a personal assistant which then we call the smartphone a complete device as a medium of communication, social as well as entertainment.

For the development of mobile phone technology there is a platform that developed into the most widely used platform to date android. Android as the most widely used smartphone OS platform with nearly 80% of users in Indonesia and around 60% worldwide (Stat Counter Global Stats, 2016) has an important role to present oriented applications that help people to improve their performance in life. Recognized or not the penetration of this mobile device is very fast, more than the PC. These devices are in the case of easier operation than the PC.

In the scope of e-learning, learning is done using electronic media that can be replaced by m-learning where the flexibility of the user to use the use of mobile learning devices generally in Indonesia where mobile device users are very much even the type of smartphone especially among students.

This can actually be used for learning, especially learning Physical Education Sports and Health. According to Law Number 20 of 2003 the national educational system has the goal to educate the life of the Indonesian nation and develop a complete Indonesian man who is a believer and devoted to God Almighty and virtuous noble character, possessing knowledge and skills, physical and spiritual moment, berkepribadain steady and independent and a sense of community responsibility and life.

Based on the field survey conducted by the author In 2 SMA in Semarang district that is SMA Negeri 1 Ungaran and SMA Negeri 1 Ambarawa prove that the majority of high school students have gadgets such as smartphones. Regarding the regulations at school in two high schools is allowed the use of communication tools as long as its use does not disturb teaching and learning activities, and even allowed when the use of gadgets to support learning better or interesting. But from both high school learning PJOK not yet take advantage of the potential existence of smartphones that have been owned by students, especially in learning PJOK learning media most often used only video or book media, and indeed the applications available in smartphone devices especially based on android support the current teaching and learning activities are still rarely developed.

Learning media development by utilizing cell phones prove very effective. Empowers teachers and students to be more up-to-date and innovative media available. And can direct students to optimize the use of the gadgets in the world of education. Learning media development by utilizing cell phones is making designs from existing Android application, intended for all cell phones berplatform Android. With reason, because the operating system Android is transformed into a system that is most widely used on Smartphones (Indrianto, 2017). Research development that departs from the potential will have more added value, when compared with the departed from the problem. Research that departs from the problem tends to solve the problem, but research that departs from the potential will develop the potential that there will be added value (Sugiyono, 2015). Therefore, the author tries to design android based programs to improve learning PJOK to be more interesting.

The author's decision is based on field observation where the potential of smartphone users among high school students has not been utilized to support teaching and learning activities let alone for learning PJOK. While the selection of android-based smartphone based smartphone android is the most popular operating system today besides the students are also more interested in using the gadget rather than reading books and the nature of android easy developed by third parties facilitate various parties to develop this android-based applications.

The author tries to solve the problems that exist in the research of how the concept of learning when using the application, the concept of the application itself and the impact of the use of the application to students.

METHODS

According Sugiyono (2015) research and development methods can be interpreted as a scientific way to research, design, produce, and test the validity of products that have been produced. And based on the above understanding Sugiyono mengaris that 4 most important things in research development, i.e., research, design, production, and testing.

As has been exposed, methodologically. Research development has four difficulty levels: researching without testing (not making and not testing the product), testing without researching (testing the validity of existing products), researching and testing in an effort to develop existing products, and researching and testing in creating products new.

The subjects of this research are high school students of Class X located in Semarang Regency. Schools that became the product test site of SMA Negeri 1 Ungaran, SMA Negeri 1 Ambarawa and SMA Islam Sudirman. The implementation of the Small Scale Test is in SMA Negeri 1 Ungaran while the Large Scale Test covers all the schools involved in the research.

Before stepping into the field test the author has done product validation. Furthermore, each test phase of the scale there are pre test and post test and assessment.

The results of the pre test and post test and overall assessment of the experts taken and obtained the final product.

RESULTS AND DISCUSSION

Small scale trial aims to find out and identify varPrior to the small-scale testing of the authors to validate products to health experts and media experts.

Validation is useful to know the product that the author made decent or not to advanced kethap next is the small-scale test and large-scale test, and **table 1** following the results of the validation.

Table 1. Result of validation

Expert	Score	Notes
Health Expert	78,6 %	Better or if possible given problem more hone student's analysis power
Media Expert	82,35 %	Considered the use of other names for apps to appear to sell when uploaded to playstore
Number of	80,475 %	Eligible for field test

The results of validation of media experts and health experts

Small-scale test conducted by the author on 20 and 27 April 2017 in the class X MIPA 4 SMA Negeri 1 Ungaran in the results of pre-test and post test compared to whether the progress of student learning outcomes after treatment with the product.

Class X MIPA 4 consists of 36 students consisting of 11 students and 25 female students at the time of pre test conducted there is 1 student who can't follow the pre test because it is following the race.

Of the 35 students who pre-tested the highest score was achieved a student named Intan with a score of 70 and the lowest value obtained by Revian Farhan with a value of 42. The result of the class X of MIPA 4 is also not too good ie 54.48 or closer to the lowest value compared the highest score.

Table 2. Results of pre test class X MIPA 4

Category	Value
The highest score	70
Lowest Value	42
Average value	54,48

The results of this post test are compared with the pre test results and see whether there is progress of the results after treatment with the product

Table 3. Post result of class X test of MIPA 4

Category	Value
Highest Value	100
Lowest Value	56
Average Value	79,2

Pre Test conducted in 3 classes in 3 schools in the interview before pre test learning healthy lifestyle has not been done by 2 schools namely SMA Negeri 1 Ungaran and SMA Islam Sudirman while SMA Negeri 1 Ambarawa has been giving health lesson but with material of Drug and HIV / AIDS and from Pre Test obtained results as follows.

Table 4. Comparison of Pre Test Results In 3 Schools

Name of School	Value Lowest	Value Lowest	Average Value
SMA Negeri 1 Ungaran	45,5	70	58,516
SMA Negeri 1 Ambarawa	45,5	78	58,806
SMA Islam Sudirman	17,5	61	41,279
Average			52,867

After done Pre test and treatment to student writer do post test where in post test writer will get final result which will known how progress obtained by student after get learning using APPJOK application product.

Table 5. Post test results in 3 schools

Name of School	Value Lowest	Value Lowest	Average Value
SMA Negeri 1 Ungaran	58	100	83,9354
SMA Negeri 1 Ambarawa	56	100	74,766
SMA Islam Sudirman	52,5	96,5	67,125
Average			75,2754

Table 6. Comparison of pre test and post test results

School Name	Category	Pre test	Post test	Progress Student
SMA Negeri 1 Ungaran	Lowest Value	45,5	58	Yes
	Highest value	70	100	Yes
	Average	58,516	83,9354	Yes
SMA Negeri 1 Ambarawa	Lowest Value	45,5	56	Yes
	Highest value	78	100	Yes
	Average	58,806	74,766	Yes
SMA Islam Sudriman	Lowest Value	17,5	52	Yes
	Highest value	61	96,5	Yes
	Average	41,279	67,125	Yes

After the students do post test, students assess the product with 12 aspects in it. And following the results of students' assessment of the product.

Table 7. Results of product assessment of students in 3 schools

School Name	Average Score	Percentage	Category
SMA Negeri 1 Ungaran	46,9	78,275%	good
SMA Negeri 1 Ambarawa	44	74%	good
SMA Islam Sudirman	47	79%	good
Average		77,091 %	good

The student's response to the product showed good result where the students in SMA Islam Sudirman showed interest in the product followed by SMA Negeri 1 Ungaran and SMA Negeri 1 Ambarawa. With a total percentage of 77.091% then the products in the student ratings are included in the good category.

The product assessment is done by the learning expert in this case the teacher from 3 schools namely Wahyu Supriyanto from SMA Negeri 1 Ungaran, Yurisa Novita from SMA Islam Sudirman and Purwanto from SMA Negeri 1 Ambarawa with the result.

Table 8. The results of the product assessment by the teacher

Teacher name	Total Score	Percentage	Category
Wahyu Supriyanto, S.Pd	62	82,6%	VERY GOOD

Purwanto	69	95,8%	VERY GOOD
Yurisa Novita P. S.Pd	65	90,2%	VERY GOOD
Average		89,5%	VERY GOOD

Prototipe Produk

Table 9. Prototipe Produk

Information	Visual
Opening	APPJOK Logo
Tittle	APPJOK
Main Menu	Program Menu: Material (Healthy Life-style, Nutrition / Nutrition, Disease due to Nutrition imbalance, and Balanced Nutrition, calorie table) Problem Exercises Nutrition Calculator About the Program
Sub-menu Material About Healthy Lifestyle	Description and description of what is a true healthy lifestyle
Sub-menu of Material Nutrition	Description of what it means of nutrition and its benefits
Sub-menu of Material Balanced nutrition	The description of what is meant is balanced nutrition. In daily practice.
Sub-Menu Due to Nutrition Imbalance	Description of the result of nutritional imbalance from excess nutrient to malnutrition
Problem training menu	Various exercise questions accompanied by results that can be seen directly
Nutrition Calculator	Users can input and view ideal weight results of the current weight category up to daily caloric needs.
About	Application Instructions for apps

Tabel 10. Story board of APPJOK products

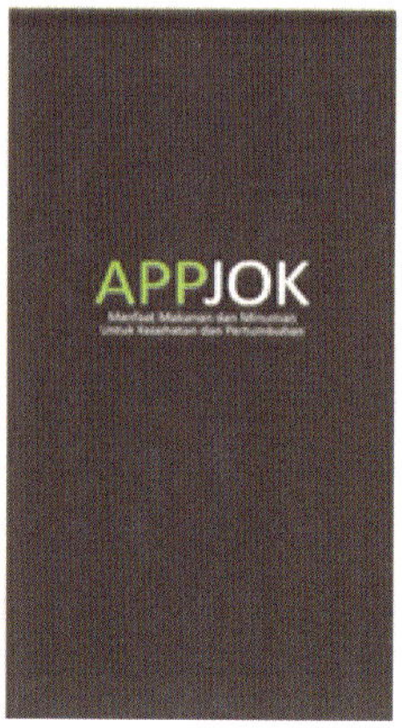

APPJOK display when first opened.

Menu view in APPJOK

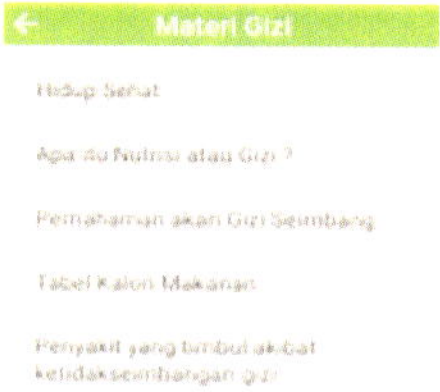

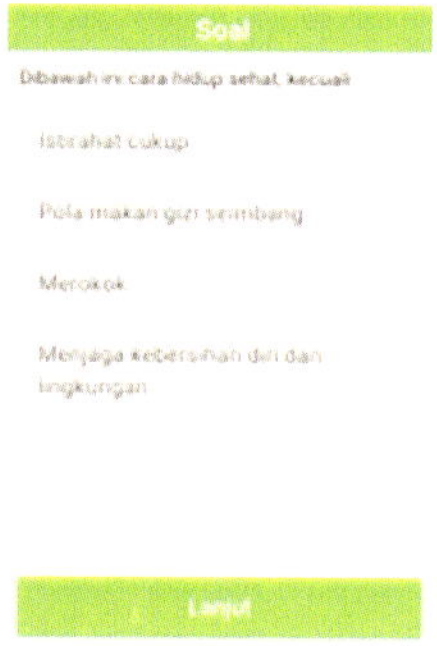

Display the exercise menu problem

Nutrition menu display

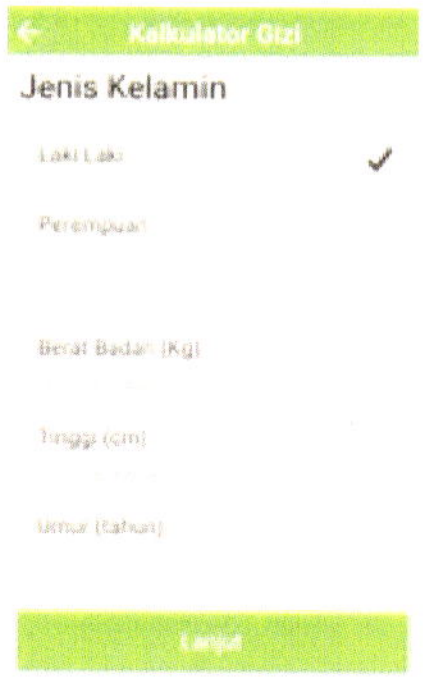

Nutrition consultation menu view

APPJOK products are application products created using Android Studio, Adobe Illustrator, and Adobe Photoshop programs. Runs in android system with specifications:

1. Android: Ice Cream Sandwich and above
2. Memory: has more than 15 MB free space

The product has limitations and advantages ie

Disadvantages: APPJOK only runs in android smartphone and offline system, the material in APPJOK is only for health materials that is the type of food that is useful for the growth of health and development.

Pros: APPJOK runs in offline system so it

does not require internet connection, APPJOK can be opened wherever and whenever without depending on server or internet connection, APPJOK has nutrition calculator feature which can calculate ideal weight, current weight category, and caloric requirement, APPJOK has practice questions that contain 5 random questions from a total of 20 questions and assessments can be seen immediately upon completion.

CONCLUSION

Based on the results of research that has been implemented and has been listed on the results of the discussion in this thesis, it can be concluded as follows:

APPJOK products may and may be appropriate for use in the learning process. It is based on data analysis on trial I and II test obtained from expert evaluation each get an average percentage of 80,475 for Health Expert and Media Expert and Learning Expert in this case teacher in 3 School get result 89,5% . The assessment of the students got an average of 77.091%.

Learning media products PJOK Android-based APPJOK with material types of foods and beverages that are beneficial to the Health of growth and development can already be practiced to the subject of trial. This is based on the results of data analysis obtained from experts and learning experts. Based on the results of research and discussion on this thesis, it can be concluded as follows:

Learning media PJOK Android-based APPJOK with food and beverage type materials that are beneficial to the Health of growth and development, as a new innovation in learning PJOK as well as participate in technological developments today where high school students have an average smartphone device that became one of the resources has not been fully utilized as a medium of learning by teachers.

On learning PJOK using APPJOK Android app students are enthusiastic because although students often use smartphones but the android apps used by teachers is a new medium for them.

REFERENCES

Darmawan, D. 2011. Teknologi Pembelajaran, Bandung: Remaja Rosdakarya.

Indrianto, D., Setyawati, H., & Kusuma, D. W. Y. (2017). App Inventor2 Learning Basketball at Grade X Senior High School. Journal of Physical Education, Health and Sport, 4(1), 9-17.

GS Stat Counter, Top 8 Mobile & Tablet System Operation(Indonesia/Worldwide) http://gs.statcounter.com/#mobile+tablet-os-id-monthly-201305-201605 diakses pada 15 Juni 2016 pukul 11:00

Sugiyono. 2015. Metode Penelitian dan Pengembangan, Bandung: Alfabeta Bandung.

Undang-undang Republik Indonesia Nomor 20 Tahun 2003 Sistem Pendidikan Nasional. 08 Juli 2003.

The Strategy of Presenting Daily Sports News "Suara Merdeka" in The Midst of Mobile Media Competition

Lina Dewi Nurutami[1✉], **Heny Setyawati**[2], **Agus Raharjo**[3],

Department of Health Physical Education and Recreation, Sport Science Faculty, Universitas Negeri Semarang, Indonesia[123]

Article History

Keywords:
Journalism; Journalistic; Pers; News, Sport

Abstract

Seeing the potential of untapped learning media. Creativity of teachers to create learning media not only for solving problems, but also exploit the potential that exists. Therefore the author tries to design an Android-based program to improve learning experience of Physical Education, Sport and Health to be more interesting. Using Pre test and Post test method in trial scale. The results showed that, (1) the results of media expert and health expert validation showed 80.475% in the "excellent" category and small-scale trials showed an average of 54.114 results in pre test and 79.2 in the post test. (2) The results of data analysis on large-scale trials in 3 schools showed 52,867 results in the test and increased to 75.2754 in the post test. (3) The students' assessment on the product was 77.091% or in the "good" category and the assessment of the learning expert was 89, 5% in the category of "very good." Learning media product of Physical Education, Health and Sport in Android-based named APPJOK with focused on subject types of foods and beverages that are beneficial to the health of growth and development can be practiced to the subject of the trial.

✉ **Correspondence address :**
Jl. Kembang Joyo, Ds. Kalidoro, Rt 02 Rw 01 No. 48, Kec. Pati, Pati District, 59117 Central Java
E-mail: dewi11nurutami@gmailcom

INTRODUCTION

For hundreds of years, print media has become a dominating medium for information dissemination. Ishwara (2011) explains that since the 1960s and 1970s every survey shows that most americans got the first news from television and car radio. This broadcast media takes over the front page function of newspapers, except for news self-developed newspapers, not available on radio or television, such as news analysis, background news or comments.

This shows that people have a tendency to switch to mass media that get a touch of technology. Because the more advanced technology, the sooner also in getting an information or news.

Handheld devices (handheld devices) is the name for a device that size fit in your hand (zaki, 2008). Viewed from the type, this device is a type of mobile device that works to support your mobile lifestyle. Mobile devices (mobile) or in english called mobile devices are small devices that have limited computing capabilities. The meaning of mobile itself is moving or easy to move and carry.

The advancement of the electronics industry contributes to the rapid development and number of mobile devices. In this case it is a smartphone. As a result, the price also decreased considering the competition among producers increasingly fierce. It affects the price of smartphones are priced cheaper. That way, smartphones can now be owned by all levels of society. With the increasingly popular smartphone, and also supported the mobile lifestyle of today, the mass media of the internet become a community favorite. The perpetrators of journalism was also active in using the internet mass media. Proven with the rise of online news sites, such as detik.com, okezone.com, tribunnews.com, and others.

Smartphones now have a major role in terms of practicality, ease, and speed of news spread. In the world of sports for example, to get information about the development of sports and sports outcomes, or even want to watch sports games that take place, we often rely on internet mass media on our smartphones. In addition, sports enthusiasts in indonesia usually have one favorite sport and want to keep up with the development of the athlete, or his favorite sports team. If we missed the sporting event or wanted to know about the developments in the world of sports, we can use our smartphone to search for news in just a few hours after it happened. We also do not have to bother out looking for newspaper merchants. Even a news site usually provides video content, thus increasingly spoiling the site's visitors.

Factors of speed and practicality that encourage readers of the segment familiar with the internet began to switch to online media to satisfy the needs of information, especially information in the world of sports. If these conditions continue to run, it will threaten the future of print media. According to sholahuddin (2013), the managers of the press also admitted it was facing a formidable challenge to defend its business. Printing press not only faces competition among print industry, but the most severe, facing new competitors in the multimedia press with its various advantages.

Print media, the newspaper, is the most ancient mass media today. Its characteristics differ greatly from the characteristics of the internet mass media. When a sporting event is phenomenal, or there is a development in the world of sports, then a newspaper can deliver it to the public the next day. That's because the information obtained by newspaper journalists through several stages, namely writing, typing, editing, and printing. News published by a newspaper is news that happened yesterday. In addition, the content contained in newspapers is just text and images.

One of the print media that still survive to this day is suara merdeka., which has editorial office at jl. Raya kaligawe no. 5 semarang, central java. Suara merdeka has the slogan "100% central java" which reflects the marketing position of the newspaper.

Based on the background and focus of the problem above, the authors formulate the problem "how is the strategy of presenting daily news coverage of suara merdeka in the middle of competition in the era of mobile media?"

The purpose of this study is to know the strategy used daily suara merdeka in presenting sports news in the middle of the competition in the era of mobile media.

METHODS

The approach used in this research is descriptive method. According Sukmadinata (2011) descriptive research is research aimed to describe or describe the phenomena that exist, whether natural phenomena or human engineering. In qualitative research pay more attention to the characteristics, quality, interrelationship between activities (Sukmadinata 2011). So in this research, researcher use descriptive research method with qualitative approach.

In this study the research subjects selected by the researcher were randomly selected sports news reporters, the head of the sports desk Suara

Merdeka on behalf of Mr. Edi Indarto, the deputy leader of the Redakasi II Suara Merdeka on behalf of Mr. Ananto Pradono, and Mr. Amir Machmud as observer, sports writer and sports news developers.

This study uses natural settings, where the implementation of this research does occur naturally, as is, in the situation, naturally. Then the sources used are primary sources and secondary sources, where the primary sources are sports reporters Suara Merdeka, head of the sporting desk Suara Merdeka, and deputy editor-in-chief of Suara Merdeka, and secondary sources are sports observers and documents or data supporting the process of presenting sports news. Further data collecting techniques include: observation as the initial data collector before the research, and interviews as the main data collection tool of this research, and documentation as a complementary data collection tool in this study.

The validity of the data using triangulation technique, while the data analysis of this research using the theory of Miles and Huberman.

RESULTS AND DISCUSSION

Suara Merdeka has two ways to get news. First through the reporter-reporter if the news in the region of Central Java. Second through its news agencies such as Antara, AFP, and Reuters if the news is national and international. In Semarang, Suara Merdeka has 2 sports reporters. The division of work coverage is one reporter covering football news and one other reporter covering non-soccer news. But basically, both should be able to all the sports. For those in the area, the assignment is shared by each bureau chief. In selecting news sources, the reporter will choose someone who is qualified and has a relationship with the field to be covered. Preparation of reporters before the interview is making the agenda of anyone who will be met, make a list of questions, then memorize it. When the interview the reporter should be ready with the interview material and should not carry or read the note.

The structure of news applied by Suara Merdeka is to use inverted pyramid, of importance, less important, less important, and so on. To compose the title of sports news, will be selected words "bombastic" by reporters and editors. For example "Barcelona Libas Real Madrid". Or with poetic words like "Rise or Add Pain". In preparing the sports news leads are actually not mandatory 5W1H for promoting leads that break down and core news to be delivered. The news body contains 5W1H along with its development. Will be selected the most attractive and interesting photo or picture that will be displayed along with the news.

In writing sports news, Suara Merdeka chose the most popular sports news in the community, trying to provide more information than what has been enjoyed by people when it was made (in depth news), including statistical data, presenting news analysis before and after the game, and write sports news with an objective perspective of subjectivity. In addition to the 5W1H element, another thing that is written is the element "next". It also features local news of Central Java so it remains close emotionally with the readers.

The development of mobile media has a negative impact and positive impact on Suara Merdeka. The negative impact is making the production of Suara Merdeka decreased from year to year. The positive impact is to make the reporters and editors in presenting the news to be more innovative, responsive, proactive, extroverted, and able to manage the actuality.

CONCLUSION

It can be concluded that the strategy of presenting daily news coverage of Suara Merdeka in the midst of competition in the era of mobile media is to present in-depth news, features, match statistics, quote of the day, news before and after game, and highlight local sports news Central Java

REFERENCES

Ishwara, L. 2011. Jurnalisme Dasar. Jakarta: PT Kompas Media Nusantara

Kusumaningrat, H., dan Kusumaningrat, P. 2014. Jurnalistik Teori & Praktik. Bandung: PT Remaja Rosdakary

Sholahuddin. 2013. Strategi Pengembangan Produk di Industri Media Cetak di Indonesia (Bertahan di tengah Persaingan dengan Media Online). BENEFIT Jurnal Manajemen dan Bisnis Volume 17, Nomor 1. Hlm. 9-17

Social Media and Website Tracking with Analytics. Detik.com. www.trackalytics.com/website/detik.com/. Diakses pada 21/05/17

Sukmadinata, N. S. 2011. Metode Penelitian Pendidikan. Bandung: PT Remaja Rosdakarya

Sumadiria, A. S. H. 2014. Jurnalistik Indonesia Menulis Berita dan Feature Panduan Praktis Jurnalis Profesional. Bandung: Simbiosa Rekatama Media

Zaki, A. 2008. E-Lifestyle: Memanfaatkan Beragam Perangkat Teknologi Digital. Jakarta: Salemba Infotek

Development of Android-Based Anatomy Edutainment Instruction Materials

Farizha Irmawati[1], Erfitra Rezqi[2], Ika Oktaviana[3]

Physical Education Program of Health and Recreation, IKIP Budi Utomo Malang, Indonesia[123]

Article History

Keywords:
Teaching Materials;
Edutaiment; and Android

Abstract

This study aims to produce teaching materials anatomy edutaiment-based android decent and effective in learning in Prodi Education Biology IKIP Budi Utomo Malang. Android-based teaching materials capable of supporting Anatomy learning with various features provided and will be more communicative and interesting to use in learning. This research is a development research using ADDIE model. Based on the validation results indicate that anatomy based edutainment and anatomy teaching materials in both categories with the validation score of material experts 89 and the validation of media experts 86.4, so it can be concluded that the teaching materials anatomy edutainment based android decent and valid for use in learning Anatomy Student Study Program Physical Education Health and Recreation IKIP Budi Utomo Malang.

Correspondence address :
IKIP Budi Utomo Malang, Jalan Simpang Arjuno No. 14B Malang
E-mail: farizha99@gmail.com

INTRODUCTION

In the current era of globalization, the development of information and communication technology can not be dammed anymore, in the side of human life in the 21st century. The speed of development of information and communication technology is clearly visible in the field of business, economy and governance with the emergence of concepts and applications in the form of e-Government, e-commerce, e-community and so forth. This phenomenon has become an easy-to-use trend and gradually shifts the methodology conventionally. In the world of education began to shift, along with the development of information and communication technology, emerging terms of E-learning, online learning, web-based training, online courses, web-based education and so forth, and also there are many educational institutions that utilize E-learning system to improve the effectiveness and flexibility of learning (Tasri , 2011).

Currently technology, information and communication has become part of the world of education that becomes a learning medium, which becomes an integral part in the learning process. This can be seen from the definition of the media is anything that can be used to channel the message from the sender to the receiver so as to stimulate the thoughts, feelings, and interests and concerns of students in such a way that the learning process occurs (Sadiman, 2007). Learning media is one component of the important learning resources of its existence also determine the success of a learning (Sadiman, 2005). Learning media is a means of communication used to convey the message, it is necessary teaching materials that are supported by a meaningful media learning and fun (edutaiment) to attract interest, increase motivation, and improve students' understanding of learning materials, of course, will be more optimal use by following the technology trends information and communication, has now penetrated up to the students that the popularity of Android is embedded in smartphones (Aziz, 2015).

One way to boost interest and motivation of students in the learning process is to maximize teaching materials and learning media that are used. Media that can be used smartphone device that is produced with the aim as a communication tool, with the facilities embedded in it can be used for learning media. By utilizing the smartphone as a medium of learning to support teaching materials, of course it creates a more communicative and interesting learning atmosphere.

This is supported by research conducted by Nuraidah which shows there is an increase in student interest in learning Mathematics by developing Edutainment based learning media in the form of android mobile games, and research conducted by Arina and Agung (2017) on the development of Interactive Materials Based on Android On Journal Material Adjustment And Journal Correction For Class XII Accounting At SMKN1 Surabaya.

Based on the results of observations on IKIP BUDI UTOMO Malang, Physical Education and Health Recreation program that the student interest in taking lessons Anatomy less than the maximum, due to several things, such as the limited accesses and support of IT-based reference resources among students IKIP Budi Utomo, where a reference source should be easily and quickly accessible to students. In addition, some of the subject matter of anatomy is difficult to understand because many use of foreign terms and media used less mengung interest student in general. The above issues illustrate the empirical and academic anxieties of this study. Therefore, this study will design easy-to-understand and IT-based teaching materials to provide substantial support for the problems faced by IKIP Budi Utomo students. It will primarily discuss a subject-matter of instruction by anatomy-based edutainment.

Based on the above background, this research is aimed to 1) to arrange Prototype of anatomy based edutainment teaching materials for students of Physical Education Study Program of Health and Recreation of IKIP Budi Utomo Malang, and 2) to know the feasibility and validity of anatomical edutainment based teaching materials for students of Education Studies Program Physical Health and Recreation IKIP Budi Utomo Malang.

METHODS

Development of subject matter of course Anatomy Edutainment based on android refers to the model of ADDIE development (Branch, 2009). The model consists of five steps: (1) analyze (analysis), (2) design, (3) development, (4) implementation, and (5) evaluation (evaluation). Stages of development carried out in this research is the stage 1) analyze (analysis), 2) design (design), and 3) development (development).

Subjects in this study were 10 students Prodi PJKR IKIP Budi Utomo Malang who had taken the course of Anatomy. This study was conducted to determine the feasibility and validity of instructional edutainment based on android for use in learning.

Validation data of validators (material and media validation) as well as data from user (student) of teaching materials will be analyzed which is used as a reference to improve and revise teaching materials as well as to analyze scores for mnegetahui level of eligibility and validity of developed materials.

RESULTS AND DISCUSSION

Android-based edutaiment teaching materials for anatomy courses are done through several stages: 1) Analyze Stage (Analysis), this stage performed basic competence analysis in accordance with the curriculum in PJKR, and translated into several indicators of learning as in **table 1.**

2) Stage Design (Design), this stage is done by determining the objectives, objectives, material framework, materials, and various references to be used. Development of edutainment based teaching materials android compiled using flash media macro software version 8.

Table 1. Basic Competencies and Indicators

Basic competencies	Indicator
1. Understand the scope of osteology	1. Explain the notion of osteology and skeleton 2. Explain the function of skeleton 3. Name the bones of the body.
2.Understand the structure and composition of the network	1. Explain the structure of the constituents of bone tissue. 2. Analyze the composition of bone tissue
3.Understanding the classification of skeletal bone framework in humans.	1. Describe the organization of the skeletal system. 2. Explain the kind, shape of bone. 3. Analyze open and closed fracture improvements.

Components of developed learning materials consist of home, profile, material and reference list. The type, color, and font size are set proportionally to be interesting for users to read. The initial display section is given the logo of IKIP Budi Utomo Malang. Examples of the initial display are presented in **picture 1**.

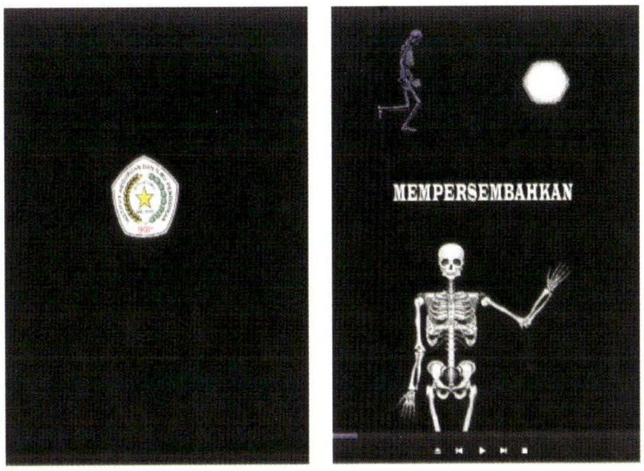

Picture 1. Initial Display of Instructional Materials.

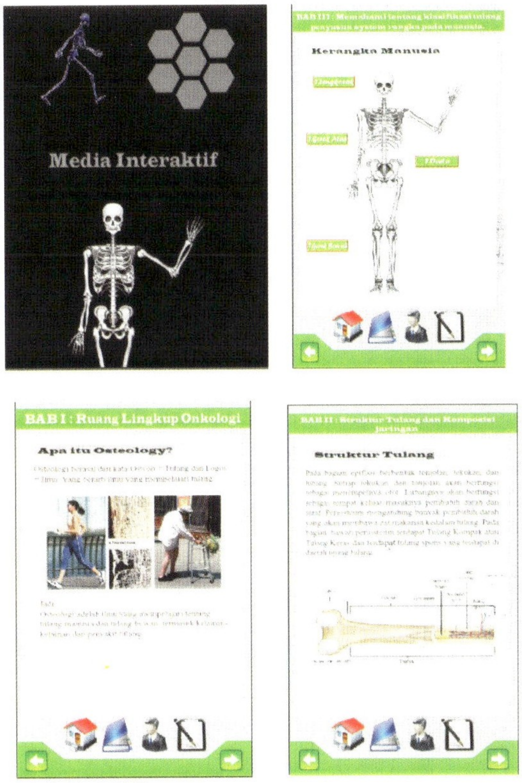

Picture 2. Display Media Edutainment

The content consists of three competencies: understanding the scope of osteology, understanding the composition and structure of the network and understanding the classification of human skeletal bone. The teaching materials contain animations allowing students to understand the anatomical material and examples in motion on the bone.

3) Development Stage (Development), this stage is done by revising the teaching materials based on the input of expert media validator and practitioner validator. Based on the results of the assessment of media expert Faris Mushlihul A., M.Komari from the State University of Surabaya, scored 89 with very interesting criteria and can be

used used without revision, and penilaiaan based on the input of expert material and practitioner Gema Fitriyadi, M.Pd, who is a lecturer of PJKR in Malang State University get value of 86,4%, with criterion have been feasible to be used. The teaching materials after being validated will be revised in accordance with the input of the validator review, then tested on 10 students of PJKR who have taken the subject of anatomy, based on the test result get the value of 91,25 with the criterion of qualification is very interesting and can be used without revision.

Development of teaching materials based on android can bridge the indicator of competence that must be achieved by students. Teaching materials are tools used to achieve competence in the form of knowledge, instructional materials (materialsal materials), and skills. In detail, the types of learning materials consist of knowledge covering facts, concepts, principles, procedures, skills, and attitudes or values (Depdiknas, 2006).

Useful teaching materials to facilitate fluency in the learning process, especially in anatomical subjects. Kusdiyanti (2011) revealed that, teaching materials that are arranged in relation to the curriculum should pay attention to certain goals to be achieved through education conducted by using textbooks concerned.

The result of the development of instructional materials based on the android on the subject of anatomy, there are revisions made in accordance with the development research procedure by considering the suggestions and input from the material content experts, media experts and instructional materials design. The result of data analysis that has been done on the development of instructional materials based on the android on the anatomy course shows the validation result of teaching materials deserves to be used as a reference to the anatomy course, with this android-based teaching material is expected to help the students in obtaining the material flexibly and effectively.

Ardhana (2002) states that development research is conducted to bridge research and educational practices. The development of research-enhanced curriculum and research-based learning (RETL), in various models, has grown very well and is believed to be the right choice for today's pattern of teaching and learning activities.

CONCLUSION

The validation results for edited android based edutainement materials according to media experts and experts are in decent category with good predicate (86.4% for media aspect and 89% for material aspect), so it can be said that teaching materials are feasible and valid for use in learning.

REFERENCE

Ardhana, W. (2002). Konsep penelitian pengembangan dalam bidang pendidikan dan pembelajaran. Makalah Disampaikan pada Lokakarya Nasional Angkatan II Metodologi Penelitian Pengembangan Bidang Pendidikan dan Pembelajaran. Malang: Universitas Negeri Malang.

Aziz, M., K. 2015. Pengembangan media pembelajaran interaktif Berbasis android untuk meningkatkan Partisipasi dan hasil belajar siswa Pada mata pelajaran PAI.

Branch, R., M. 2009. Instructional Design: The ADDIE Approach. Speingger Science Business Media, LLC .

Departemen Pendidikan Nasional. 2006. Direktorat Jendral Manajemen Pendidikan Dasar Menengah.

Kusdiyanti, H. (2011). Pelatihan Pengembangan Bahan Ajar Kearsipan Berbasis Potensi Lokal dalam rangka Program pemberdayaan Siswa Binaan Labsosdik di SMK se-Malang.

Tasri, L. 2011 .Pengembangan bahan ajar berbasis web. Jurnal medtek: volume 3, nomor 2, oktober 2011

10

The "Happy Bouncing Ball" Game for The Learning of Table Tennis for Grade V Primary School Students

Moch Fahmi Abdulaziz[1], Harry Pramono[2], Anirotul Qoriah[3], Bagus Ginanjar MS[4]

Jurusan Pendidikan Jasmani Kesehatan dan Rekreasi, Fakultas Ilmu Keolahragaan, Universitas Negeri Semarang[1234]

Article History

Keywords:
Happy Bouncing Ball; Ping-pong; Modifications

Abstract

Physical education, health and sports is an integral part of the overall education, aiming to develop physical fitness, skills of motion, critical thinking skills, social skills, reasoning, emotional stability, moral action, aspects of healthy living patterns and the introduction of clean environment through physical activity, sport and health selected planned systematically in order to achieve the goals of national education. Physical education, health and sports are the attempts to embody the whole person in the school, either from a basic to intermediate education level. Table tennis is one of the Physical education learning material taught in elementary school. However, the reality in the learning process has not been implemented optimally because the table was not proportional to the number of students. Thus the need to win and the modifications to the game, make students more actively in learning. The problems that plagued the school made teacher's creativity in developing models of learning a new, yet fun and in accordance with the objectives of the learning that has been set. Modification of the learning game of ping-pong was one of the efforts that must be realized. Learning the ping-pong game through the happy bouncing ball game was expected to make children more actively engaged in a variety of pleasant situations and conditions, while following the learning of table tennis game.

Correspondence address:
Gedung F1 Lantai 2 FIK Unnes Kampus Sekaran, Gunungpati, Semarang, 50229
E-mail : moch.fahmiabdulaziz12@gmail.com

INTRODUCTION

Physical Education

Physical education is part of overall education. Physical education is aiming to achieve the educational process through motion and physical activity. In fact, physical education has an important role in the development of the quality of education in Indonesia.

Physical education is an educational venture by using the large muscles activity up to the educational process taking place is not hampered by health problems and the growth of the body. As an integral part of the overall educational process, physical education is an effort that aims to develop the area of organic, neuromuscular, intellectual, and social (Ateng, 1992:4).

According to Supandi (1992:1) physical education is a process of systematic interaction between the student and the environment in physical development through governance effectively and efficiently towards the formation of the whole person. Thus, physical education is an integral part of the overall education that support the development of students through physical activity or human movement. It is then organized systematically in the form of teaching-learning activities to meet the needs of the growth and development of the physical, mental and social.

Sharman in Nadisah (1992:15) suggests that physical education is part of the education (in General) that goes through activities that involve motion mechanism of human body and generate patterns of behaviour on the individual concerned.

While according to the definition of the terminology (committee of terminology, 1951) in Nadisah (1992:17) health education is the process of granting learning experiences with a view to influence knowledge, attitudes and behaviour with regard to the health of the individual or group.

According to Rusli Lutan (2001) that physical education is a series of lessons that provide a real contribution in everyday life in an attempt to improve the growth and development of physical as well as spiritual learners. Therefore the Organization of physical education should be further developed more optimal so that learners will be more innovative, skilled, creative, and have the physical freshness and healthy living habits and have knowledge and understanding of human motion.

According to Samsudin (2008:2) suggests that physical education is a process of learning through physical activity designed to improve physical fitness, develop motor skills, knowledge and behaviour of healthy and active living, an attitude of sportsmanship, and emotional intelligence.

So based on some of the opinions above about the sense of physical education, can be summed up that physical education is a process of education done through physical activity and created to enhance the growth and development of the entire physical realm, namely: psychomotoric, cognitive and affective student.

According to Adang Suherman (2000:23), in general, physical education objectives can be classified into four categories, namely:

a. Physical Development

Goals related with the ability to perform activities that involve the physical powers of the various organs of the body of a person.

b. Development of motion

This objective relates to the ability of doing the movement effectively, efficiently, smoothly, beautifully, perfectly.

c. Mental development

This objective relates to the ability to think and interpret the overall knowledge about physical education into their surroundings so as to allow the growing and development of knowledge, attitudes, and responsibility.

d. Social Development

This goal relate students' ability in adjusting themselves to a community group.

Table Tennis

The development of the table tennis is now like a fungus. Table tennis quickly spread in all areas, caused the game's rated sports community as a recreational sport for leisure, sports achievement, an educational tool as well as the media to socialize. This was confirmed by the opinion of Hodges (2007:1) stating that the game of table tennis is a racquet sport which is popular in the world and the number of participants occupying second place.

The popularity of table tennis can also be due to the game's many privileges, such as can be played by everyone ranging from children to adults either male or female, doesn't require a vast place, the tool used is light and easy to use, the price of the equipment was very affordable by all people, this game can also serve as a mean of recreation that can become entertainment.

Table tennis game was very popular in the society. This game can be played by children, teenagers or even adults, as well as a recreational sport.

Modification of Learning

In accordance with the basic competence of table tennis material especially for large classes, it is mentioned that students can practice basic techniques of small ball games with rules modified to foster cooperation, sportsmanship and honesty. In the process of learning table tennis in meet some things, among others:

1. The tools and facilities are in minimal use.
2. The rules of the table tennis game are used in accordance with the actual rules or rules in the game of table tennis.
3. Tend to many students when following the lesson just sit around and not actively follow the table tennis lesson
4. The learning table tennis game provided by the teacher is still not packaged in the form of modifications, so that found students who feel unhappy, bored, and lazy to move.

Learning physical education through table tennis sports has not been effective as a medium of motion learning. The learning materials of table tennis games have nōt been able to make children move effectively. During the learning time table tennis game students only make a few minute movement because they have to take turns. This situation results in the limited time the child is in motion, so the learning of motion is not optimal

Based on the above description, it is expected that the role of teachers in modifying the table tennis game in order to create a model of learning in the form of a new game that aims to attract students so that students do not feel bored quickly, more motivated and passionate in following the process of physical education.

The development of learning model of Penjasorkes is one of the efforts to help solve the limited problem of teaching and learning facilities of Penjasorkes in schools. The development of the Penjasorkes learning model conducted by Penjasorkes teachers can bring an innovative learning atmosphere, with the creation of fun learning and can motivate learners to have more opportunity to exploit the movement widely and freely, according to their level of ability. By modifying learning media of physical education will not reduce student activity in doing physical education. But just the opposite by modifying the learning and approaches in the form of games as an example, the process of learning physical education will be more fun. Teachers can reduce or increase the complexity and difficulty of teaching tasks by modifying the equipment used to perform that skill. For example, the weight-lighter, large-small, high-low, long-short equipment used. (Rusli Lutan 2001) states that "Modifications in the subject of physical education are necessary, increasing the likelihood of success in participating and being able to move correctly."

METHOD

This research is a development research that aims to produce a model of learning table tennis through mini table tennis for elementary school students (SD).

The steps used in this study use seven main steps, namely:

1. Conduct preliminary research and information gathering. Includes field observation and literature review.
2. Develop the initial product form (in the form of a happy bounching ball game rules).
3. Evaluation of experts by using an expert Pengas and two learning experts, as well as small group trials, using questionnaires and consultations and evaluations that are then analyzed.
4. First product revisions, product revisions based on results from expert evaluation and small group trials. This revision is used for improvements to the original product made by the researcher.
5. Field trials.
6. The final product revisions are made based on the results of field trials.
7. The final result of the table tennis model through the happy bouncing ball game for grade V elementary school students (SD) generated through field test revision.

RESULTS AND DISCUSSION

Modification of the learning
The Happy Bouncing Ball game

The Happy Bouncing Ball game was played in the school courtyard and 1 set of table tennis. The field was divided into 3 posts include: post bouncing bomb, post, post relay bouncing bouncing pong.

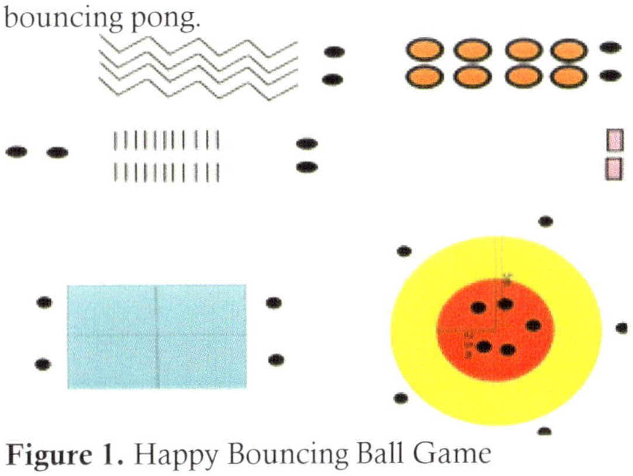

Figure 1. Happy Bouncing Ball Game

Description ;

	= Students		= Running Track
	= Basket		= the limit of players outside and inside
	= Jump Line		
	= Zig-zag line		= Area Players Inside
	= The Line Raised		= Table

Bouncing Estafet

Bouncing ball game relay dibet and ran towards the area of the friend who had been waiting in front of him. The player must run and follow the player hurdles ahead of him. How to feed the ball like the movement hit in table tennis, and a friend who can control all received ball with bat and continue on across the line that was already prepared. Finally the players must be able to place the ball into the basket already supplied to earn points.

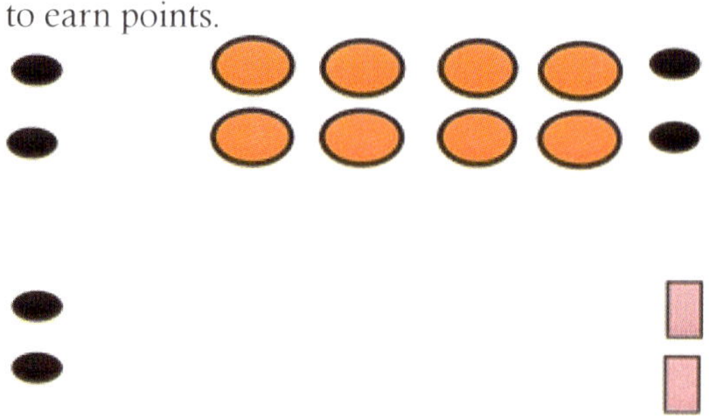

Figure 2. Field relay and bouncing description

Description:

	= Students		= Running Track
	= Basket		= Jump Line

How to play Bouncing Relay

a. The Group raced past the line that was already prepared by reflecting the ball above the bat and followed the line.
b. After the line passed, gave the ball to the next friend by hitting the ball towards his friend using the drive in table tennis.
c. The next player received the ball by using the bat, and continued his journey.
d. Finally Players hit the ball with the use of the technique drives the ping-pong balls into the baskets already provided.
e. This game lasted for 10 minutes
f. Students must walk following the path that already exists, if not breaking in countdown points.
g. Points were earned when the last ball can enter into the basket that was already prepared.
h. The bouncing ball fell in the middle of the journey must be reset at the beginning of the line.

Bouncing Bom

What is meant by bouncing ball bouncing game is bomb dibet, then complementary opponents who are inside the circle. The ball hit the opponent's body into points. The opponent can avoid and beat back the ball using the bat, to protect themselves. This game lasted for 2 minutes once alternately for 10 long play. The most points became the winner.

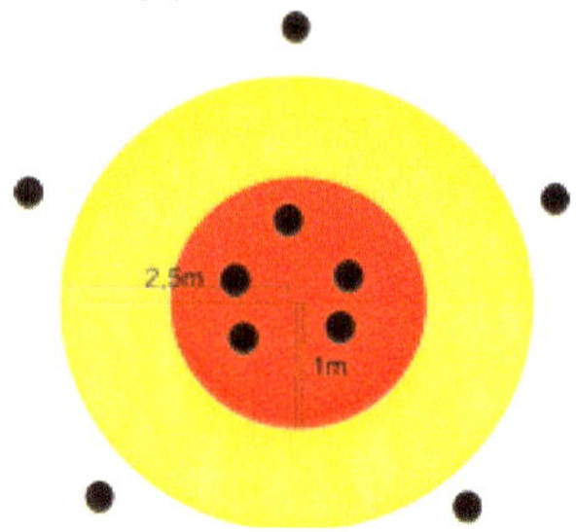

Figure 3. bouncing bombs and field description

Description:

	= Students		= the limit of players outside and inside
	= Area Players Inside		

How to play Bouncing Bomb

a. There were two groups that play in one game, bomb bouncing inside a circle, a 1 was outside of the circle.
b. Group that was within the circle was in charge of protecting themselves by using bat from the opponent's bombs.
c. Group outside hoops was in charge of finding as many points by opponents that were bombed in the circle.
d. For 2 minutes once changed place four times, the game lasted for 8 minutes.
e. The most Points was declared the winner.
f. Ball on head did not earn points.
g. Hit the ball must use the technique drive on table tennis, if they did not comply did not count points.

Bouncing pong

What is meant by bouncing pong was a game using the table as bouncing media field. The balls reflected on the bat once, then in the opponent area, the ball went into the opponent's area can directly restored or reflected. The table used was part of the long side. Calculation of points was the same as the game of table tennis.

Figure 4. Field pong and bouncing description

Description:

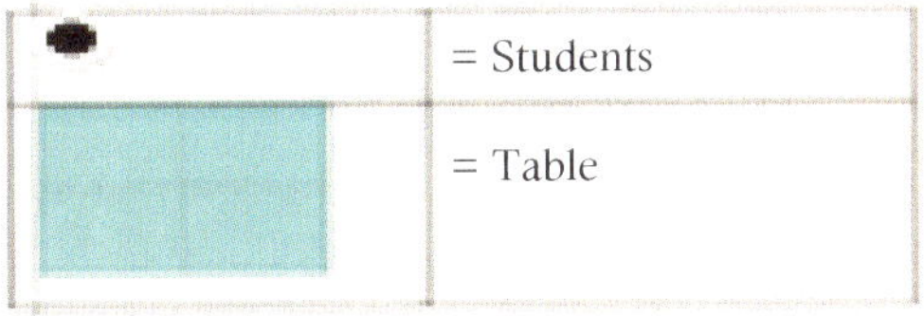

How to play Bouncing Pong

a. The game was like a game of ping-pong, but used half the table to play.
b. Students may reflect as much dibet ball once and hit back to the opponent.
c. Calculation of this game using the three times victory by using the relaypoint system 11 points
d. At the time the service was touching the net, the service being restarted.
e. The ball entered the opponent's desk in the field considered points.
f. Ball that struck out of the opponent's desk turned out, without touching the opponent, considered the points made.
g. Controlling the ball must not be more than 2 bounce on the bat.

Measures in play

Before doing the happy bouncing ball game, students must first master the techniques of table tennis game. Thus there were several processes that should be mastered, in order to play happy bouncing ball. Exercises to do amongst other students; bounce ball, squash, and playing in pairs.

Bounce ball

This exercise aimed to promote or hold the adjustment between the player with the ball, and the bat was also adapted at using the tools and had a good feeling/subtle related to the bat and bounce his ball (Muhtar and Sulistyo, 2009:3.2).

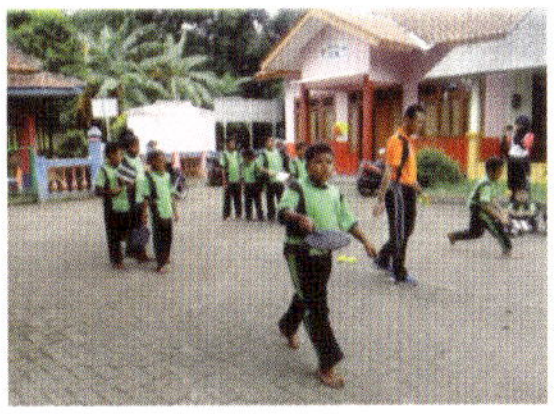

Figure 5. Bouncing ball

1. Bouncing Ball over using the bat.

Initially conducted separately, for example, by the side of the forehand or backhand side, then can proceed with a combination of forehand and backhand.

2. Reflecting the ball onto the floor.

This exercise can also be varied, ranging from exercise bouncing to the floor in place, then while walking forward, backwards, left or right.

3. The overall Regulatory

a. Students were divided into six groups, each group had 5 members.
b. The referee drew a group a match.
c. Every post was played simultaneously, with the command listened to the referee set each post.
d. After each post already found the winner, the Group took turns to the next post and continued the game posted.
e. Postal Order was Bouncing bomb, Relay, and Bouncing Bouncing Pong
f. This game will last until the last post.
g. The Group stated three bouncing post won the game when they got points.

Play Equipment

1. The ball in the game three to use post bouncing ball this was using a lightweight tonnis.
2. The Bat
   Bat used for game three of the post it was bouncing modifications to bat using the square board with a side of 20 cm and 15 cm long handle.

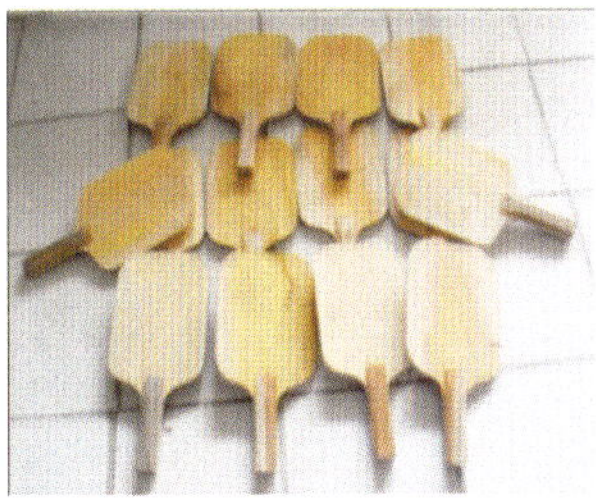

Figure 6. Bat the game modification of table tennis

Advantages and disadvantages of the "Happy Bouncing Ball" game

1. The advantages of this game were:
   a. the Happy bouncing ball game can be

played by all students
b. can be played at schools that did not have a ping pong table
2. Weaknesses of products produced were:
a. Required a spacious place to play , and required a lot of bet.

CONCLUSION

The end result of this development research is the product of table tennis model through the game of happy bouncing ball based on the data during the small scale test (N = 15) and field trials (N = 30).

This happy bouncing ball game model can be accepted by all students because in this game the students have been able to move actively and understand the rules that apply. The game model is good in accordance with the level of students' needs in the move, in accordance with the level of development, and is in accordance with the growth rate of students.

REFERENCES

Anni, C. T. 2006. Psikologi Belajar. Semarang: UPT MKK UNNES

Ardi, S. W., Hartiawan, U., & Pujianto, A. (2013). Pengembangan Model Pembelajaran Tenis Meja Lantai Dalam Penjasorkes Pada Siswa Kelas VI SD Puri Kecamatan Pati Kabupaten Pati. ACTIVE: Journal of Physical Education, Sport, Health and Recreation, 2(3).

Ateng, A. 1992. Asas Dan Landasan Pendidikan Jasmani. Departemen Pendidikan Dan Kebudayaan Direktorat Jenderal Pendidikan Tinggi

Damiri, A. dan Kusmaedi, N. 1992. Olahraga Pilihan Tenis Meja. Departemen Pendidikan Dan Kebudayaan Direktorat Jenderal Pendidikan Tinggi Proyek Pembinaan Tenaga Kependidikan

Darsono, M. 2001. Belajar dan Pembelajaran. Semarang: CV IKIP Semarang Press

Fakultas Ilmu Keolahragaan, 2011. Buku Panduan Penulisan Skripsi FIK UNNES. Semarang

Hamalik, O. 2005. Kurikulum dan Pembelajaran. Bandung: PT Bumi Aksara

Kertamanah, A.2003.Teknik Dan Taktik Mahir Permainan Tenis Meja. Jakarta:PT Raja Grafindo Persada

Kurniawan, P. B. (2013). Peningkatan Hasil Belajar Tenis Meja Melalui Pendekatan Permainan Bouncing Ball Siswa SMP. ACTIVE: Journal of Physical Education, Sport, Health and Recreation, 2(7).

Kusuma, O. Y. J. (2014). Model Pembelajaran Keseimbangan Melalui Permainan Estafet Bola di Lingkungan Persawahan. Journal of Physical Education Health and Sport, 1(2), 93-97.

Larry, H. 2007.Tenis Meja Tingkat Pemula. Jakarta:PT Raja Grafindo Persada

Lutan, R dan Suherman, A. 2000. Perencanaan Pembelajaran Penjaskes. Jakarta: Departemen Pendidikan Jasmani

Ma'mun, A. dan Saputra, Y. 2000.Perkembangan gerak dan belajar gerak. Jakarta: DEPDIKBUD.

Muhtar, T. dan Sulistyo, W. 2003. Tenis Meja (Mata Kuliah Pilihan 1). Jakarta: Universitas Terbuka

Nadisah. 1992. Pengembangan Kurikulum Pendidikan Jasmani dan Kesehatan. Bandung: direktorat jenderal pendidikan tinggi

Rusli Lutan, 2000. Strategi Belajar Mengajar Penjaskes. Jakarta: Departemen Pendidikan Jasmani

Samsudin. 2008. Pembelajaran Pendidikan Jasmani Olahraga dan Kesehatan SD/ MI. Jakarta: Litera

Saputra, Y. M. 2003. Pembelajaran Atletik di Sekolah Dasar. Jakarta: Depdiknas.

Sudarmono, M. 2010. Pengembangan Model Pembelajar melalui Permainan Sepakbola Gawang Ganda bagi Siswa SMP Ajibarang Kabupaten Banyumas Tahun Ajaran 2009/2010. Skripsi. UNNES.

Suherman, A. 2000. Dasar-Dasar Penjaskes. Departemen Pendidikan Nasional Direktorat Jenderal Pendidikan Dasar dan Menengah

Sukirman,Dkk. 2004.Matematika.Jakarta:UT

Supandi. 1992. Strategi Belajar Mengajar Pendidikan Jasmani Kesehatan. Departemen Pendidikan Dan Kebudayaan Direktorat Jenderal Pendidikan Tinggi

Tim Abdi Guru. 2007. Pendidikan Jasmani Olahraga dan Kesehatan, Jakarta. Erlangga.

Widya, M. D. A. 2006. Gerak- Gerak Dasar Atletik Dalam Bermain. Jakarta: PT Raja Grafindo Persada

11

The Association Between Physical Self Concept, Sport and Gender In Algerian Adolescents

Farid Mouissi, **Martin Hofmeister**
Farid Mouissi
APSSES Laboratory,Institute of Physical Education and Sports, University of Chlef, Algeria
Martin Hofmeister
Consumer Centre of the German Federal State of Bavaria, Department Food and Nutrition, Germany

Article History

Keywords:
Physical Self Concept; Gender; Sport; Physical Activity; Algerian.

Abstrak

This study aims to clarify the impact of sport specialty in physical self concept and gender, and also the difference in the dimension of the physical self concept. A sample of research is made up of 169 sportsmen in different disciplines from Chlef's sport league with an average age of 18.3± 2.45 (soccer , volleyball, athleticism). The Physical self-description questionnaire (PSDQ) was used to measure the concept of physical self-according to multidimensional perspectives. The research results have demonstrated that the kind of sport discipline practiced by high level players has an impact on their understanding of their physical selves, and the second results might assert the general approximation which we are about to speak about. Gender issue influences self-esteem in relation to individuals, yet in the field of sport, we realize that males and females are equal at the level of all other dimensions of the questioner.

Correspondence address:
APS,Society,Education and Health,APSSES Laboratory, BP, 151University of chlef, 02000, Algeria.
E-mail: f.mouissi@univ-chlef.dz/mouissif@yahoo.fr

INTRODUCTION

The self-concept is becoming one of the most important crucial variables for psychological domain, being a concept that allows us not only to judge the personality and behavior of the person but also to predict his conduct. It has been considered by Carl Rogers as pillar in understanding the human personality (Rogers, 1959). This is what led many studies to deal with the concept of the self analytically even it is done under different terminology such as self-esteem, self-perception and self-fulfillment and many other terms that revolves around the same context. It would be quite difficult to find another concept that has been given so much importance (Guérin, Famose, 2005).

Through this concept we might possibly explain the behavior of individuals and predict their future actions. It might also reflect the different representations which these individuals might have about themselves. This concept has become so important as to be labeled water of life (Fortes, 2003). It has been deployed in fighting against violence, psychological illnesses, addiction, educational failure and sports (Ninot, 2003).

In fact, it does not only reflect the behavior of the individual and its characteristics, but also their emotions through self-evaluation of its different sides and aspects, which has been acquired as a consequence of his interaction with the environment (Lau et al., 2008).

According to Rosenberg (1979), it is that evaluative side of the self or the feeling of self-satisfaction or rejection of what we wish to become. Given the importance gained by this concept, it might have been crucial to have researches in the field of psychology include this concept in the study of the psychological life of the sportsman due to its connection with impulsiveness, achievement, control and anxiety and many other psychological characteristic features (Ferreira, Fox, 2004; Klomsten al., 2004). Therefore, this concept has been studied together with many other sport terminologies. The results of these studies have demonstrated that the concept of positive self as related to the individual leads to a high physical performance, hence a good sport results (Levy, Ebbeck, 2005)

Research studies have also pointed to the existing connection between the concept of the self and the participation in physical and sport activities (Marsh, Jackson, 1986). The individuals who are distinguished by the concept of positive self are more inclined to practice physical and sport activities. Besides, this concept is related to physical ability through its proper means of measurement. The study of Marsh et al. (1986) has demonstrated that the participation of the individual in a given training programme increases his level of self-esteem. In addition to this, comparative study between sportsmen and non-sportsmen has asserted that the estimation of the physical self, together with the dimension of physical competence, is higher in sportsmen (Marsh et al., 1995). The concept of physical self has gone through the same stages which have been undergone by the concept of general self.

The concept of physical self and its relationship with gender variable: Many studies referred to the relationship that exists between the concept of the physical self and gender variable (Alsaker, Olweus, 1993; Babic et al. 2014; Block, Robins, 1993; Bolognini et al., 1996; Kling et al., 1999; Maïano et al., 2006; Marsh, 1998; Marsh et al., 2015). Research results have confirmed the existence of divergences in the concept of physical self between males and females: it's in the advantage of males at different levels (Marsh et al., 2015). Studies, which has been performed by Maïano et al. (2006) on a group of young French people using the physical self perception profile have shown that the results of males were far more variable than that of females at multiple dimensions, especially the dimension of sport competence.

As Marsh (1998) remarked, overall aim of the comparative studies in relation to the concept of the self between the two sexes is concentrated on the degree and not the formula of the concept itself. And this is what we have remarked in the tools used in measuring the concept of the self and physical self in particular, where we do not find tools of measurement special for males and females. The difference that exists between the results related to the concept of the self requires the finding of a paradigm that might explain the structure of the concept of the self for both males and females (Famose, Guérin, 2002). The results of these differences between males and females are related to many issues, the most important ones are: the nature of physical activity practiced in different countries including the European ones. The overall activities practiced are of male character, i.e. activities characterized by power and intensity, and this is what does not match the female nature (Maïano et al., 2004).

Still, the conception developed by the individual as a result of his interaction with the environment to which he belongs about the kind of body and the industrial culture has imposed a new paradigm in regards to the image of body that females should seek. And as a result of social comparison, the evaluation of the physical self will be negative. This is what Marsh et al. (1995) referred to when he said that the reason for negative self-esteem for females is caused by the differences that exist between the concept held by females and the culture that imposes a new mode.

For this reason our present research about gender profile and its relation with the concept of physical self as related to high level players puts as the center of its concern the following problematic:

Does gender variable influence the concept of physical self?

Do the practiced physical activities have influence on the concept of physical self?

METHOD

A sample of research is made up of 169 sportsmen (136 males, 33 females) in different disciplines from Chlef's sport league with an average age of 18.3 years ± 2.45 (soccer, volleyball, athleticism). According to the problematic of the present research, and as we try to proof the paradigmatic aspect of this pattern and its connection to some variable that characterized sportsmen and women, the convenient method to our research study is the method of comparative, it is also known as the description and interpretative method paradigm that does not only stop at the level of the relationship and the difference that exist between variable, but to interprets this connection and differences, it also measures the degree of these connection and the disparities that exist between the variable of the our research topic.

The 70-item Physical self-description questionnaire (PSDQ) - designed by Herbert W. Marsh and others in 1994 - was used to measure the concept of physical self-according to multi-dimensional perspectives: health, coordination, physical activity, body fat, sports competence, appearance, strength, flexibility, endurance, and two global measures of self-concept (Global Physical Self-Concept and Global Self-Esteem). Each specific subscale is represented by 6 or 8 items. The PSDQ has been translated and modified to fit the Algerian environment in a previous study done by the researcher (Mouissi et al., 2010).

Data analysis: Before statistical analyses were performed, Kolmogorov-Smirnov test was used to test normality of data distribution. All results are expressed as means ± standard deviation. Major study variables were tested using student's t-test and one-way ANOVA. Value of less than 0.05 was considered statistically significant. Statistical analyses were performed using SPSS software version 20.0.

RESULTS AND DISCUSSION

The results of this investigation are summarized in Table 1 and 2. The research results have demonstrated that the kind of sport discipline practiced by high level players has an impact on their understanding of their physical selves. Since the internal logic of each sport influences the extent of their physical self-perception. Therefore, the underlying dimensions of this concept change and alter with it the concept of general self because it is of hierarchical nature (**Table 1**).

Table 1. To verify the first hypothesis according to which there are disparities in the concept of physical self between sportsmen and the different practiced disciplines: results of the one-way ANOVA

Discipline	Mean	Standard deviation	Value
Health	31.82	6.97	7.94**
Coordination	26.03	4.66	5.99**
Physical activity	24.82	5.48	1.65
Obesity	28.39	7.17	15.75**
Sport Competence.	25.94	5.87	3.91**
Appearance	23.04	6.09	3.65**
Strenght.	23.44	5.33	1.32
Flexibility	24.57	5.25	6.44**
Endurance.	26.04	5.94	6.90**
Physical self-satisfaction	27.63	6.31	8.42**
Self esteem	32.12	5.70	6.23**

Significance 0.01**, 0.05*

Gender issue influences self-esteem in relation to individuals, yet in the field of sport, we realize that males and females are equal at the level of all other dimensions of the questioner.

Table 2. To verify the second hypothesis according to which gender influences the concept of physical self in sportsmen: results of t-test.

Discipline	Gender	N	Mean	Standard deviation	Value
Health coordination	Female	33	31.91	8.63	-0.21
	Male	136	31.78	6.05	
Physical activity Obesity	Female	33	26.00	4.82	0.029
	Male	136	26.04	4.59	
Sport Competence. Appearance	Female	33	25.06	5.65	0.16
	Male	136	24.71	5.41	
Strenght. flexibility	Female	33	3176	5.93	3.75**
	Male	136	26.75	7.16	
Endurance. Physical self-satisfaction	Female	33	27.09	6.75	1.69
	Male	136	25.38	5.33	
Self esteem health	Female	33	22.55	7.18	-1.01
	Male	136	23.28	5.50	
Coordination Physical activity	Female	33	23.48	6.37	0.55
	Male	136	23.41	4.78	
Obesity Sport Competence.	Female	33	24.82	5.91	0.76
	Male	136	24.46	4.92	
Appearance Strenght.	Female	33	23.61	6.97	-3.79**
	Male	136	27.22	4.99	
Flexibility Endurance.	Female	33	29.82	7.19	3.47**
	Male	136	26.57	5.57	
Physical self-satisfaction	Female	33	33.48	6.60	2.09*
	Male	136	31.46	5.11	

Significance 0.01**, 0.05*

Throughout the results of the first hypothesis that points to the influence of the type of specialization and the nature of sport discipline on self-esteem and its different dimensions, we find that it has been realized. Results pointed out the existence of differences between results that correspond to the kind of practiced sport discipline in exception to two dimensions: the dimension of power and that of physical activity. Studies focused on this dimension pointed to the differences between groups (males, females), (practitioners, non-practitioners) (Crooker et al., 2000; Daley, Buchanan, 1999; Lindwall, Lindgren, 2005; Schneider et al., 2008), yet it didn't study the differences between these groups of sport practitioners themselves. Going back to the definition referred to previously, we find that the concept of the self in general terms develops through the opinions and judgments of other, and especially these who are considered as important persons by the individual. In other words, it is that concept that develops as a result of other's judgments. As we know that in the physical activities there are special characteristic features to each type of sport, or there is an internal logic that governs this type as mentioned by Pierre PARLEBAS.

This is what makes these sportsmen estimate themselves physically in different way. The kind of sport practiced compels the sportsman to distinguish himself in a given physical aspect. It is considered as the most important element for that kind of sport. Judo player, for instance, who practices this sport in heavy weight category, is characterized with high level obesity in comparison with the rest of sportsmen, yet his self-esteem will be positive. This is because the characteristics of this kind of sport discipline pushes towards this kind of self-acceptance. The individual understanding of physical self is related primarily with the dimension which is most important, being acquired through the opinions of the others that surround him, such as the coach, the public audience and what is already imposed by the physical activity itself.

Concerning the second hypothesis, the results might assert the general approximation which we are about to speak about. Gender issue influences self-esteem in relation to individuals, yet in the field of sport, we realize that males and females are equal at the level of all other dimensions of the questioner. And this is due to the fact that females are about to practice physical activities that are not different from that practices by males, except that we have noticed that the differences were pointing to close dimensions: the dimension of obesity and that of continuity. This is caused by the importance given by females to the dimension of obesity. Given the social culture prevalent now makes girls develop a negative opinion about obesity. Concerning the second dimension which is continuity, it is related to the non-concern given by females to this kind of physical abilities because of its tiring and intense nature. The difference that exists between males and females is caused by the nature of the psychological structure that characterizes each sex. Females give more importance to their physical appearance because the development of their physical selves is controlled by the social perception of women. Society gives more importance to the image women more than that of men, and this is what pushes them to develop conceptions and understandings about themselves that differ from the one that can be found in men (Bariaud et al., 1999). A limitation of this study was the cross-sectional nature of the data.

CONCLUSION

The results of this study have referred also to the fact that the concept of the physical self is related to its underlying physical dimensions as related the practiced physical activity, and this is what provides us with new data about judgment in self-construction and the psychological dimension of sportsmen according to the nature of physical activity. The psychological preparation of sportsmen is influenced, at the level of the conception of the self, by the nature of the practiced physical activity itself. It is impossible to generalize the different psychological theories in the psychological preparation of high level players in different sport disciplines.

Conflict of interest

The authors declare that no conflicts of interest exist.

REFERENCES

Alsaker FD, Olweus D. Global self-evaluations and perceived instability of self in early adolescence: a cohort longitudinal study. Scand J Psychol 1993;34(1):47-63.

Babic MJ, Morgan PJ, Plotnikoff RC, Lonsdale C, White RL, Lubans DR. Physical activity and physical self-concept in youth: systematic review and meta-analysis. Sports Med 2014;44(11):1589-1601.

Bariaud F, Rodriguez-Tomé H, Cohen-Zardi MF, Delmas C, Jeanvoine B. Effects of puberty on the self-concepts of adolescents. Archives de Pédiatrie 1999;6(9):952-57.

Block J, Robins RW. A longitudinal study of consistency and change in self-esteem from early adolescence to early adulthood. Child Dev 1993;64(3):909-23.

Bolognini M, Plancherel B, Bettschart W, Halfon O. Self-esteem and mental health in early adolescence: development and gender differences. J Adolesc 1996;19(3):233-45.

Crocker PR, Eklund RC, Kowalski KC. Children's physical activity and physical self-perceptions. J Sports Sci 2000;18(6):383-94.

Daley AJ, Buchanan J. Aerobic dance and physical self-perceptions in female adolescents: Some implications for physical education. Res Q Exerc Sport 1999;70(2):196–200.

Famose JP, Guérin F. La connaissance de soi en psychologie de l'éducation physique et du sport. Paris: Editions Armand Colin; 2002.

Ferreira JP, Fox KR. Self-perceptions and exercise in groups with special needs: preliminary results. In: Ferreira JP, Gaspar PM, Ribeiro CF, Teixeira AM, Senra C (Eds.). Physical activity and promotion of mental health. University of Coimbra, Portugal; 2004. p. 33-40.

Fortes M. La dynamique de l'estime de soi et de soi physique: Un regard nouveau sur la variabilité et le fonctionnement des modèles hiérarchiques. Thèse de doctorat STAPS. Université Montpellier I; 2003.

Guérin F, Famose JP. Le concept de soi physique. Bulletin de Psychology 2005;58(1):73-80.

Kling KC, Hyde JS, Showers CJ, Buswell BN. Gender differences in self-esteem: a meta-analysis. Psychol Bull 1999;125(4):470-500.

Klomsten AT, Skaalvik EM, Espnes GA. Physical Self-Concept and Sports: Do Gender Differences Still Exist? Sex Roles 2004;50(1):119-27.

Lau PWC, Cheung MWL, Ransdell LB. A structural equation model of the relationship between body perception and self-esteem: Global physical self-concept as the mediator. Psychol Sport Exerc 2008;9(4):493-509.

Levy SS, Ebbeck V. The exercise and self-esteem model in adult women: the inclusion of physical acceptance Psychol Sport Exerc 2005;6(5):571–84.

Lindwall M, Lindgren EC. The effects of a 6-month exercise intervention programme on physical selfperceptions and social physique anxiety in non-physically active swedish girls. Psychol Sport Exerc 2005; 6(6): 643-58.

Maïano C, Ninot G, Bilard J. Age and gender on global self-esteem and physical self-perception in adolescents. Eur Phys Educ Rev 2004:10(1):53-69.

Maïano C, Ninot G, Stephan Y, Morin AJS, Florent JF, Vallee P. Geographic region effects on adolescent physical self: an exploratory study. Int J Psychol 2006;41(2):73-84.

Marsh HW. Age and gender effects in physical self-concepts for adolescent elite athletes and non-athletes: A multicohort-multioccasion design. J Sport Exerc Psychol 1998;20(3):237-59.

Marsh HW, Jackson SA. Multidimensional self-concepts, masculinity, and femininity as a function of women's involvement in athletics. Sex Roles 1986;15(7):391-415.

Marsh HW, Richards G, Barnes J. Multidimensional self-concepts: the effect of participation in an outward bound program. J Pers Social Psychol 1986;50(1):195-204.

Marsh HW, Richards GE, Johnson S, Roche L, Tremayne P. Physical Self Description Questionnaire: Psychometric properties and a multitrait-multimethod analysis of relations to existing instruments. J Sport Exerc Psychol 1994;16(3):270-305.

Marsh HW, Perry C, Horsely C, Roche L. Multidimensional self-concepts of elite athletes: How do they differ from the general population? J Sport Exerc Psychol 1995;17(1):70-83.

Marsh HW, Morin AJ, Parker PD. Physical self-concept changes in a selective sport high school: a longitudinal cohort-sequence analysis of the big-fish-little-pond effect. J Sport Exerc Psychol 2015;37(2):150-63.

Mouissi F, Lezaar S, Ninot G, Rouab A, Torki A, Bouabdellah S. La version algérienne du PSDQ. Revue académique des études sociales et humaines 2010;4:57-63.

Ninot G. Note de synthèse en vue de l'obtention de HDR. Du niveau inter individuel à la dynamique interindividuelle de l'estime de soi. UFR-STAPS - Université Montpellier I; 2003.

Rogers CR. A theory of therapy, personality, and interpersonal relationships, as developed in the client-centered framework. In: S. Koch (Ed.). Psychology: A Study of a Science: Vol. 3. New York, NY: McGraw-Hill; 1959. p. 184-256.

Rosenberg M. Conceiving the self. New York: Basics Books; 1979.

Schneider M, Dunton GF, Cooper DM. Physical activity and physical self-concept among sedentary adolescent females: An intervention study. Psychol Sport Exerc 2008;9(1):1-14.

12

Effect of Ladder Drill Exercise on Speed, Surrounding, and Power Leg Muscle

Ketut Chandra Adinata Kusuma[1], I Kadek Happy Kardiawan[2]

Department of Sport Coaching Education, Faculty of Sport and Health, Universitas Pendidikan Ganesha, Indonesia[12]

Article History

Keywords:
Ladder Drill; Speed; Agility; Power of Leg Muscle

Abstract

This study aimed at finding the effect of ladder drill training upon: (1) run speed, (2) agility, and (2) power of leg muscle. This study is an experimental research. This study utilized one group pre test-post test design. There were total people as the subject of this research. Data collection technique used 30-meter sprint test to measure run speed, Illinois agility test to measure agility, and vertical jump test to measure power of leg muscle. Data analysis technique which was used for normality test, homogeneity test/F-test, and T-test with significant level 5% by using SPSS 16.0.0. Based on the finding, there was effect of ladder drill training upon run speed with sig value=0.007, agility and power of leg muscle with sig value=0.000. Based on the data analysis, it could be concluded that there was significant effect of ladder drill training upon run speed, agility and power of leg muscle.

Correspondence address :
Jalan Pulau Selayar Gang 12 Nomor 4 Singaraja, Bali
E-mail: chandra_ketut@yahoo.com[1], happy.kardiawan@yahoo.com[2]

INTRODUCTION

A very popular sport, at present, is futsal. Futsal is a game played in an indoor and outdoor field, with a length of 25-42 meters and a width of 15-25 meters, by five players per team and it is arguably this sport is a combination of football, basketball, and handball. Futsal is a very fast and dynamic game because it uses a relatively small field and there is almost no room to make mistakes. Therefore, futsal players are required to have excellent physical condition. Excellent physical condition is a very supportive appearance of a player. Poor physical condition, of course, will be bad for the performance of techniques and tactics.

According to Sajoto (1995) there are ten kinds of physical conditions that need to be developed, such as strength, endurance, muscular power, speed, flexibility, agility, coordination, balance, accuracy, and reaction. In futsal game, physical condition is one of the components that absolutely must be trained. Because, futsal players who have better physical condition, then some techniques needed in futsal can be applied well too. From some components of physical condition in futsal sport, among others, endurance, speed, agility, and power are the components that must be trained properly, of course, without leaving other physical components (Lhaksana, 2011).

Speed is the ability to move the body from one point to another or to work on a repetitive activity that is the same and continuous in the shortest time (Nala, 1998). Judging from the motion system, speed is the basic ability of central nervous system mobility and muscle device to display movements at a certain speed. Speed is a combination of three elements, namely reaction time, the frequency of movement per unit of time, the speed of a certain distance.

Agility is the ability to change rapidly the direction of the body or parts of the body without disturbance of balance (Depdiknas, 2000). Meanwhile, according to Nala (1998) agility is the ability to change the position of the body, the direction of body movement quickly while moving, without losing balance or awareness of orientation to body position. Thus, agility is one element of physical condition that plays an important role, especially in futsal game, especially when dealing with opponents. A player must be able to move quickly to change direction or break away.

Power is the ability of a person to exercise maximum strength, with his efforts being deployed in short time (Sajoto, 1988). Power is needed in this sport because with a small field model, the movement and repulsion of the athlete's feet must be fast and strong. The connection with the characteristics of futsal game, which is required to have speed, agility, and power, then the training method applied must be effective. Effective in the sense that by one method can train the three physical components or more simultaneously and in accordance with the characteristics of the futsal game itself. In recent years a training method has been developed to improve speed, coordination, agility, and power. The method is known as ladder drill, which is an excellent form of training to improve speed, coordination, agility, and overall power (Tsivkin, 2011). The method of ladder drill is a method that matches the characteristics of futsal game that prioritizes speed and agility. The point is in the agility exercise that the athlete is required to run fast, turn fast, without losing balance. So it can be said that agility training can also indirectly train speed.

The problems that I encountered during observation on 22 to 24 February 2017, when the futsal performance coaching schedule, the movement looks without and with a ball, players very slow. The game transition from defending to attack is not exploited by using speed. Movement without a ball or movement with a fastball must be supported by agility and power. Limb muscle power works when the player performs a prefix during short speed movements. While the transition survives to attack requires running speed.

Based on this, the authors are interested to reveal the effect of ladder drill training on the running speed, agility, and leg muscle power of the students of the Faculty of Sport and Health Undiksha who programmed program the Futsal Performance Class. Previous research related to ladder drill practice has also been revealed by Purnamadinata (2015). The results showed that there was a significant influence on agility and leg muscle power after futsal extracurricular students at SMAK 2 BPK Penabur Bandung were given ladder drill training for 8 weeks.

METHODS

This type of research is quasi-experiment. The design of this study using one group pre test-post test design. This design has no control group, and the subject is not placed randomly because there is only one group.

T1 x T2

The subject of this study were 30 males and a student of Faculty of Sport and Health Undiksha who programmed the Futsal Performance Class. The research instrument used a 30-meter sprint test to measure running speed, Illinois agility test to measure agility, and vertical jump to measure leg muscle power. Data analysis using t-test at 5% significance level, but before testing the hypothesis first tested normality using Kolmogorov-Smirnov test and Levene's Test Of Equality Error Variance test for homogeneity.

RESULT AND DISSCUSION

The normality of data distribution is tested to ensure that the study subjects are normally distributed. To know the normality of data distribution, then used the formula Kolmogorov-Smirnov at significance 0,05. If sig> 0.05 data is normally distributed, otherwise if sig <0.05 the data is not normally distributed. Based on the analysis that has been done by using SPSS 16.00 for Windows results obtained like the following table.

Ho: the variance in each group is homogeneous
Ha: the variance in each group is not homogeneous

With the test criteria used is accept Ho if the value of p> 0.05 where the data has the same variance if the resulting significance number more than 0.05. Summary of data homogeneity calculations using SPSS 16.00 for Windows can be seen in the following **table 1.**

Table 1. Normality of Data Distribution Test

	Kolmogorov-Smirnov[a]		
	Statistic	df	Sig.
Hasil Pretest Speed	0.078	30	0.200*
Hasil Posttest Speed	0.156	30	0.061
Hasil Pretest Agility	0.107	30	0.200*
Hasil Posttest Agility	0.135	30	0.168
Hasil Pretest Power	0.099	30	0.200*
Hasil Posttest Power	0.126	30	0.200*

Based on **table 1** above, it is seen that for all variables of significance on the Kolmogorov-Smirnov test is greater than 0.05. Thus, all distributed data is normal.

The homogeneity test of variance is done by grouping based on the given test model. The homogeneity test of variance between groups was performed with the help of SPSS 16.00 for Windows using Levene's Test Of Equality Error Variance. The statistical hypotheses tested in the homogeneity testing are as follows.

Table 2. Summary of Homogeneity Test of Variances Variances

	Levene Statistic	df1	df2	Sig.
speed	3.402	1	58	0.070
agility	0.014	1	58	0.906
power	0.382	1	58	0.539

Based on **table 2** of Levene's test results show that for test results with a significance level of running speed is 0.070, the agility is 0.906, and leg muscle power is 0.539. So, it can be concluded that the variance in each group is homogeneous.

The research hypothesis has been sug-

Table 3. Summary of Paired Samples Test Result

Paired Samples Test

		Paired Differences					t	df	Sig. (2-tailed)
		Mean	Std. Deviation	Std. Error Mean	95% Confidence Interval of the Difference				
					Lower	Upper			
Pair 1	Pretest Speed - Hasil Posttest Speed	0,17433	0,33013	0,06027	0,05106	0,29760	2,892	29	0,007
Pair 2	Pretest Agility - Hasil Posttest Agility	1,00000	0,66490	0,12139	0,75172	1,24828	8,238	29	0,000
Pair 3	Pretest Power - Hasil Posttest Power	-8,40000	4,23125	0,77252	-9,97997	-6,82003	-10,874	29	0,000

gested that there is the influence of ladder drill results on the speed of running, agility, and leg muscle power. Hypothesis testing using t-test with the help of SPSS 16.00 for Windows. The result of analysis with t-test is presented in **table 3.**

Based on **table 3** we get significant value = 0.000 then p <0,05. These results serve as a basis for making decisions. The decision taken is rejecting Ho and accept Ha. These results suggest that there is an influence of ladder drill training on the speed of running, agility, and leg muscle power. It can be concluded that there is a significant influence between ladder drill training on running speed, agility, and leg muscle power.

Based on the first hypothesis testing, there was a significant effect of ladder drill training on running speed. Ladder drill training is an excellent form of training to improve the speed, coordination, and agility of the foot as a whole (Tsivkin, 2011). The ladder drill training is a training by using a fitness tool in the form of a ladder where an athlete will run, jump and jump by moving his legs quickly over the stairs so as to help develop the speed and agility of the athlete (Schirm in Triharsono, 2013). Based on the results of research Chandrakumar and Ramesh (2015) also showed that training of ladder drill able to increase significantly speed and agility. Running speed is needed by every player because the character of futsal game is so fast in rolling the ball to each side of the field. Thus, the practice of using a ladder drill is very effectively used to increase the speed of an athlete's run.

The results of research Hadi, et al. (2016) also showed results of increased agility after being given ladder drill training. Agility is one component of physical condition that is needed in playing futsal, because with the size of a long futsal field 25-42 meters, and width of 15-25 meters, each player must be able to move quickly and change direction without losing balance.

Based on the first hypothesis testing it turns out there is a significant influence of ladder drill training on leg muscle power. Power is the result of the multiplication of force and the time of execution (P = F x T). A combination of strength and speed, shown when athletes make leaps, punches, throws and other explosive moves that require full exertion. ladder dill is a practice of various different foot movement patterns through staircase exercises placed on the ground/floor where an athlete is required to jump, move right to left quickly. Talking about jumping and moving from right to left quickly, of course, it is not far from the agility and power of the limbs. These two components are factors that support the futsal game with the agile movement to give the ease of a futsal player moving freely in the field. This is also supported by the explosive movement of a futsal player in snatching the ball or doing a good shooting. Purnamadinata (2015) through the results of his research shows there is a significant influence on agility and leg muscle power after futsal extracurricular students in SMAK 2 BPK Penabur Bandung given ladder drill training for 8 weeks.

CONCLUSION

Based on the results of data analysis and discussion above it can be concluded that ladder drill training affects the speed of running, agility, and leg muscle power. So it is expected that futsal club coaches and futsal extracurricular teachers can implement the exercises to increase the running speed, agility and leg muscle power of the players/students.

REFERENCES

Chandrakumar dan Ramesh. 2015. "Effect of ladder drill and SAQ training on speed and agility among sports club badminton players". International Journal of Applied Research, Volume 1, Nomor 12 (hlm. 527-529).

Depdiknas. 2000. Pedoman dan Modul Pelatihan Kesehatan Olahraga Bagi Pelatih Olahragawan Pelajar. Jakarta: Departemen Pendidikan Nasional.

Hadi, et al. 2016. " Pengaruh Latihan Ladder Drills Terhadap Peningkatan Kelincahan Siswa U-17 Di Persatuan Sepakbola Jajag Kabupaten Banyuwangi". Jurnal Pendidikan Jasmani, Volume 26, Nomor 1 (hlm.213-228).

Lhaksana, J. 2011. Taktik dan Strategi Futsal Modern. Jakarta: Be Champion.

Nala, N. 1998. Prinsip Pepelatihan Fisik Olahraga. Denpasar: PPs Universitas Udayana.

Purnamadinata, I. 2015. Pengaruh Latihan Ladder Drill Terhadap Kelincahan dan Power Otot Tungkai. Tersedia pada http://repository.upi.edu/14430/ Diunduh pada tanggal 25 Oktober 2016.

Sajoto, M. 1995. Peningkatan dan Pembinaan Kekuatan Kondisi Fisik. Semarang : Dahara Prize.

Sajoto, M. 1988. Pembinaan Kondisi Fisik dalam Olahraga. Jakarta : Ditjen Dikti, Depdikbud.

Triharsono, P. 2013. Pengaruh Pelatihan Ladder Drill dan Tingkat Kelentukan Terhadap Kecepatan Lari. Tesis (Tidak diterbitkan). Pascasarjana Program Studi Pendidikan Olahraga, Universitas Negeri Surabaya.

Tsivkin, T. 2011. Tersedia pada http://www.sport-fitness-advisor.com. Diunduh tanggal 28 Oktober 2012.

13

Model Development of Volleyball Thrower

Agung Wahyudi

Jurusan Pendidikan Jasmani Kesehatan dan Rekreasi, Fakultas Ilmu Keolahragaan, Universitas Negeri Semarang, Indonesia

Article History

Keywords:
Development; Ball Thrower; Volleyball

Abstract

The purpose of this research is to create ball thrower which is utilized for motor skill practice for volleyball athletes. This research utilized qualitative approach, and major data gained through observation, interview and documentation. The procedure used was research and development model by Borg and Gall, which contains of 10 steps as follow: (1) information research and collection, (2) planning (3) developing product' initial form, (4) initial field test, (5) major product revision, (6) major field test, (7) operational product revision, (8) operational field test, (9) final product revision, (10) dissemination and implementation. Ball thrower tool model can be used for motor skill practice, safe and secure as well as improving practice result. Volleyball AW_2016 Launcher tool models can be used to exercise the skills of volleyball athletes for motion.

Correspondence address :
Gd. F1, Lt. 2, Kampus FIK Unnes, Sekaran, Gunungpati, 50229
E-mail: agungwahyudi@mail.unnes.ac.id

INTRODUCTION

Indonesia Volleyball Association (PBVSI) (1995:1) mention that the archetypal game of volleyball i.e. reflecting sphere (mem-volley) continuously passes over the net. Whereas the aim of the game of volleyball according to Indonesia Volleyball Association (PBVSI) (2005:1) is skipping a ball over the net to be able to touch the opponent's Court and flooring to prevent your opponent from the same business. According to Dieter Beutelstahl (2008:8), the technique is a procedure that has been developed based on practice, and aim at solving a certain movement problems in the most economical and useful. Further, skill techniques according to Cecile Reynaud (2011:23) are grouped into two, namely: 1) the engineering skill attack which consists of serving, passing, and attacking, and 2) engineering skills survive consisting of block and dig.

Various basic engineering skills must be learned and mastered to be able to volley the ball according to the technical principle of volleyball. Through a long and continuous exercise, volleyball athletes learn, master and improve motion skills serve, pass/dig, set, spike, and the block was needed in the tactics and attacking volleyball sports game.

The observation result from the aspect of volley ball exercise facilities and infrastructure showed that no one uses the technique skill tools based on the innovation of science and technology of sport. Interviews on aspects of facilities and infrastructure show that athletes and trainers use building walls (for those who use indoor volleyball courts) to practice motion skills of serve, pass, and spike. Interviews with coaches or club officials also confirmed that coaches or clubs does not have the equipment to practice motion skills due to cost factors or expensive equipment prices. Based on observations on aspects of the exercise, the exercise of athletes in learning the skills of volleyball can be done by using the ball feedback from the coach. Coach hits the ball when athletes practice forearm / under pass, set-up, over-head pass, block and spike skills in each training session. Coach does a lot of hits to meet the needs of passing ball during athletes practice volleyball skills. In accordance with the results of interviews with trainers and athletes, motion skills should be trained by using a repetition model of movement (drilling) which is performed with the help of a passing ball of the trainer. Repetition of movements should focus on the search for a form of movement, rectification of the motion of errors often done by the athlete, and the habituation of movement or technique. Besides the passing ball of the trainer, passing ball is goes on by paired exercises or using building walls.

The problem arises is the result of passing ball frequently changes, the height, the target, and the speed of the ball, and it is affecting the results of athletes training in learning the skills of motion, so it is necessary to produce a tool that can produce bursts of ball with constant speed and accuracy. This tool will help to practice volleyball skills.

Furthermore, it is necessary to create the environment and pay attention to the factors that support the quality of athlete training, so that athletes can learn, practice, repeat the movement and able to master the techniques of attacking skills and also the defense technique. The quality of exercise is not only dependent on the trainer, but many factors can affect the performance of the athlete. Bompa (2009: 8) states that the factors that affect the quality of the exercise include: a) trainer knowledge and personality, b) facilities and equipment, c) supporting science, and d) matches or competitions. The training facility is a supporting factor that determines the quality of the exercise, including equipment or equipment, so as to create a quality workout, it should pay attention to the adequacy of equipment or equipment in the exercise.

Elite sports can not develop independently, requiring the synergy of all stakeholders to ensure the sustainable development of sport. The lack of sustainable coaching is against the demands of the elite sport that will only succeed if it has fulfilled long-term coaching principles. Rusli Lutan (2013: 33) states that as a system, elite sports coaching involves a number of key components and research results reveal at least 10 major components, including sports infrastructure: training facilities, and scientific research: input of sports science and technology. The function of science and technology of sports is to seek innovation in coaching and in the development of science and technology, the existing technology makes sports activity is no longer a difficult activity.

According to Ministry of Youth and Sports (2014) thesedays, science and technology is seen as something difficult and is in the clouds. Science and technology should be earthed in the way each sport immediately apply the science and technology, because there is interaction between the trainers in the field with the scientists to improve the performance of athletes. If many sports technology innovations are realized in research, then the future is not impossible results can be one way in supporting sports coaching.

Through sports technology research is expected to technological innovation in sports field will develop. This has been done by many countries that have advanced in the field of sports achievement.

METHOD

This research uses a research and development approach because it fits with the purpose of research, that was the development of a model of a ball thrower for volleyball athletes. While the selected model is Borg and Gall. With that understanding, the series of research and development steps are conducted cyclically, and at each step to be passed always refers to the result of the previous step until finally obtained a product.

Borg and Gall (1983:775) describes a series of stages were taken in this model, such as research and information collecting, planning, develop preliminary form of product, preliminary field testing, main product revision, main field testing, operational product revision, operational field testing, final product revision, and dissemination and implementation.

RESULTS AND DISCUSSION

Research results were the form of product model tool Launcher volleyball. This product is called a model tool Launcher volleyball AW_2016, is a work system that aims for the sake of ball exercises for athletes in the study of motion skills receive-serve, pass/dig, set-up, block and spike volleyball. Model capabilities the tool Launcher volleyball are: being able to throw as many as 900 times/h, pebbles while letting stand the used 3 hours continuously, can provide precise and steady pebbles while letting, maximum 98.3 km/h pebbles while letting speed.

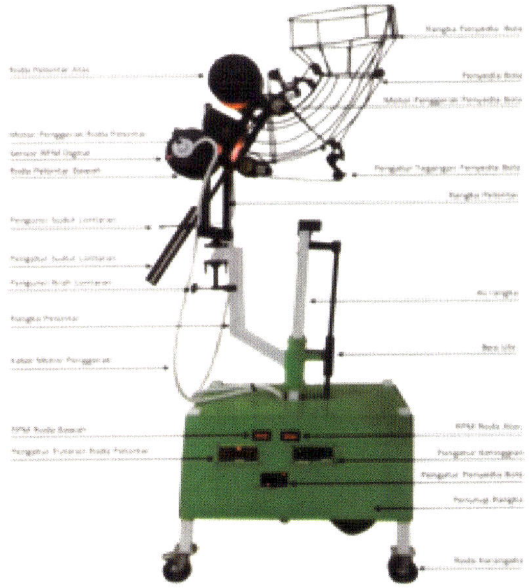

Figure 1. Product Research: Activating Tools Model Volleybal

Volleyball AW_2016 Launcher model can meet the needs of pebbles while letting the ball to exercise the skills of volleyball, motion can be arranged on an angle, direction, and velocity of pebbles while letting, can be used to learn the skills of motion exercises receive serve, pass/dig, set-up, block, and spike volleyball, and economical.

Based on the test results of expert/experts, test a small group, large group testing, test the effectiveness of the model as well as the results of the analysis of the data shows that the model of the tool Launcher volleyball meets the criteria of a valid, practical and effective. The resulting research product revealed useful, safe and comfortable in rehearsal learn volleyball skills of motion. Interview results indicate that the model is a tool useful for volleyball practice Launcher volleyball. The highest answer the respondent showing the product model can help in the process of exercise coaches volleyball retrieved from the capabilities of the tool ball. Model tool able to catapult balls are run continuously and so has the nature of drilling to meet the needs of pebbles while letting during exercise. Fulfillment needs pebbles while letting the balls used for athletes in the study of motion skill or technique of volleyball. This condition used coaches and athletes in the meet the needs of practice. Thousands throw products generated ball Launcher used athletes to repeat the movement as the process of exercise, this is what is termed the drilling. The repetition of movement by using the results of pebbles while letting the ball to learn various skills of volleyball game technique or motion. Model tool Launcher volleyball volleyball drills used for secure, most respondents and convincing answer is the absence of physical contact or touch between models and athletes during Launcher tool used in the process of practice. It is derived from the ability of the products can be adjusted the position, the type of target, and pebbles while letting pebbles while letting. In addition, the ability of the model with an adjustable ball direction angle, pebbles while letting pebbles while letting, and typically a factor terhindarnya physical contact during volleyball practice used in the process. The ability of speed, direction, and angle of the roll can be a factor model tool Launcher volleyball comfortable use. Ball speed selection with pebbles while letting results 0-98 km/h, and right on target result of setting direction and angle makes the results of pebbles while letting may be used to fulfill rehearsal tactics and attack. Results of pebbles while letting the balls used for athletes practicing receive serve, block, and pass/dig for tactics to survive. Practice set-up and spike is attacking tactics that can be trained with this ball Launcher tool model. The influence of indirect use of the ball Launcher tool model product is related to physical conditions. This refers to the relatively fast repetitions in each athlete's motion due to appearance of the pebbles while letting the product model tool Launcher. This situation demands the stamina of athletes who are good to always show the appearance of exercise as the demands of exercise. This meaning that the model tool Launcher volleyball is a model designed and developed on the basis of a strong theoretical foundation, and can be implemented practically in the classroom/field.

CONCLUSION

Based on the steps of development in this research, the research has met the target of capaiannya which is an end product that is produced through a systematic development process. The products generated through research is a new product model in the tool Launcher volleyball. Volleyball AW_2016 Launcher tool models can be used to exercise the skills of volleyball athletes for motion.

REFERENCES

Beutelstahl, D. Belajar Bermain Bolavoli. Bandung: Pioner Jaya, 2008.

Bompa, Tudor O. G., Haff, G. Periodization: theory and methodology of training. (USA: Human Kinetics: 2009).

Borg & Gall. Educational Research. (USA: Von Hoffman Press: 1983).

Kemenpora. Lokakarya Penerapan Iptek Olahraga Menuju ASIAN Games Incheon. http://kemenpora.go.id/index/preview/berita/8483/2014-02 (diakses pada tanggal 28 Nopember 2014).¬

Latar, I. M. (2015). MENINGKATKAN KETERAMPILAN BOLAVOLI MAHASISWA PENJAS DENGAN METODE LATIHAN. Journal of Physical Education Health and Sport, 2(1), 1-10.

Lutan, R. Pedoman Perencanaan Pembinaan Olahraga. Jakarta: Asdep Iptekor Kemenpora, 2013.

Maksum, A. Metodologi Penelitian Dalam Olahraga. Unesa University Press: 2012.

PBVSI. Jenis-Jenis Permainan Bolavoli. Jakarta: Sekum PP. PBVSI, 1995.

Peraturan Permainan Bolavoli. Jakarta: PP. PBVSI, 2005.

Pikiran Rakyat. Sports Science di Indonesia Mulai Berkembang. Pikiran Rakyat Online. http://www.pikiran-rakyat.com/node/260453 (diakses pada tanggal 28 Nopember 2015).

Reynaud, C. Coaching Volleyball Technical and Tactical Skills. (United State: Human Kinetic, 2011).

Viera, B. L. dan Fergusson, B. J. Bolavoli Tingkat Pemula. Jakarta: PT. Raja Grafindo Persada, 2004.

14

The Development of Biometric Sensors to Net Sports Volleyball

Devi Fatma Nurlina[1], Imam Santosa[2], Supriyono[3]

Department of Health Physical Education and Recreation, Sport Science Faculty, Universitas Negeri Semarang, Indonesia[123]

Article History

Keywords:
Development; Biometric Sensors; Volleyball

Abstract

The objective of this research is to design biometric sensor designs for the net of volleyball to detect failures occurring on the net. The approach used in this research is Research and Development (R & D) method. Research subjects were athletes and volleyball referees. Expert volleyball volleyball results one is better with the total score of 85, the validation of the volleyball of two is good with the number of score 87, for the electro expert one expressed well with the total score of 86, the two electro experts stated both with the number of scores 88. The conclusion of this study Produces a net biometric sensor product for the net of volleyball in 2017 in a volley ball beast worthy of use in a volleyball match, for athletes referees and coaches may recommend trying as a means of detecting errors occurring on the net of the volleyball.

Correspondence address :
Dk. Kepatihan Rt.02 Rw.02 Ds. Tersono Kec. Tersono, Batang District, 51272 Central Java
E-mail: devifatma049@gmail.com

INTRODUCTION

Athletics for elementary school different from Sports achievements accomplished through the process of coaching and development programmatically, tiered and sustainable, with the support of science and technology keolahragaan. This is in line with the opinion of the Adang Suherman "sports achievements are sports that nurture and develop the sportsman programmatically and sustainable through the competition to reach the achievements with the support of science and technology (Science and Technology) ". (Act of the Republic of Indonesia Number 3 Year 2005 About National Keolahragaan System. 2007.)

Boal volleyball as the industry that must be supported by adequate infrastructure and one of the referees must be right in deciding the offence in the match. Volleyball game presided over by a referee, the referee is an important part of a game. Referees who are not usually good quality is often a problem that invited protests for a player, a coach, nor the audience could trigger riots.

In a match of volleyball that has already led to systems of digital technology, for example in digital scoresheet volleyball that serves to display the results of the matches, the turnover of players, determine the libero, connected to a central server to report print out. In this modern era needed a tool supporting the game of volleyball.

Based on the findings of field researchers surveying directly into referee-referee in Central Java region especially in Kabupaen stem. Based on the interviews to the referee about leading a game of volleyball. It turns out in a match of volleyball referees requires high concentration, because every game should lead to good terms at the time the ball takes place it is expected the referee did nothing wrong. In the main it is a-class players nationwide, automated boalnya fast that requires high concentration. At the time of the match referee's task was not as heavy as any field umpire their games should be run with the hot weather or rain. Constraints when officiating usually when fastballs in front of the net. To overcome such barriers may be the creation of tools for the referee in front of the net.

Based on consideration of the author's wish to develop a model design tool which gives ease for the referee, in taking decisions when it comes to the net. This tool was developed in the form of biometric sensors to net sports volleyball comes a warning alarm and warning lights. According to the opinion of the referee for this tool used in the game of volleyball is still using manual compliance PBVSI i.e. using the net in General. While the sensors to the pre-existing but has not been used during the game Area, national, and international level. The expectation that later with the presence of the biometric sensor development products for net sports volleyball, the net can be grown in all regions of Central Java and the surrounding area.

The sensor is a detector that has the ability to measure some kind of physical quality that occur, such as pressure or light. The sensor will then be able to convert the measurement into a signal that someone will be able to read. Most sensors can be used when this is really going to be able to communicate with electronic devices that will do the measuring and recording. (Sam Rafiuddin, 2013). A product is anything that can be offered go to market to get attention, purchased, used or consumed that can satisfy the desires or needs. Product quality is the hallmark of the whole as well as of one product or service on its ability to satisfy the needs expressed. (kotler dan Amstrong 2001).

Formulation of the problem is how the development of biometric sensors to net sports volleyball year 2017.

The purpose of this research development produce a biometric sensor development for net sports volleyball year 2017..

METHODS

The design of the penilitian used is using the model-based development research (research-based Development). According to Sugiyono (2010) model of research and development (research and Development) is research used to produce a particular product and test the effectiveness of these products.

The subject of the test classifies into two test subjects are as (1) an expert volleyball experts mean in question was a volleyball referee role to determine whether the biometric sensors to net sports volleyball is already appropriate material and the truth. (2) electrical electrical expert expert on research is a Lecturer/expert in terms of addressing the usual electro. Validation is done using the now about the design and effectiveness of biometric tools series tools. Product tests in the subjects of the research are 12 athletes and 2 referee program Porma in FIK UNNES, whereas in a free trial of the use of the research is the 12 athletes and 11 referees in matches Pom Rayon I Jateng. The design of biometric sensor development products for the volleyball net developed by researchers is product specification. Pproduct designed to help alleviate the performance of the referee. The basic ingredients of products made of the electrical components are cheap and there are plenty of electrical at market. On the net it is a tool that was developed is indeed being a solution, but the sensor cannot be obstructed by an object such as a shirt.

How this research data analysis using qualitative approaches and methods of model development.

The draft design:

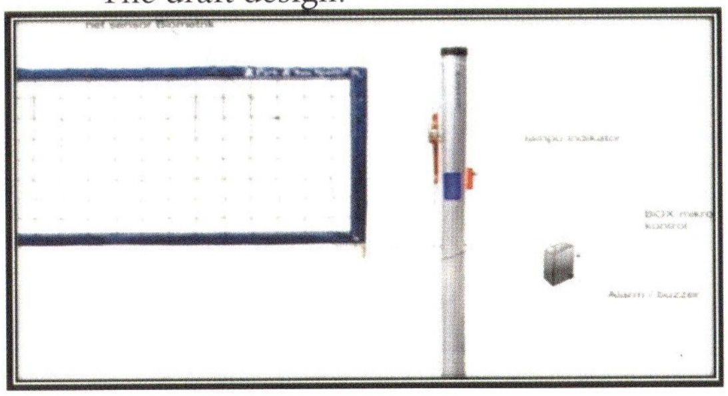

Image design of products: net the top white band lined with aluminium foil as a conductor kesensor. For the light is placed on the net to overlook the referee two will be transmitted to an electronic circuit through cables and Sockets. For micro box controls that are in his or her electronic circuits contain alarm or buzzer and placed on the table scorer.

The way it works at the moment there is a touch of the hand of the flow sensor voltage of about 0.5 mV to 1 mV later reinforced by an op-amp amplified 1000 times strengthening so that it becomes a voltage that is able to drive the relay so that the relay could trigger turn the strobe lights and buzzer, so the referee can figure out which team touched the net.

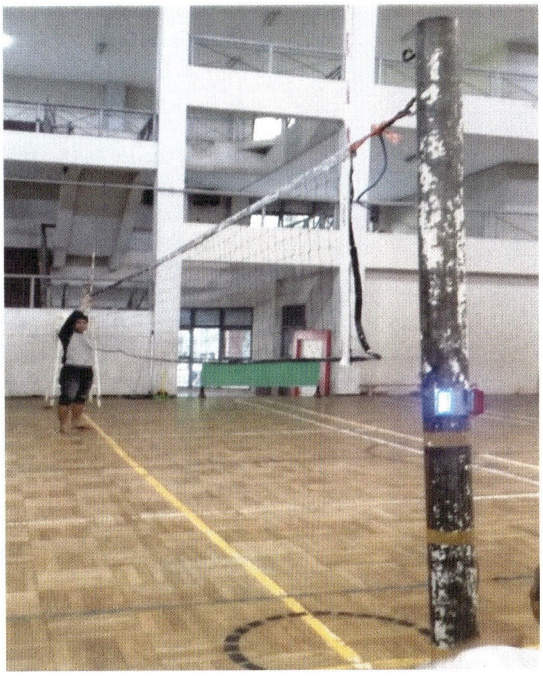

RESULTS AND DISCUSSION

Small scale trial aims to find out and identify various problems such as weakness, deficiencies, or effectiveness of the product when used by players. Data obtained from this test is used as the basis for performing the revision of the product before use on field trials. Data obtained from filling the questionnaires by the experts is the initial data to state whether the biometric sensors product net worth used and effective use of volleyball matches. Data obtained from the results of interviews conducted by researchers to the respondents or subjects of a test used to evaluate a product before it is used in a tested wide scale usage.The **table 1** details the results of the inter-

Table 1. Details the results of the interviews

Substances	The results of the interview the volleyball player						Conclusion
	1	2	3	4	5	6	
Security	V	V	V	V	V	V	The product is safe
Usability	V	V	V	V	V	V	Comfortable products
Measure	V	V	V	V	V	V	The size corresponds to the size of the White Ribbon.
Sound	-	-	V	-	-	-	A little disturbing the concentration of players
Comfort to match	V	-	V	-	-	V	The product can't be used a means in the match
The next match for usability	-	-	V	-	V	V	The product can't be used in the next match

views have been done researchers in small-scale trials II volleyball player is as follows:

By looking at the **table 1** above, then the results obtained by researchers in small-scale trials are as follows, As many as six players of volleyball stated:

1. The product is safe to use in volleyball match
2. Comfortable products already used for volleyball matches
3. The product is in compliance with the White Ribbon size
4. The product is a little annoying when the game of volleyball players
5. The product can not be used for means of volleyball matches.

Free trial of wide scale trials widely conducted at Gor UIN information in the POM RAYON 1 Jateng. The number of athletes and referees are used in wide-scale trials were 12 athletes and referees from several regions in Central Java

Table 2. Wide-scale trial

Substances	The results of the interview the volleyball player						Conclusion
	1	2	3	4	5	6	
Security	V	V	V	V	V	V	The product is safe
Usability	V	V	V	V	V	V	Comfortable products
Measure	V	V	V	V	V	V	The size corresponds to the size of the White Ribbon
Sound	V	V	-	-	V	V	A little disturbing the concentration of players
Comfort to match	V	V	-	V	V	V	The product can not be used a means in the match
The next match for usability	-	V	V	V	V	-	The product can not be used in the next match

Based on the analysis of the results of research and discussion in this thesis, then do some revision include :

Net product changes on the development of biometric sensors to net sports volleyball originally regular net in General and in the modifications into the biometric sensor net to net sports volleyball.

1. The White Ribbon Changes the top of net in aluminum foil your, 2. The Sound is still pretty much the same, 3. At the time of the match does not interfere with the referee. Research Development made by share stages. The research starts from the initial product validation tests of the product i.e. small-scale trials and scale great that produced bulk products where the product can be used kebermanfaatannya, researcher involves 4 validator with the expertise of each i.e. electrical expert and expert material consisting of national volleyball referees. The tests are performed in a scale kesil Porma FIK UNNES and large scale trials are conducted in a Pom Rayon I Central Java. Product validation is performed using instruments in the form of the now know the extent to which these tools are said to be worth to tested. Kuesoner/question form used in the research process as data validation and test the effectiveness of products. At the same time do some checking, such as documentation, interviews and discussions on more than one source in the same way i.e. observation and expert on experts. For assessment using the assessment have been developed application of science and technology sport, Deputy Minister of youth and sports of the Republic of Indonesia in 2011. The results of the expert assessment expert volleyball one with a score of 85, two volleyball experts with a score of 87, expert electrical expert one by a score of 86, two electrical experts with a score of 88, the results of the evaluation by the respective experts obtained a score above 85 that goes criteria good and proper.

Research results based on the analysis of the trial data, description of implementation in the trunk and Semarang to tiredness the tool how far this tool could diguanakan in a match, free trial of effectiveness, observation techniques (observation), interview, documentation and discussion. A description of the results of the selection of products, researchers developed a biometric sensor net development products, and based on a needs analysis and specifications owned on the net. The initial draft description, in the making of the initial design, the researcher operates on the criteria that have been used by kemenpora in the selection and research for innovative technology works competition participant sports in the year 2011. IE: aspects of Orisinilitas, the innovative aspect of the benefit Aspects, economic aspects, security aspects, aspects of Comfort.

The initial product was designed aiming used to practice volleyball player, about the toughness of this tool as seen from accuracy, tension, if exposed to the armor can sound or not. Mechanical tests, speed of reaction or response from the tool, the tool ball conflict can stand what do not. For a free trial of the weather, the extent to which the tool if it is exposed to wind or rain, whether it could survive for long. When the sensors used can cause problems for an audience or not. The possibility for error diet, lights and the sound is not turned on. Just note the referees one and two. How to uninstall install tool, takes how long. Heat and water resistant for how long. The possibility of system error.

Validation of the product early, before the tested biometric sensor development for the sport of volleyball net in advance need validation by the appropriate experts with specialist research field. The validation is done by means of a team of experts to observe the biometric sensor product is accompanied by the evaluation sheet along with pieces of suggestions and input.

Data validation, data obtained from the evaluation sheets or kuesoner charging by expert expert. The results of the expert assessment expert volleyball one with a score of 85, two volleyball experts with a score of 87, expert electrical expert one by a score of 86, two electrical experts with a score of 88, the results of the evaluation by the respective experts obtained a score above 85 that goes criteria good and proper.

The initial draft of the revision of a product, based on the advice of the expert's expert on the development of biometric sensors to net sports volleyball year 2017 then carried out a revision of the product **tabel 3**.

Table 3. Revision of the product

The Revised Section	The Reason The Revised	Repair advice
Sound too loud	Interfere with the concentration of the players	So that sounds just the referee
Hook lights to pillars	Since each different diameter pole	Replaceable wear rope krek.
Nylon on the net given the thin cable between team A and team B	Too complicated in installations, takes a long time	We recommend that you just dihilangi
Colour light yellow	Less glowing moments in the pool	Replaced the colors brighter

Effective product development of biometric sensor failure detection diet is based on the results of tests on a large scale. Effective products in question include the effectiveness of the use of the time, the effectiveness of the performance of the referee, and the effectiveness of automated products.

At the time of the discussion to implement biometric sensor development for the sport of volleyball net that already are considered final, researchers presenting expert expert. This activity aims to deliver development results (process procedures and products) to the users and the professional discussion to find out the extent to which research success is achieved. From the results obtained by researchers in field interview that the referee declares the tool is very helpful to the referee about the officiating in the match turns out volleyball volleyball referee requires high concentration and the constraints which often happens by the referee when the ball-the ball quickly in front of the net, to overcome the barriers may be created if there are tools that can help referees in a game. Presiding umpire stated a tool that researchers make it very helpful to referees Moreover, when the concentration is reduced or when the referee did not see the occurred error when on the net.

From the results obtained by researchers when the documentation is the real test, the tool is already working with a either a flame and lights as a warning sign when the player touches the net, but after the researchers observed when running game referee each has a duty which should be the referee was watching this tool but referee focus with tugasnnya let alone when the player is in front of the net and jellies should focus the referee saw it, so these tools there is no scrutiny of the referee at all. As for the cue in the regulations volleyball referee must be memorized and can be implemented in accordance with the existing errors in field. This gesture is performed only once, done by hand signals to designate one kesalaan who did a turn, pointing to the designated service while giving the sign points from mistakes made one squad.

From the results obtained from expert kuesoner expert in electronics and ball volialat this is already good, and athletes when performing tests of athletes stated that the tool safely used at the time of the match, the athlete also feel comfortable when the tool is used the time of the match. Atletpun do not feel bothered the existence of such a device, but some athletes expressed the tool worthy of use in the match and claimed it has not been feasible to use in the game.

In this case the application tool that all referees declare the tool is already good and athletes declared safe and convenient tool is used when the match. But the results are more even inversely proportional, the tool has not been beneficial for the referee. Because it could not focus on the tool. The tool is also not to increase sportsmanship are high because a lot of constraints on when the match takes place and could cause unrest for the audience as well as a coach. Then it uses to facilitate the performance of the referee as observed many problem for referees itself, must change the rules of considered and many more about the tool. See the conclusions of these tools can not be used to help improve the performance of the referee. This tool also can not be used as a means for doing volley ball game.

CONCLUSION

Based on the results of analysis and discussion, then the conclusions that can be drawn from this research is produce net product using biometric sensors in refereeing volleyball is worthy to be used in the game of volleyball. To referee the athletes and coaches can recommend to try as a tool to detect errors that occur at the top of the net on a volley ball match. See the limitations of this product, in order to be further developed with the biometric sensor net product is to match the expected.

REFERENCES

Kotler dan Amstrong. 2001. Tentang teori produk

Peraturan Resmi BOLAVOLI 2015-2016

Soegiyono. 2010. Metode Penelitian Pendidikan:Pendekatan Kualitatif dan R&D, ALFABETA, VC. Jl gegerkalong Hilir No.84-9 Bandung

Soenyoto, T. 2013. "Pengembangan Prototype Alat Jamur (Mushroom) Cabang Olahraga Senam Arstistik Putra Jawa Tengah". Disertasi Program Pascasarjana Universitas Negeri Jakarta

Syam, R. 2013. Dasar-Dasar Teknik Sensor. Makasar. Fakultas Teknik, Universitas Hassanuddin

Undang-undang Republik Indonesia Nomer 3 Tahun 2005 Tentang Sistem Keolahragaan Nasional. 2007. Jakarta: Kementrian Negara Pemuda dan Olahraga Republik Indonesia.

The Influence of Learning Approach and Eye-Hand Coordination Against The Results of A Free Throw in Basketball Games

Pramoda Wardana[1] ✉ ,M.Furqon Hidayatullah[2], Kiyatno[3]

Prodi Ilmu Keolahragaan Program Pascasarjana,Universitas Sebelas Maret Surakarta, Indonesia[123]

Article History

Keywords:
Free Throw; Basketball; Hand-Eye Coordination; Direct and Indirect; Experimental Research

Abstract

The purposes of this recearch were to examine the influence of direct and indirect learning approaches on free throw result in basketball, the difference of free throw result played by students with good and poor hand-eye coordinations, and the interaction influence of learning approach and hand-eye coordination on the result. This research applied experimental method with 2x2 factorial design. The population within this study was male students in 5th semester of the major program. Purposive Random Sampling was used as the sampling technique. 40 students were taken as the samples, in which students with good and poor hand-eye coordinations were equal. The analytical technique of this study belonged to ANOVA to use SPSS 22 and 5% significancy. Study result showed the difference of significant influence between direct and indirect learning approaches on free throw result, for p-value = 0,045, smaller than 0,05; the difference of increase in the result from students with good and poor hand-eye coordinations, for p-value = 0,035, smaller than 0,05; and the interaction of learning approach and hand-eye coordination on the result, for p-value = 0, 012, smaller than 0,05.It is concluded that there were differences of the significant influence between the learning approaches on free throw result, the free throw result from students with good and poor hand-eye coordinations, and there was an interaction influence of learning approaches and hand-eye coordination on the free throw result.

✉ **Correspondence address:**
Kampus Pascasarjana UNS Jl. Ir. Sutami No. 36A Kentingan Surakarta 57126
E-mail: wardana_pramoda@yahoo.co.id

INTRODUCTION

The development of the sport was rapidly grown and not only played in the community or clubs, but also among professionals. But further, the sport was also entered into the realm of education in Indonesia, especially in the educational curriculum of physical education in schools, incorporate the skills of the game was as one of the great ball skills. The game was taught from the primary school level, and at the level of SLTA (Senior High School). The game that had been incorporated into the educational curriculum not only studied in schools, but also into the education curriculum in higher education, particularly for the Physical Education Department. This game was also played between the campus and always became a very prestigious match.

In addition to the Foundation of SME activities (Student activity units) at various colleges, skill games was also studied by students who attended the sport. As any student of the semester 5 FKIP University Surakarta Development Shoots POK were given material skills basic techniques of the game. Although they set out from the background of the ability of different sports, but it had become a liability for the entire students to master the skills of the game. It is considering they are prepared to become a teacher of physical education should be colonised a wide range of sports, including the skill. As had been mentioned before that the game was taught at the most basic level of education up to the secondary level, so there should be no reason for prospective educators or teachers of the sport not being able to master the techniques of the game. In addition to be prepared to be a teacher, students of University of Surakarta Development Shoots POK must be ready to become a coach if the team where he taught will join in a match.

The game was a complex game, which was involving elements of strength, speed, endurance, explosive power, flexibility, coordination and other physical conditions. Mastery of the domain motion in the game was also one of the important elements. The player should also have supporting elements in order to play well. In addition to support the above elements of mastery in the game, was to have the basic techniques that must be mastered by players. The basic techniques were, among others, passing, dribbling, shooting, and pivot. The basic technique must be controlled by a player because with a good mastery of the basic engineering, a player will also be able to play outstanding. In the game, shooting technique was the most important technique, because the object of the game was given scoring. So the only way to print numbers in the game was by doing the shooting. The good shooting ability will provide a lot of numbers anyway. The game was divided basically into three types of shots, namely standing shoot, jump and shoot and lay up shoot. Variation in doing the shots can be done by a player in accordance with the situation and condition of the time the game takes place. The variation range of the shot was done so that while doing the shots a player will be able to outwit opponents and enter more numbers.

The difficulty of doing free throw themselves was visible in the teaching and learning activities on University students FKIP POK Shoots Development Semester 5 who got the courses. In the activities of the study, errors were still found when doing free shots or free throw techniques. Errors that often occured during a free throw were often right on target and the ball was not going on the air or the ball did not touch the basketball hoop. In addition, students also often looked unfocused when they will do this shot and they were less doing shots with a relaxed attitude. The direction of the shot was not appropriate on targets were probably influenced by the bad eye-hand coordination from students themselves. A good coordination will probably produce a good accuracy anyway and vice versa. Strong suspicion that in order to achieve a high degree of accuracy in conducting free throw then eye-hand coordination was an important component of the alleged. In addition to those factors the errors may also occur due to inappropriate learning approach on students themselves.

See the various constraints that were found above, it was necessary to apply in a method or approach to learning that can be applied to students. The learning approach was how a teacher or teachers used steps or learning methods to deliver the materials, with the goal of learning that the material can easily be mastered by students or student body. With the right learning approach, the students were expected to be able to properly understand what had been delivered by a teacher, be it from lecturers or lecturers' assistant. In the world of learning, there were lots of approaches that can be applied to deliver a material and the effectiveness of each learning approach will be different. Learning can be centered on the teacher as its main source or can also be centered to students or pupils, while the teacher just purely as intermediaries.

Examined the elaboration of the background issue which had been discussed above, as well as saw some factors barrier to learning activities in a free throw then the author chose the title "The Different Influence of the Learning Approach and Eye-Hand Coordination Against the Results of a Free Throw In the Game (Experimental study of Direct and Indirect learning methods on students of semester 5, PKO FKIP University Development Shoots Surakarta)".

Based on the background of the problem, identification of the problems and limitations of problem then the problem can be formulated as follows; Is there any difference between the influence of direct and indirect learning methods against the results of the free throw was?, is there any difference in the results of the free throw among the students who have high and low hand-eye coordination?, is the influence of the interaction between the learning approach and eye-hand coordination against the results of the free throw?

The Study of Theory

The game was a great ball game developed in a city in America and was becoming a very popular sport of many people. According to Gede Eka (2015:262) the game was played by two teams, each consisting of 5 players. According to the Firm Chinese Indonesian surname (2016:42) the game was a sport ball played by a group consisting of two teams each consisting of 5 people and each competed for scoring points by inserting the ball into the opponent's basket. The goal of each team is to score a number to the opponent's basket and try to prevent the other team to score. While according to Sucipto, Dian Budiana, Lukmanul Hakim Lubay and Jajat Darajat (2010:23) "a team sport is played in a manner of reflecting balls, and shooting the ball into the opponent's basket. Each team consists of five people and attempting to insert the ball into the basket of his opponent and prevent the opposing squads enter into our basket ball ".

Learning Approach

According to Ngalimun (2016:8) as for the term approach (approach) in learning according to Sanjaya (2007) have similarities to the strategy. A different approach is actually better with the strategies and methods. The approach can be defined as a starting point or point of view toward the learning process. Term approach refers to the view of the occurrence of the process which is still very common. Therefore, strategies and learning methods used can be sourced or depending on the approach in learning. Further explained the term approach refers to the view of the occurrence of an approach centered on the teacher (teacher-centered approaches) and student-centered approach (student-centered approach). Teacher-centered approach to lowering the direct learning strategies (direct instruction) deductive learning, or learning expository. Whereas, the approach of learning based on student learning strategies lowers discovery and inkuiri as well as inductive learning strategies.

According to Fathurrahman (2007) method literally means way. In general usage, refers to a method as a means or procedure used to achieve a particular goal. In relation to learning, a method is defined as a means of presenting learning materials on learners to achieve the goal that has been set. Thus one of the must-have skills that a teacher is learning skills in choosing the method. Election methods directly related to teachers ' efforts in showing the teaching to suit the situation and conditions so that the achievement of the objectives of teaching gained the most.

According to Suprijono (2009:45-46) "a Model of learning is the cornerstone of the practice of learning results decrease educational psychology and learning theory that is designed based on an analysis of the implementation of the curriculum and its implications on operational level class". Learning can be defined as a pattern that is used for the preparation of curriculum, managers of the material, and give instructions on the teacher in the classroom.

Direct Learning Approach

According to Ngalimun (2016:9-10) "a direct Learning Strategies is learning that many directed by the teacher. This strategy is effective to specify the information or skill development stage by stage. " Direct learning is usually an deductive. According to Tite Juliantie dkk (2013:41) "directly learning can be defined as a model of learning where the teacher is transforming the information or skills directly to students and learning oriented on purpose and distukturkan by the teacher".

According to Suprijono (2009:46-47) direct or direct instruction learning known as active teaching. Direct learning is also called a whole-class teaching. The mention refers to the style of teaching where the teacher is involved actively in carrying content on learners and teach it directly on to the whole class. According to Zhang Dongbo (2011) Limited direct effect is working good in depth as an indicator of knowledge and understanding of the causes of the limited vocabulary understanding.

Indirect Learning Approach

Indirect learning is a learning centered on the pupil students. The teacher's role shifted from a lecturer to become the facilitator ", according to Ngalimun, (2016:10). Indirect learning approaches according to Samsudin (2008:30-32) "is a diverting task control learning on student learning, where teachers are no longer in control of the learning in full but gives in completely on the students to get together to do it."

Indirect learning strategies often called inductive inkuiri, memecahan problems, decision-making and discovery. Contrary to the approach of learning direct, indirect learning generally are generally centred on learners, though despite the two strategies complement each other.

Hand-Eye Coordination

According to Rogram (2015:17) "Coordination is the ability to do work or movement quickly and efficiently". The coordination of various factors of harmonious relations States that happen to a movement. The ability of koordinatif is a good basis for learning ability is sensomotorik, the good level of coordination will be more rapid and effective movement difficult to get done anyway.

The sense of coordination, according to some experts like according to Suharno (1993:61) that "coordination is the ability of athletes to link several motion into one movement intact and aligned". Barrow and McGee cited by Harsono (1988:220) provides a limitation regarding the coordination of "the ability to combine a variety of movements into one or more special motion patterns". Thus the conclusions and opinions of the coordination is the ability of two or more organs of the body that moves with a certain movement patterns.

Broer and Zernicke in Harsono (1988:221) explained that coordination is the ability to combine multiple motion without tension in the correct order and do complex movements smoothly without excessive energy expenditure. Thus the result is movement efficient, smooth, seamless (smooth) and well-coordinated.

Based on the opinion of the above, it is clear that coordination of the formulation is one of the important elements for motion motor skills. Good level of coordination or whether someone's motion coordination is reflected in his ability to perform a move smoothly, precisely and efficiently. A student with a good coordination is not only able to do a skill perfectly, but also fast and easy can do the skill that was new to him. Besides it can also change rapidly from one motion to another motion patterns so that her movements became more efficient. Students who do not cooperate well usually do gerakan-gerakannya rigidly, with tension and with excessive energy is so inefficient.

Energy Exercise System Coordination

A good exercise to improve coordination is to do a wide variety of gestures and skills. Students who have a specific sport specialties, preferably involved in skills in different branches of sports or other sports. Students have a lot to be trained with new skills from his branch or branches in other sports. If not, will not develop coordination and ability to learn new gestures will decrease. In coaching skills, difficulty and complexity of the movement must be constantly enhanced. The easiest coordination developed in young children at the time of adaptability nervous system better than the staff of adults (Bompa in Harsono, 1988:222).

Factors affecting Coordination

In addition to paying attention to the signs of exercise coordination, the problems should be noticed in this exercise, as the notion is innervated resiproke a race that coincided with the arrival of the one negative and the other positive. Synergistic muscles and antagonistic working together harmoniously to produce a good coordination. Agility, balance and kelentukan needs to be improved as well as possible to support the coordination of high quality. Almost all sports require coordination, complex movements even though levels of difficulties and their needs vary for each sport. Train the ability should since early age in motion as the basis of enrichment process skills at the junior and senior students.

Influence of the differences between direct and indirect learning approach against the results of the free throw was.

Learning approach with direct and indirect learning approach on deployment in the field, especially in the emphasis of physically and mentally. The advantages of direct learning approach to learning is planned and it is easy to use. On the approach of learning direct, given learning-oriented application technique free throw was. Thus, students can directly develop techniques that are taught in accordance with the game environment. Whereas the indirect approach to learning, training oriented given the ability of mastering the technique free throw was. The emphasis tends to be on increasing exercise the ability to shoot the ball into the basketball hoop continuously on every practice session until a set time limit. Advantages of indirect learning approach is encouraging the interest and curiosity of the students, creating alternative problem solving, encouraging creativity and skills development, and better understanding.

From the explanation above by observing that there are advantages and disadvantages to each approach to learning, then it can be suspected that between direct and indirect learning approach will give a different result against the influence of the free throw was. And the most influential was the exercise by using an indirect approach to learning.

The difference between the results of the free throw was a student who has a eye-hand coordination is high and low.

Hand-eye coordination that is owned by every student is not all the same, there are high and some are low. High low hand-eye coordination that is owned by a student will certainly have an effect on the reaction arm muscles student concerned. This is due to the hand-eye coordination is one of the dominant elements in movements that require a high level of eksplosifitas.

From the description above, it can be presumed that the difference eye-hand coordination is high and low can give different effects against the results of the free throw was. And the most influence on the results of the free throw was is a student who has a high hand-eye coordination.

Influence of the interaction between the learning approach and eye-hand coordination against the results of the free throw was.

Indirect learning approach is not particularly in need of eye-hand coordination capability are high, since the delivery of the material gradually and the teacher as a facilitator then tend to be gradual process to increase the explosive coordination. While the use of direct learning approach will require eye-hand coordination is higher, because the learning process a lot delivered by guru then it is more effective to increase strength, muscle endurance, coordination and muscle formation.

For students who have a low hand-eye coordination in applying the learning approach of direct disadvantage. Eye-hand coordination with low student will be hard to adapt to the needs of the eye-hand coordination. Indirect learning approaches more appropriate use for students who have hand-eye coordination that is low to master free throw was.

From the above description, it can be presumed there is interaction between the learning approach and eye-hand coordination against the results of the free throw was.

METHOD

Research methods used in this research is a method of experimentation using 2 x 2 factorial design.

The large samples used in this study is 40 students, obtained by purposive random sampling techniques. According to Sudjana (2002:148) purposive random sampling technique of population to be sampled should comply with the provisions to meet the research objectives. These provisions are:

1. Gender male and 5th semester student majoring in Sports Education Coaching Faculty of teacher training and educational sciences UTP Surakarta.
2. Interested to follow the research with iklas.
3. healthy physical and spiritual.
4. Willing to sample and conduct treatment research.
5. Have the capability of free throw good or less, based on the results of observation and information

The sampling technique used was Purposive Random Sampling, the samples taken as many as 40 students, composed of 20 students who have a high level of eye-hand coordination, 20 students who have a low level of eye-hand coordination.

From a number of students who have such provisions, then hand-eye coordination was obtained by tests of throwing tennis balls, data capture results such hand-eye coordination is used for grouping, namely coordination which has samples of eye-high hand and eye coordination that has a sample-low hand. Next ranked, from the results of the rank was divided into three groups, the level of eye-hand coordination in high, medium and low. 20 students who have a level of eye-hand coordination are not included, so the large samples used in this study were 40 student son consisting of 20 students who have high hand-eye coordination, and 20 students who have hand-eye coordination. Next 20 students who have high hand-eye coordination and have eye-hand coordination low each divided into two groups in a way to be drawn (random), i.e. 10 students getting preferential treatment by direct learning approach and 10 students as a group get indirect learning approach.

Engineering analysis using ANOVA using SPSS program 22 and 5% significance.

RESULT AND DISCUSSION

The first hypothesis in this study stated that "the differences Influence the learning approach of Direct and Indirect Learning approach, there are the results of Free Throw in the game of basketball." Based on hypothesis testing first it turned out that there was a difference between the real influence of a group of students who were given the learning approach of direct and indirect learning approach (p-value = 0,045 < 0.05). Direct learning approach group had an average final result of free throw of 5.950, better than indirect learning approach which had the results of a free throw of 4.100.

Learning by direct approach in improving the results of free throw in the game of basketball was a pattern of learning used by providing learning materials free throw learned directly without going through the stages of a certain distance. In practice, learning free throw with the direct approach was as follows: (1) the student was given a learning material about free throw with the actual movement patterns. (2) implementation of teaching and learning activities carried out directly on the actual field.

Based on the results of the analysis of the data indicated that there was a distinction between direct and indirect learning approach against the results of the free throw, in this research, direct learning approach had better results than the indirect learning approach, it can be seen from the results of direct learning approach score that is 5.950 and indirect learning approach score that is 4.10.

The second hypothesis in this study stated that "there is a difference in the results of Free Throw In the game of basketball between students who have high and low hand-Eye coordination". Hand-eye coordination was one of the supporting factors in the success of a person in his free throw movement in the game of basketball, free throw motion was the complex movement and needed harmony in the motion. Learning the techniques of free throw not regardless of how a student was able to perform the task with the right moves. The truth movement will affect the level of energy expenditure. If students were wrong or not able to do the movement correctly then they will waste their energy. This condition will affect the result to be achieved.

The most important factor that affects the quality of the student in carrying out the tasks of motion exercises correctly and effectively was hand eye coordination. The precision mastery of motion of a person's professional basketball player to perceive a function of the organs of the human body which were closely related to the motion of the body as well as members of the active or passive body. The movement associated with the basic movements of the free throw.

Students who have a high hand eye coordination would be easier to perform motion given in learning, with the precision of the type of learning that was done will be able to provide faster results compared to those with less hand-eye coordination.

The results of the analysis of the data indicated that there was a difference between students who have a high hand eye coordination compared to the low hand eye coordination, it was in accordance with the above theory that the high ratio of sit and long limbs will show the precision of a person to perform the duties of the motion correctly, quickly and effectively. The more the students have high hand eye coordination so that students will be able to carry out all types of learning properly and accurately in accordance with the harmony of motion and the rate of energy expenditure was needed.

The third hypothesis in this study stated that "there is interaction between the Learning Approach and Eye-hand Coordination Against the results of a Free Throw In the game of basketball". In total there were influences of interaction on both a variable approach to learning, i.e. the achievement of outcomes free throw is influenced directly by the learning approach and eye coordination hand. The achievement of the results of the free throw, directly influenced by the level of coordination of eye difference factors in the hands of students.

The research results indicated that the interaction of learning approach with hand eye coordination against the results of the free throw. This was evidenced from the value of H0 was accepted at = 0.05. This can be proved by the results of the analysis of variance calculation 2 factors i.e. because p-value = 0.012 < 0.05. Learning approach for direct and indirect learning approach with the hand-eye coordination level against the results of the free throw, meaning there was significant influence interactions between them or there was an interaction between the two.

This can be explained that the approach of learning direct will have good results when given to the student who has a high hand-eye coordinating learning approach and indirect will have better results when given to students who have a low level of eye-hand coordination.

CONCLUSIONS

From the results of testing a hypothesis can be drawn conclusions that there was a difference significant influence between the direct and indirect learning approach against the results of a free throw in the game of basketball. The direct learning approach gave a better influence than indirect learning approach. The average increase in their respective direct learning approach and indirect learning approach was 5.950 of 4.100.

There was a difference in the results of free throw in the game of basketball between students who have a high hand eye coordination and students who have a low hand eye coordination. Students who have a high hand eye coordination had better results compared to students who have a low hand eye coordination. The average increase in high and low hand-eye coordination was 6.00 of 4.050.

There was a direct interaction between the learning approach and eye-hand coordination against the results of a free throw in the game of basketball.

Direct learning approaches had better outcomes when treatment was given to students who have high hand eye coordination.

Indirect learning approaches had better outcomes when treatment was given to students who have a low hand eye coordination.

REFERENCES

Annarino, Anthony A., Cowell, Charles C. & Hazelton, Helen W. 1980. Curriculum Theory and Design in Physical Education. 2rd Edition. St. Louis: The CV. Mosby Company.

Brooks, G.A. & Fahey, T.D. 1984. Exercise Physiology Human Bioenergetics and its Aplication. Canada: Jhon Wiley & Sons Inc.

Bompa, T., and Carrera, M. 2015. Conditioning Young Athletes. United States of America: Human Kinetics.

Darmawan, G. F. B. (2015) Cabang Olahraga Bola Basket. Graha Ilmu Yogyakarta.

Deborah, A. Wuest & Charles, A. Bucher. 1995. Foundations of Physical Education and Sport. 12th Edition. St. Louis, Missouri: Mosby-Year Book, Inc.

Dongbo Zhang Keuko Koda (2011) Contribution of morphological awareness and lexical inferencing ability to L2 vocabulary knowledge and reading comprehension among advanced EFL learners: testing direct and indirect effects. Springer Science Bisness Media B.V 2011.

Fathurrohman, P. dan M.Sobry Sutikno. (2007). Strategi Belajar Mengajar Melalui Penanaman Konsep Umum & Konsep Islami Bandung: PT. Refika Aditama

Gagne, Robert M. 1985. The Condition of Learning. 4th Edition. New York: CBS College Publishing.

Good, Thomas L. & Brophy, Jere E. 1990. Educational Psychology: A Realistic Approach. 4th Edition. New York: Longman.

Grace, J. Craig. 1983. Human Development. 3rd Edition. Englewood Chiffs: Prentice-Hall, Inc.

Harsono. 1988. Coaching Dan Aspek-Aspek Psikologis Dalam Coaching. Jakarta: Ditjen Dikti.

Harsono. (2015) Kepelatihan Olagraga. Bandung: PT. Remaja Rosdakarya.

Imanudin, Iman.(2008). Ilmu Kepelatihan Olahraga. FPOK, UPI Bandung.

Juliantine, Tite, dkk (2011). Model-model pembelajaran Pendidikan Jasmani. FPOK. Bahan Ajar. Bandung. FPOK UPI

Johnson, B. L. & Nelson, J. K. 1986. Practical Measurement for Evaluation in Physycal Education. New York: Macmillan Publishing Company.

Kosasih, D. (2008). Fundamental Basketball. Semarang: Karangturi Media

Kirkendall, D. R. Joseph, J. R. Robert, E. J. 1987. Measurement and Evaluation for Physical Educators. Illionis: Human Kinetics Publishers. Inc.

Maulana, F. (2015). Perbandingan Latihan Set Shoot Pada Area Free Throw Dengan Menggunakan Repetisi Berubah Set Tetap Dan Repetisi Tetap Set Berubah Terhadap Hasil Free Throw Pada Peserta Ekstrakurikuler Bola Basket Putra Sma Negeri 1 Kajen Kabupaten Pekalongan. ACTIVE: Journal of Physical Education, Sport, Health and Recreation, 4(3).

Muhadjir. 2005. Teori dan Praktek Pendidikan Jasmani Untuk Kelas I SMP. Jakarta: PT. Ghalia Indonesia.

Mulyono, B. A., 1999. Tes dan Pengukuran Dalam Pendidikan Jasmani Olahraga. Surakarta: Universitas Sebelas Maret Press.

Ngalimun. (2016) Strategi dan Model Pembelajaran. CV. Aswaja Pressindo. Jogjakarta

Oliver, S. (2007). "Strategi Public Relations". Penerbit Erlangga. Jakarta

Sajoto. 1995. Peningkatan dan Pembinaan Kondisi Fisik Dalam Olahraga. Semarang: Dahara Prize.

Salim, A. (2006). Teori dan Paradigma Penelitian Sosial Yogyakarta : Tiarawacana

Singer, Robert N. 1980. Motor Learning and Human Performance (An Application to Motor Skills and Movement Behaviors). New York: Macmillan Publishing Co. Inc.

Sucipto. et al. (2010). Modul Permainan Bolabasket. Bandung: FPOK UPI

Sudjana. 2002. Desain dan Analisis Eksperimen. Bandung: Tarsito.

Sugiyanto. 1997. Perkembangan Gerak. Surakarta: UNS Press.

Suharno, H. P. 1993. Ilmu Coaching Umum.Yogyakarta: IKIP Yogyakarta Press.

Sutanto, T. (2016). Buku Pintar Olahraga. Pustaka Baru Press,Yogyakarta

Thomas. J. P. & Nelson. J. K. 2001. Research Methods in Physical Activity. Second Edition. Champaign Illinois: Human Kinetic Publisher.

Wahyuni, M. E., & Mulyono, A. (2015). Pengembangan Media Pembelajaran Dribble Bola Basket Menggunakan Job Card Bagi Siswa Kelas VII SMP. Journal of Physical Education Health

16

The Development of "Drilling" Machine For Sepak Takraw Practice

Isnaini Nurul Hidayah[1]✉, Bambang Priyono[2]

Department of Health Physical Education and Recreation, Sport Science Faculty, Universitas Negeri Semarang, Indonesia[12]

Article History

Keywords:
Pelontar; Sepak Takraw; Drilling; Development

Abstract

This study aimed at finding the effect of ladder drill training upon: (1) run speed, (2) agility, and (2) power of leg muscle. This study is an experimental research. This study utilized one group pre test-post test design. There were total people as the subject of this research. Data collection technique used 30-meter sprint test to measure run speed, Illinois agility test to measure agility, and vertical jump test to measure power of leg muscle. Data analysis technique which was used for normality test, homogeneity test/F-test, and T-test with significant level 5% by using SPSS 16.0.0. Based on the finding, there was effect of ladder drill training upon run speed with sig value=0.007, agility and power of leg muscle with sig value=0.000. Based on the data analysis, it could be concluded that there was significant effect of ladder drill training upon run speed, agility and power of leg muscle.

✉ **Correspondence address :**
Dk. Kuniran, RT 06, RW 02 Jatilawang, Wonosegoro, Boyolali District, 57382 Central Java
E-mail: indahfitri195@gmail.com

INTRODUCTION

Sepak Takraw is a game that uses a ball from rattan. The rattan ball is kicked from foot to foot, feeding the comrades and hitting or turning off the ball on the opponent's field. So the idea of Sepak Takraw is making the ball falling down on the opponent's field and try or make sure the ball does not fall down on our field. (Darwis, 1992)

Across the country in Southeast Asia, the ball used in Sepak Takraw was originally made of hand-woven rattan, a material easily accessible in a hand-embroidered area, a highly accessible material in the region. Generally, the ball has a diameter of 5 inches and is mostly played by the villagers by the way they stand in a circle and bump each other. Historians mentioned that the use of rattan balls was first about 500 years ago. However, due to reduced rattan, new regulations were set to protect the presence of rattan. In addition, rattan balls are also more easily damaged and broken in the game nets. Then comes a synthetic ball in the same shape as a rattan ball and is still woven with a hand. (Engel, 2010)

The development of Sepak Takraw in Semarang is now increasing, this is due to the increasing number of achievements of Sepak Takraw in Semarang. The unity of Sepak Takraw is a place or means to develop the ability of an athlete of Sepak Takraw. Such as Association of Sepak Takraw "PPLOP" Central Java Province and the Student Activity Unit Sepak Takraw University of Semarang which makes it easier to improve the skills and techniques of players. To get good skills, from the beginning the athlete has been given basic engineering training, so that with the basic techniques that the player will be able to develop the next skills of Sepak Takraw.

To be able to play Sepak Takraw well, then the athlete must have the ability and good skills. A very important and very necessary ability is the basic ability in Sepak Takraw. The ability is kicked by using the legs, playing the ball with the head, playing the ball with the chest, playing the ball with the thighs, playing the ball with the shoulder. The basic competence of one another is an inseparable unity. Without mastering basic skills or basic techniques, Sepak Takraw cannot be played well. Basic techniques can be mastered well when the basic techniques are learned and trained properly and continuously. (Darwis, 1992). Effect of single leg push off exercise on the result of power of foot at the athlete of sepak takraw daughter of Central Java. This gives the idea that the single leg push off exercise can increase power, where the power in the legs at tekong measured by the speed of a tight ball obtained athletes sepak takraw daughter of Central Java while serving. Football basic technique movement takraw dominated in the form of football takraw done with one foot, then the foot of the pound should have sufficient muscle strength to maintain the balance. Of course, not just one leg is trained (

The development of techniques in sepak takraw has been widely developed in accordance with the variations of exercise. Drills practice method is a variety of exercises done by individuals or groups for the development of techniques in accordance with what is to be achieved. The importance of the drills exercises model is also presented by Harsono (1998). He stated that each exercise should contain useful drills and clear directions and objectives.

The drills exercise model is a varied, patterned, systematic and continuous pattern of specialized training for skills development. Hanif (2015) submitted to improve the basic skills of the receiver of the ball, first needed drill exercise. The form of drill exercise is repetitive motion repetition, where the intensity of the athlete in moving becomes increasingly increasing, and is expected to be able to be directed to form the basic attitude of the athlete in motion. In addition, this exercise can also automate the motion of athletes, and will thoroughly improve the quality when attacking the opponent.

There are still many trainers who train athletes using drilling methods using hand throws, re-throw using tennis racquets, and re-throw using wooden rackets. To create an achievement athlete required intensive training, the success of the drilling exercise should also be supported by various factors, such as infrastructure facilities, this is because the trainer must follow the increasingly sophisticated technological developments. Therefore, the absence of machines in the exercise becomes one of the factors lack of facilities and infrastructure in drilling practice.

Observations made on March 16, 2017, at "PPLOP" Sepak Takraw of Central Java obtained the result that drilling exercises still use hand throws, punches using tennis racquets, and punches using a racket made of wood. Burhan Basyiruddin, one of the graduate students at Universitas Negeri Jakarta, tried to create a football launcher for Sepak Takraw. He has created a machine in the training process for trainers. Based on these considerations, the authors want to develop a model that provides convenience for trainers in training drilling Sepak Takraw. This machine will be developed in the form of ball launcher machine with a speed of one second per four meters and is equipped with the direction of the ball that can be adjusted in the direction of the player, the ball out automatically using the button, the price is economical and can be taken anywhere without the load is too heavy and high size.

The machines used in doing drilling exercises, currently, still use the trainer power and require more energy. According to the trainer, this machine can be a new innovation and is needed to facilitate the trainer in doing drilling exercises. This machine is also expected to streamline the practice time.

The problem is How to design Product Development of Drilling Machine In Sepak Takraw Training?. The purpose of this research is to develop the Drilling Machine In Sepak Takraw Training.

METHODS

The research design used is a research-based development model (Research and Development). According Sugiyono (2010) research and development model is the research used to produce a specific product and test the effectiveness of the product.

The test subjects classified the subjects of trials into three, among others (1) sepak takraw experts, among others, Sepak Takraw coach of Central Java who plays a role to determine whether the product of this development is appropriate material and truth. (2) electro expert.

Validation is done by using a questionnaire about the design of Electro circuit machines and the effectiveness of the machine. The last one is the engine expert. Validation is done by using a questionnaire about the design of machine circuit machines and the effectiveness of the machine. In the experiment of the research, the subject product was 6 athletes of Student Activity Unit of Sepak Takraw Faculty of Sports Science, Universitas Negeri Semarang, while the trial use of this research is 15 athletes in "PPLOP" Central Java.

The data collection techniques in this study were Observation, Interview, Documentation, and Expert Validation. Data analysis used qualitative approach and model development method.

The product developed is a drilling machine in Sepak Takraw practice in the form of a ball throwing machine. This drilling machine aims to simplify the role of trainers in drilling exercises as a substitute for the ball throwers that have been done manually by the coach, either using a racket or hand throw. This ball launcher machine can also facilitate and ease the trainer in drilling drills.

This ball-throwing machine uses a dynamo to launch the ball, it also consists of a ball storage container that can be filled with 6 balls and can be set the speed, the direction, and the launcher also connect to electricity. This ball-throwing machine is also equipped with the frequency control of the number of balls that come out from the machine in every second and can adjust the ball to the desired player.

This drilling machine is a ball thrower machine that is made to simplify and help the trainer to train drilling in Sepak Takraw. During this time, coaches still use hand throws, throws using tennis racquets, and throws using specially designed wooden rackets. The design of products made are as follows **picture 1**:

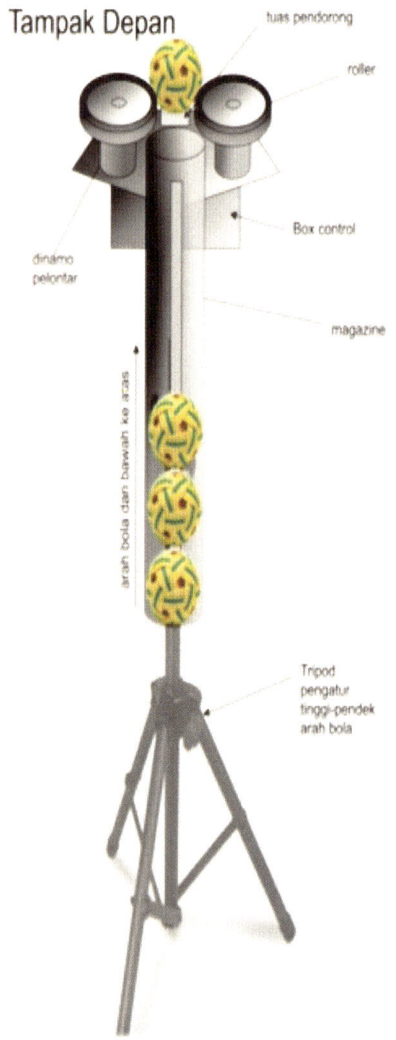

Picture 1. Machine Design

The development of this ball-launcher machine is the development of science and technology conducted in the field of sports to facilitate the trainer during drilling exercise for athletes. Drilling exercises generally use tennis rackets and hand throws. This time the researchers made the development of the ball launcher machine that automatically works if pressed the button will release the ball with an average speed of 4 MPs.

The development of this thrower machine is equipped with switches and red and yellow LED lights as the setting out the ball automatically. If the switch is touched by an iron ring associated with the chain, then the ball automatically comes out one by one.

The product developed is a ball launcher for sepak takraw. The machine designed specifically to launch the ball automatically by pressing the button installed in the pipe.

RESULT AND DISSCUSION

This small-scale trial was conducted at Student Activity Unit Sepak Takraw Faculty of Sports Science, Universitas Negeri Semarang with respondents 6 athletes and aims to identify and identify various problems such as weakness, deficiency, or product effectiveness when used for measurement. Data obtained from these trials are used as a basis for revising the product before it is used in field trials. The data obtained from the questionnaires by experts is a preliminary data to indicate whether the development product can be used for drilling practice on sepak takraw. Data obtained from the interviews conducted by the researcher to the respondent or the trial subjects were used to evaluate the product before it was used in a large-scale trial. **The table 1** details of the results of a small-scale test interview on athletes are as follows:

Table 1. Rincian hasil wawancara

Content	Interview Results					
	1	2	3	4	5	6
Safety	V	V	V	V	V	V
Comfortability	V	V	V	V	V	V
Speed	V	V	V	V	V	V
Drilling Practice	V	V	V	V	V	V
Usefulness to play	V	V	V	V	V	V
Usefulness to practice	V	V	V	V	V	V

The results obtained by researchers in small-scale trials I are as follows. A total of 6 athletes stated:

1. The product is not safe to use for beginner player training
2. Uncomfortable product used for beginner player training
3. The product does not fit the needs of athletes related to the speed of bursting the ball
4. The product can not be used as drilling practice
5. The product can not be used for training
6. The product can not be used for further training

Small-scale trials II were conducted with the same respondents and the same number of 6 athletes.

The results obtained by researchers in small-scale trials II are as follows. A total of 6 athletes stated:

1. The product is safe to use for beginner player training
2. The product is comfortable to use for beginner player training
3. The product is in accordance with the needs of athletes related to the speed of the ball
4. Products can be used as drilling exercises
5. The product can be used for exercise
6. The product can be used for further practice.

A large-scale trial was conducted at PPLOP sepak takraw Central Java with a total of 15 athletes, along with details of interviews on large-scale trials. A total of 15 athletes stated:

1. The product is safe to use for beginner player training
2. The product is comfortable to use for beginner player training
3. The product is in accordance with the needs of athletes related to the speed of the ball
4. Products can be used as drilling exercises
5. The product can be used for exercise
6. The product can be used for further practice.

Research development is done by sharing the stages. The research started from the initial product validation of product trial that is a small-scale test and big scale so that mass-produced product where the product can be used its usefulness, the researcher involves three validators with their respective expertise ie electro expert, engineer, and sepak takraw expert. Small-scale trials were conducted at Student Activity Unit sepak takraw FIK UNNES (Universitas Negeri Semarang) and large-scale test conducted at PPLOP sepak takraw Central Java. Validation of the product is done by using questionnaire instrument to know how far this tool is said to be worthy to be tested. Questionnaires used in the research process as product validation data and effectiveness test. At the same time, other checks such as documentation, interviews, and discussion of more than one source, in the same way, are observed and expert experts. For assessment using the appraisal that has been developed the deputy of Implementation of Science and Technology Science, Ministry of Youth and Sports of the Republic of Indonesia in 2011. Expert assessment results sepak takraw with a score of 78, experts electro with a score of 77, engineers with a score of 91, each expert obtained a score above 77 that enter the good and appropriate criteria.

The results of the study based on the analysis of data description of trials conducted in Semarang. For the effectiveness of the tool then the tool is tested its effectiveness by using observation, interview, documentation, and discussion. Researchers create a new innovation in the form of the development of ball throwing tool. In the initial design, the researchers focused on the criteria that have been used by the Ministry of Youth and Sports in the selection and research for the participants of innovative sports technology competition in 2017. Before being tested on a small scale, the development of drilling tools in sepak takraw practice first need to be validated by expert experts in accordance with this field of research. To validate the resulting product, the researcher involves the experts consisting of 1 coach of sepak takraw Central Java, namely Bambang Edy, M.Pd., Engineer, Drs. Supraptono, and Electrical experts, namely Tatyantoro Andrasto, S.T., M.T

Validation is done by the expert team by observing drilling tool development product in sepak takraw practice when doing drilling along with evaluation sheet along with suggestion and input sheet. The evaluation sheet is a questionnaire that contains aspects of product quality. The suggestion sheet is used as a revision as well as input is given to the researcher regarding the developed tool

The evaluation result is the value of product quality aspect of the development of drilling tool in sepak takraw practice using the scoring range of 100 (1-10 scale). Questionnaire evaluation sheet for drilling tool development in sepak takraw practice

The data obtained from the evaluation sheet or questionnaire by the experts is the determination of the next step in developing the drilling tool in the sepak takraw practice in order to be used for small-scale trials and field trials (large-scale trials). The following is the result of filling out evaluation sheets from sepak takraw experts, engineers, and electro-experts.

Revise the initial draft of the product, based on the advice of an expert on the development of the athlete's endurance sensor when kicking, the product revision is made with the following details:

1. The machine can be used, but RPM must be added to get the ball out faster;
2. Added ball charge

The effectiveness of this product is based on the results of large-scale trials. The effectiveness of the product includes the effectiveness for the measurement and effectiveness of automatic production.

At the time of discussion to implement the development of drilling tools in sepak takraw that have been considered final, the researchers present the experts. This activity aims to convey the development outcomes (the process of procedure and production) to the users and professionals through discussion to know the extent to which research success is achieved.

Based on the steps of research and development to produce a product that has been done, then obtained the final product in the form of a ball-launcher machine for sepak takraw. This development product can be used for drilling practice on sepak takraw.

The indicator of the success of this product was in the form of analysis from observation result, interview, documentation, and discussion with the expert team that is sepak takraw expert, engineer, and electro. According to product trial that has been done got the result that product development of drilling tool in sepak takraw can and effective use for exercise. The results of large-scale trials showed that the product is working properly, athletes and trainers can also see the results of measurements made.

This research was a research of the development of drilling tool in sepak takraw which was structured according to the stages that have been determined.

CONCLUSION

Based on the results of the analysis and discussion, the conclusion that can be drawn from this research is to produce a ball-launcher machine for sepak takraw that can be used for training. Seeing the limitations of this product, it can be further developed for the athlete's endurance gauge product when kicking to fit as.

REFERENCE

Darwis, R. 1992. Olahraga Pilihan Sepak Takraw. Jakarta: Depdikbud.

Engel, R. 2010. Dasar-dasar Sepak Takraw. ASEC Internasional: PT Intan Sejat

Hanif, A., S. 2015. Kepelatihan Dasar Sepak Takraw. Jakarta: PT Raja Grafindo Persada.

Harsono, 1988. Coaching dan Aspek-aspek Psikologis Dalam Coaching. Semarang : Dahara Prize.

Purwaditia, P, & Suripto, A., W. (2017). Pengaruh Metode Latihan Pliometrik Terhadap Power Tekong Pada Atlit Putri Sepak Takraw. ACTIVE: Journal Of Physical Education, Sport, Health And Recreation, 6(1), 10-16.

Sugiyono. 2010. Metode Penelitian Pendidikan (Pendekatan Kuantitatif, Kualitatif dan R& D). Bandung: Alfabeta

Women in Sport Coaching: Challenges, Stress and Wellbeing

Fraser Carson[1], **Clara McCormack[2]**, **Julia Walsh[3]**

Deakin University, Australia[123]

Article History

Keywords:
Women In Coaching; Well-Being; Stress; Hegemonic Masculinity.

Abstract

With a lack of women in leadership positions in sport, there are limited role models for women pursuing coaching careers and a number of traditional gender ideologies to overcome. Female coaches therefore face unique challenges, which can be vastly different to their male counterparts. This integrative review focused on the challenges that women face in the coaching domain and the impact that these can have on their well-being. Only four articles focused solely on female coaches since 2000. Despite the lack of literature several key themes have been identified. The main stressors relate to work-life balance, prolonged periods away from family, and a need to prove they are better than male coaches. Coping strategies focused on proactive anticipation and planning, and communication with others. There is also a lack of support for female coaches and inadequate salary to assist continued engagement. Developing female coaches through mentoring and gender specific coach education programs may counteract these issues.

Correspondence address :
E-mail: f.carson@deakin.edu.au

INTRODUCTION

Female sports coaches face distinctive challenges that cannot be easily removed from the profession (Jennifer et al., 2012). These include a traditionally male-dominant domain, lack of social networks and role models, and reported conflict between coaching and personal responsibilities (LaVoi & Dutove, 2012). Traditional social constructed gender ideology in sport has dictated that femininity is associated with more nurturing roles such as teaching, while masculinity is associated with competition and demonstrating sporting dominance (Williams, 1995). This has created barriers for females both entering coaching and their continued and prolonged engagement with coaching (Norman, 2012). Opportunities for women to enter the coaching field are limited (Cutler & Jackson, 2002). It is rare to see a women hired to work with male athletes, whilst it is common for men to coach women (Knoppers, 1992). For women who do make it in such a male-dominated environment they are left isolated and unsupported (Norman, 2012). All of these experiences can impact on female coaches' stress levels, sometimes leading to burnout (Durand-Bush et al,, 2012), which links to their well-being.

There are numerous studies on well-being, stress, and burnout from an athlete perspective (Cronin & Allen, 2015; Lonsdale et al., 2009; McKay et al., 2008; Mellalieu et al., 2009) and how it can impact their performance, but limited investigation on sports coaches. Thelwell et al., (2008) stated that coaches are performers in their own right, and although their performance is a different kind to that of their athletes, they still need to cope with the stressors of competition (Olusoga et al., 2014). Coaches have performance-related stressors, which relate to their athletes' and their own performance (i.e. athlete preparation; opposition analysis; competition performance) (Olusoga et al., 2010). Coaches also have a number of organizational challenges (i.e. resources; finance; selection) that they must manage (Thelwell et al., 2008). The coach's ability to cope with these stressors is of importance as it can impact personal well-being and the ability to coach at high standards (Levy et al, 2009).

These stressors are not gender specific, rather common within sports coaching. However, women in coaching experience a number of additional stressors as compared to their male counterparts. Firstly, for women the coaching pathway has limited illumination and the struggle to become a coach starts early in their careers due to male hegemonic policing of sport and the sport workplace (Norman, 2012). Second, in many cases the female coach is still the primary caregiver in the home (or perceived to be) causing increased strain on the work-home interface (Dixon et al., 2007). The third issue is isolation, there is a dearth of female role models in sport coaching for women to model and engage with and limited opportunity to form networks of support and learning (Norman, 2012; Shaw & Allen, 2009).

The purpose of this integrative review (Whittemore & Knafl, 2005) is to explore the evidence on women's experiences as sport coaches, the challenges they face and how this can affect their own well-being. The review focused on results from a thorough search of three electronic databases (SPORTDiscus; PsycINFO; and Google Scholar), conducted between March 2017 and June 2017. The search terms identified as relevant to this review comprised of: coach*; women; challenges; stress; coping; well-being. Inclusion criteria were established to ensure results were relevant, which included peer-reviewed published articles, written in English, between January 2000 and June 2017. Articles were reviewed for appropriateness, via 1) the full title and keywords, 2) the abstract, and 3) the full text content (Bocarro, Greenwood, & Henderson, 2008). A total of 34 articles were identified. The methodology of these articles were read to identify the sex of the participant coaches, with 21 articles focused on women in coaching. Further analysis of the full text of this articles identified four studies related to stress and wellbeing.

DISCUSSION

Challenges for female coaches

Female coaches perceive a number of challenges within their role, which include: lack of support, job insecurity, inadequate salary, difficulties in working with parents / spectators, and coaching at evenings and weekends (Kubayi et al, 2017). While these challenges are not unique to female coaches, women in coaching positions do face greater challenges than their male counterparts (Lewis et al., 2018). Knoppers (1987) seminal work on gender and sports coaching recognised that many studies utilise an individual model, with the assumption that the workplace is shaped by those who work in it. The results of these occupational studies identified a number of characteristics that prevented women from flourishing. Knoppers concluded that greater opportunities for women in coaching, additional control over the coaching environment, and an increased proportion of women in leadership positions were crucial to overcome the barriers created.

Women who work in male-dominant environments are encouraged to "act like men", dress like men and to be assertive, while men are taught to be sensitive to the needs of women (Schlesinger & Weigelt-Schlesinger, 2012). This could impact female coaches more than male coaches given the traditional gendered ideology in the male-dominated sport environment (Fielding Lloyd & Meân, 2011). Roffey (2001) and Fox (1999) sought to explain the barriers female coaches faced, with perceptions of a strong old boys' network, lack of opportunity, lack of compensation, and discrimination mentioned by female coaches as common factors. Norman (2010) supports this, with coaches in her investigation believing to have fewer opportunities for development than their male counterparts. Similarly, female coaches are under more pressure to assert themselves over male coaches for employment and had to cope with less financial reward than male coaches in similar positions (Caccese & Mayerberg , 1984). The development of pathways for women coaches (Lewis et al., 2018), the perceived support by the organisations specifically for women coaches (Vinson et al., 2016), and informal networking (Norman, 2012) are three key organisational constraints that influenced the experience of female coaches.

Navigating a path as a female coach is challenging at each stage of the career (LaVoi & Dutove, 2012). Entry is difficult; the workplace is built upon gendered ideology, and the bar set for success is higher than for male counterparts (Norman, 2010). Female coaches have reported that they feel they need to prove they are better than their male colleagues to stay in the profession (Pastore & Judd, 1993). For the female coach there is a fine line between challenge and negative stress and impact on sense of control, job satisfaction and overall wellbeing.

Stressors and coping

All coaches face significant internal (i.e. meeting personal performance objectives; work-life balance; prolonged time away from family) and external (i.e. athlete performance; insufficient preparation time; managing financial support) demands in their coaching and personal life (Norris et al., 2017). At times, they perceive these demands to be greater than their resources that can resulted in experiences of stress. Commonly coaches identified themselves as stressed at least once in their career (Durand-Bush et al., 2012), and have experienced chronic stress leading to symptoms of burnout in their career (Lundkvist et al., 2012).

Specifically for female coaches stressors included the pressure of having numerous roles and responsibilities (LaVoi & Dutove., 2012), early mornings and long days/weeks (Olusoga et al, 2009), and work-life conflict (Dixon et al., 2007). Women can experience greater stressors from the competing values of work and family than their male counterparts (Jennifer E Bruening et al., 2012). This may be an implication of traditional gender ideology, where women usually have greater responsibility to child care (Dixon et al., 2007). Bruening & Dixon (2007) argued that the promotion of a 'sacrifice everything to win' culture in sports coaching exacerbates work-life conflict.

Durand-Bush et al.'s (2012) found that female coaches used various coping strategies in response to stressful situations. They indicated that female coaches prevented stressful experiences by proactively anticipating, learning and exerting adaptive control when possible. Specifically the most common strategies employed to prevent stress included: preparation/planning; self-evaluation/reflection; and communication with others.

Female coach wellbeing

Research into psychological and occupational wellbeing of sports coaches is scarce. Key findings, irrespective of gender, from the research have identified competence and autonomy to be influential to coach wellbeing (Stebbings et al, 2011). Similarly increased job security, development opportunities, and work-life balance promote positive wellbeing for coaches (Stebbings et al, 2012). For women in coaching this is a major concern, especially as they are recognised to have a disproportionate work-life balance, a lack of trust from their organisation, a lack of security in their role, and few opportunities to network (Norman et al., 2016). Female coaches had much greater scores in emotional exhaustion and significantly lower scores in personal accomplishment than male coaches (Caccese & Mayerberg, 1984). Kilo & Hassmén, (2016) reported that female coaches had higher levels of exhaustion and reduced accomplishment compared to male counterparts.

Strategies and Interventions

Greater success has come from taking an organisational approach (Kanter, 2008). More recently, Kilo & Hassmén (2016) showed that organisational factors play an important role for understanding and avoiding burnout in sport coaches. Olusoga et al. (2009) suggested that addressing stressors proactively at an organisation level may reduce levels of coach burnout. Bentzen et al (2017) concur with this recommending organisations support coaches in balancing work and personal lives to encourage self-motivation and longitudinal engagement. Norman (2012) provided an alternative approach focusing on the inclusion of socio-cultural education programs that provided women clear understanding of current context and history of the situation.

She suggests taking this approach allows women in coaching to be better prepared for the challenges they will face. Norman (2012) recommended that female coaches should be provided with support programs that could assist in the promotion of equitable salaries, the fair treatment of female coaches, and alleviate all forms of discrimination.

Stebbings et al. (2011) suggest professional development that focuses on perceived and actual competence via training through courses, feedback, and goal setting, will enhance a coach's perception of competence. Coaches who perceive they were provided continued opportunities for professional development reported greater psychological needs satisfaction (Stebbings et al., 2012). Conversely, if coaches were not provided with professional development opportunities, they felt that they were being prohibited from developing their coaching skills, leading to a sense of lack of competence. It is important to position this professional development as relevant to all coaches and not to problematize women as not having the knowledge and skills required to coach (Vinson et al., 2016).

CONCLUSION

A number of challenges and stressors experienced by coaches are independent of gender. These include: interpersonal relations between coach and athlete; team/athlete selection; perceived insufficient preparation time; and long hours consistent with coaching. At the same time several factors are identified that appear to have greater impact on female coaches. Findings suggest prolonged time away from family, particularly when the female coach is the primary care giver, can increase perceptions of stress and subsequently impact the well-being of these women. Further there is a continual need to prove they are better than other male coaches, with added stress coming from a self-imposed belief that their failure would negatively impact the whole female coach profession.

Proactive anticipation, preparation and planning are key for women (and men) in coaching. Identification of known stressful events and following pre-designed plans enables women in coaching to manage their own well-being more effectively. Reflection, self-evaluation and discussion with others is also key. However, the lack of social networks and role models providing effective support can make this more difficult for women.

There also appears to be a consistent lack of support for female coaches. There is a strong male hegemony traditionally in sports coaching and some discrimination of women in the profession. Women are also underrepresented in leadership positions in sports organisations, resulting in an inability to encourage gender diversity in the recruitment of coaches. Cultural matching, the phenomenon of selecting people similar to you, increases the likelihood that males in leadership roles are more likely to recruit male coaches. This hegemonic masculinity makes it more challenging for women to develop within the coaching domain. Sports organisations need to address this as a means to promote prolonged engagement of women in sports coaching. Development of gender specific networking groups and coach education programs, which also explain how coaching has come to the current status quo, may begin to address these issues (Norman, 2012).

REFERENCES

Bentzen, M., Lemyre, N., &켄ttä, G. 2017. A Comparison of High-Performance Football Coaches Experiencing High-Versus Low-Burnout Symptoms Across a Season of Play: Quality of Motivation and Recovery Matters. International Sport Coaching Journal, 4(2), 133-146.

Bocarro, J., Greenwood, P. B., & Henderson, K. A. 2008. An integrative review of youth development research in selected United States recreation journals. Journal of Park and Recreation Administration, 26(2), 4.

Bruening, J. E., & Dixon, M. A. 2007. Work-family conflict in coaching ii: Managing role conflict. Journal of Sport Management, 21(4), 471-496.

Bruening, J. E., Dixon, M. A., Burton, L., & Madsen, R. 2012. Women in coaching: The work-life interface. In P. Potrac, W. Gilbert, & J. Denison (Eds.), Routledge Handbook of Sports Coaching (pp. 411-423). London, UK: Taylor and Francis.

Caccese, T. M., & Mayerberg, C. K. 1984. Gender differences in perceived burnout of college coaches. Journal of Sport Psychology, 6(3), 279-288.

Cronin & Allen, J. B. 2015. Developmental experiences and well-being in sport: The importance of the coaching climate. The Sport Psychologist, 29(1), 62-71.

Cutler, M. M., & Jackson, A. L. 2002. A"glass ceiling" or work/family conflicts? The Journal of Business and Economic Studies, 8(2), 73-82.

Dixon, M. A., & Bruening, J. E. 2007. Work--family conflict in coaching i: A top-down perspective. Journal of Sport Management, 21(3), 377-406.

Durand-Bush, N., Collins, J., & McNeill, K. 2012. Women coaches' experiences of stress and self-regulation: A multiple case study. International Journal of Coaching Science, 6(2), 21-43.

Fielding Lloyd, B., & Meân, L. 2011. 'I don't think I can catch it': women, confidence and responsibility in football coach education. Soccer and

Society, 12(3), 345-364.

Fox, C. 1999. Women's perceived access to elite coaching positions in Australian sport. The Sport Educator, 11(2), 25-27.

Kanter, R. M. 2008. Men and women of the corporation: New edition. New York, NY: Basic Books.

Kilo, R. A., & Hassmén, P. 2016. Burnout and turnover intentions in australian coaches as related to organisational support and perceived control. International Journal of Sports Science and Coaching, 11(2), 151-161.

Knoppers, A. 1987. Gender and the coaching profession. Quest, 39(1), 9-22.

Knoppers, A. 1992. Explaining male dominance and sex segregation in coaching: Three approaches. Quest, 44(2), 210-227.

Kubayi, A., Coopoo, Y., & Morris-Eyton, H. 2017. Work-related constraints in sports coaching: Perceptions of south african female coaches. International Journal of Sports Science and Coaching, 12(1), 103-108.

LaVoi, N. M., & Dutove, J. K. 2012. Barriers and supports for female coaches: An ecological model. Sports Coaching Review, 1(1), 17-37.

Levy, A., Nicholls, A., Marchant, D., & Polman, R. 2009. Organisational stressors, coping, and coping effectiveness: A longitudinal study with an elite coach. International Journal of Sports Science and Coaching, 4(1), 31-45.

Lewis, C. J., Roberts, S. J., & Andrews, H. 2018. 'Why am I putting myself through this?'Women football coaches' experiences of the Football Association's coach education process. Sport, Education and Society, 23(1), 28-39.

Lonsdale, C., Hodge, K., & Rose, E. 2009. Athlete burnout in elite sport: A self-determination perspective. Journal of Sports Sciences, 27(8), 785-795.

Lundkvist, E., Gustafsson, H., Hjälm, S., & Hassmén, P. 2012. An interpretative phenomenological analysis of burnout and recovery in elite soccer coaches. Qualitative Research in Sport, Exercise and Health, 4(3), 400-419.

McKay, J., Niven, A. G., Lavallee, D., & White, A. 2008. Sources of strain among elite UK track athletes. The Sport Psychologist, 22(2), 143-163.

Mellalieu, S. D., Neil, R., Hanton, S., & Fletcher, D. 2009. Competition stress in sport performers: Stressors experienced in the competition environment. Journal of Sports Sciences, 27(7), 729-744.

Norman, L. 2010. Feeling second best: Elite women coaches' experiences. Sociology of Sport Journal, 27(1), 89-104.

Norman, L. 2012. Developing female coaches: Strategies from women themselves. Asia-Pacific Journal of Health, Sport and Physical Education, 3(3), 227-238.

Norman, L., Didymus, F. F., & Rankin-Wright, A. J. 2016. Understanding occupational wellbeing and women sports coaches. Executive report retrieved from Leeds, UK: Sports Coach UK

Norris, L. A., Didymus, F. F., & Kaiseler, M. 2017. Stressors, coping, and well-being among sports coaches: A systematic review. Psychology of Sport and Exercise, 33, 93-112.

Olusoga, P., Butt, J., Hays, K., & Maynard, I. 2009. Stress in elite sports coaching: Identifying stressors. Journal of Applied Sport Psychology, 21(4), 442-459.

Olusoga, P., Butt, J., Maynard, I., & Hays, K. 2010. Stress and coping: A study of world class coaches. Journal of Applied Sport Psychology, 22(3), 274-293.

Olusoga, P., Maynard, I., Butt, J., & Hays, K. 2014. Coaching under pressure: Mental skills training for sports coaches. Sport and Exercise Psychology Review, 10(3), 31-44.

Pastore, D. L., & Judd, M. R. 1993. Gender differences in burnout among coaches of women's athletic teams at 2-year colleges. Sociology of Sport Journal, 10(2), 205-212.

Roffey, K. 2001. Reasons for shortages of female coaches. The Sport Educator, 13(2), 39-40.

Schlesinger, T., & Weigelt-Schlesinger, Y. 2012. 'Poor thing' or 'wow, she knows how to do it' – gender stereotypes as barriers to women's qualification in the education of soccer coaches. Soccer and Society, 13(1), 56-72.

Shaw, S., & Allen, J. B. 2009. The experiences of high performance women coaches: A case study of two regional sport organisations. Sport Management Review, 12(4), 217-228.

Stebbings, J., Taylor, I. M., & Spray, C. M. 2011. Antecedents of perceived coach autonomy supportive and controlling behaviors: Coach psychological need satisfaction and well-being. Journal of Sport and Exercise Psychology, 33(2), 255-272.

Stebbings, J., Taylor, I. M., Spray, C. M., & Ntoumanis, N. 2012. Antecedents of perceived coach interpersonal behaviors: The coaching environment and coach psychological well- and ill-being. Journal of Sport & Exercise Psychology, 34(4), 481-502.

Thelwell, R. C., Weston, N. J. V., Greenlees, I. A., & Hutchings, N. V. 2008. Stressors in elite sport: A coach perspective. Journal of Sports Sciences, 26(9), 905-918.

Vinson, D., Christian, P., Jones, V., Williams, C., & Peters, D. M. 2016. Exploring how well uk coach education meets the needs of women sports coaches. International Sport Coaching Journal, 3(3), 287-302.

Whittemore, R., & Knafl, K. 2005. The integrative review: updated methodology. Journal of Advanced Nursing, 52(5), 546-553.

Williams, C. L. 1995. Still a man's world: Men who do women's work. Berkeley, CA: Univ of California Press.

18

Badminton Long-serve Skill's Level of Physical Education Male Students in the Universitas Islam Riau

Novri Gazali[1], **Romi Cendra**[2]

Jurusan Pendidikan Jasmani Kesehatan dan Rekreasi, Fakultas Keguruan dan Ilmu Pendidikan, Universitas Islam Riau, Indonesia[12]

Article History

Keywords:
Service Skills; Badminton; Technique

Abstract

This study was aimed to determine the skill level of the student badminton long service Penjaskesrek Riau Islamic University. Type of this research is quantitative descriptive research. The population in this research is a student of Penjaskesrek Riau Islamic University year of active 2015/2016 generation force totalling 236 overall students from 8 class. While the samples taken in this study are male students who numbered 40 people. Sampling techniques in the study using a purposive sampling technique, namely by taking a sample based on certain considerations. The instruments used in this study is a long service badminton service test of Nurhasan. Data analysis method used is descriptive statistics, statistics is intended for gathering data, presenting data and specify a value. The results of research is poured into 5 categories that is very good, good, enough, less and less once. Based on the data analysis that has been done, the result shows that it can be concluded that this research is the level of long service skill of students of Penjaskesrek Islamic University of Riau category enough, that is 16 students with percentage of 40% from 40 students.

Correspondence address :
Jl. Sukajaya, Desa Tarai Bangun, Kabupaten Kampar, Riau, Indonesia
E-mail: novri.gazali@edu.uir.ac.id / romicendra@edu.uir.ac.id

INTRODUCTION

Badminton is a favorit sport by people around the world, including Indonesia. This can be seen by the large number of people who participate in any badminton activities held, whether regional, national to world games, such as Thomas and Uber Cup or Olympics. Badminton sports can be played from children to adults, both indoors and outdoors.

To get a high achievement, in badminton, it takes some conditions (ability) to be fulfilled because an athlete not only rely on talent but also must have excellent physical condition skills, techniques, tactics, and mental good. Based on the four elements, the technical factor is the most basic completeness (Islahuzzaman, 2010).

The basic technique of badminton is the main thing that must be mastered by every player in playing badminton, among others: 1) How to hold the racket, 2) Wrist Movement, 3) Footwork, 4) Concentration (Tohar, 1992)

For badminton players, after mastering the basic techniques, it is required to master the technique of hitting shuttlecock. Technique to hit shuttlecock aims to fly shuttlecock to the opponent's field, including: 1) Serves, 2) Lob Serve, 3) Dropshot, 4) Smash, 5) Drive, and 6) Return Serves (Tohar, 1992).

After both techniques are mastered, the badminton player needs to master the hit-pattern, which is a sequential and continuous hit that combines one technique with another and do it repeatedly, thus making a form of circuit that can be played harmoniously and integrated. Do the easy pattern first, then go to the difficult one.

Seeing from the various techniques in badminton, Serve is a very important technique to be mastered by the players. Serves aim to fly shuttlecock to other field diagonally as game opener. Serve is an important blow in badminton game because it becomes the initial capital to win the game, in other words a player can not get scores if can not do the Serve well, so Serve is the first technique learned.

There are four kinds of Serves, including: Short Serves, Lob Serves or Long Serves, Drive Serves, and Flick Serves. Based on the four kinds of Serves on badminton, Long Serve is mostly used in single game to earn points. It is performed by flying the highest shuttlecock and falling to the rear of the opposing field (Tohar, 1992).

The purpose and intent of using Long Serve is to push the opponent's position to the back line, so that the front field becomes empty (Tohar, 1992). So the shuttlecock of the opponent can be directed to the front of the net. In addition, Long Serve blows are very appropriate to do when the opponent is exhausted, because the opponent is forced to move in a wider area and spend more power.

Long Serve includes the type of underhand stroke, which is a blow with a racket swing from bottom to top. Long Serve is commonly used for badminton games on a single party, so that the rate of shuttlecock can soar backwards and there will be a long rally. Shuttlecock at full power to dive sharply downward with Long Serve's target area is the back border of the opposing field, the border between the back border for a single game and the back border for a double game with mid-bound and edge for a single game.

Long Serve test skills can be used to measure the capabilities of Serve mastery that soar backward in the opponent's field area. Badminton players who have good long serve skills are also expected to have supportive skills, including strength, muscle endurance, and precision, so that they can survive the long game until the end of the game.

Physical Education is one of the existing study program in the Universitas Islam Riau precisely in Pekanbaru City, Riau Province. This Study Program has one of the objectives of producing qualified physical education graduates. For that students are required to have quality in sports, one of them is badminton.

Based on the results of observations on badminton courses, the ability of long serve students of Physical Education at the Universitas Islam Riau looks less. While serving, the shuttlecock falls in three quarters of the opponent's field, so the opponent will easily smash. From the results of these observations, it is deemed necessary to be given a long test to see clearly the ability of Physical Education students at the Universitas Islam Riau.

In improving skills in badminton, every player should try to improve his skills and master basic techniques in badminton games, one of which is the serve technique. In badminton, serve is the initial capital to win the game. In other words, a player can not get points if he can not serve well (buku pedoman praktis bermain bulutangkis, 2001).

Purnama in Yane (2016) said serve is a very decisive movement in the beginning of value acquisition, because players who serve well can control the course of the game, for example as an early strategy of attack. According to Dinata (2004), in badminton, there are three types of serve, namely: a) short serve, b) long serve, and c) flick serve. However, the serve usually is combined into a type or form of forehand and backhand. Each of these types varies according to the game situation in the field.

As mentioned by Grace cited by Subarjah (2001), serve is the main movement to start the game. Serve includes one of the motion skills performed with a racket swing from bottom to top. As in tennis, serving in badminton plays an important role, because the victory in the rally is preceded by serve. Serve is probably the single most important movement. It is difficult for players to get points consistently, without adequate serve.

Based on some opinions above, it can be concluded that the serve is the initial capital to win the game. In other words, a player can not get points if he can not serve well. It is difficult for players to get points consistently, without adequate serve. In badminton, there are three types of serve, namely: a) short serve, b) long serve, and c) flick serve. However, usually serve is combined into two types, namely forehand and backhand.

According to Poole (2005), serve is a very decisive move in the early points acquisition, because players who serve well can control the game, for example as an initial strategy of attack. In performing long serve in badminton, the player must perform in accordance with the rules. The provisions are among others:

a. The height of the shuttlecock when it encounters the racket head is below the waist.
b. The head of the racket should be downward.
c. Both feet are in the serve field, not touching the center line or the front line.
d. There is no double movement (when the racket is swung up to encounter the shuttlecock is a one-time move).
e. Racket movement must be continued without any interrupted time.

Long serve type on badminton is widely used in single game. Long serve is the movement to hit the shuttlecock as high, and fall into the back line of the opponent's field (Tohar, 1992). According to Wicaksono (2008), how to do long serve is :

a. Shuttlecock must be struck with full force to allow the shuttlecock to float high and fall perpendicularly behind the opposing field line.
b. In doing a long serve, while hitting the shuttlecock, both legs are hip-width apart and both feet are always in contact with the floor.
c. For the racket swing movement is performed backward, forward and after hitting, must be done perfectly and followed the movement of the center point of weight from the hind leg to the front leg which must be continuous and harmonious.
d. Get used to always concentrate before hitting the shuttlecock.

METHODS

This was quantitative descriptive research that aimed to get a real picture or reality of the state of the object of research. It was supported by data in the form of numbers obtained from the data collection, such as tests and measurements. In this study, researcher would like to know the level of long serve skill from male students of Physical Education of the Universitas Islam Riau in the year of 2015/2016. Data were analyzed to determine the extent of skill level of long serve in badminton.

Data collection techniques used test and measurement techniques. The test instrument in this study used a long serve test (Nurhasan, 2001). This test aimed to measure accuracy in hitting a shuttlecock toward a specific target with a long serve technique. While the validity of this test amounted to 0.54 and reliability 0.77.

Population in this research was physical education male students of the Universitas Islam Riau in the year of 2015/2016 as an active year, around 236 students from 8 classes participated. While the samples were 40 male students. Sampling technique was purposive sampling technique which is taking sample based on certain considerations. In this study the researcher took five samples of each class that got the best score on badminton courses.

Data analysis was descriptive statistics, these statistics were intended to collect data, present data, and determined the value. Furthermore, the data was analyzed as a discussion of the problems addressed by reference to the standard of long serving ability in badminton.

The results were shown in five categories that are excellent, good, fair, less, and poor. To determine the category using the formula from Sudjana (2007), as for the formula in table 1.

Table 1. Category Formula

No	Rumus Kategori	Kategori
1	$X \geq M + 1.5\ SD$	Baik Sekali
2	$M + 0.5\ SD \leq X < M + 1.5\ SD$	Baik
3	$M - 0.5\ SD \leq X < M + 0.5\ SD$	Cukup
4	$M - 1.5\ SD \leq X < M - 0.5\ SD$	Kurang
5	$X < M - 1.5\ SD$	Kurang Sekali

Source : Sudjana (2007: 42)

RESULTS AND DISCUSSION

This research was conducted for two months, from October to November 2017 at GOR Badminton Pandau at 8 am every Saturday.

Based on the data collection with a sample size of 40 people, then the data were analyzed using descriptive statistics. From the measurements that have been done to Physical Education students, it turns out that from 40 athletes being sampled, there are 6 people or 15% belonging to excellent service level, 6 people or 15% are good, 16 or 40% , 12 people or 30% are categorized less, and poor level was no one. For more details can be seen in **table 2.**

Based on **table 2**, the data analyzed with the following calculation, at excellent level, there are 6 people; at a good level, there are 6 people; at a fair level, there are 16 people; at the less level, there are 12 people; while at the poor level, no one. So from the five categories, the most results were at the fair level, it could be concluded that the long serving level of badminton from physical education male students of the Universitas Islam Riau is categorized as fair.

Ma'mun and Saputra (2000) argue that the attainment of a skill was influenced by many factors. These factors are generally divided into three main things, namely the factors of teaching and learning process, personal factors, and situational factors (environment).

These three factors are believed to have been a major determinant of achieving a degree of success in learning skills.

A new skill can be mastered or acquired when studied or trained with certain requirements, one of which is a continuous learning or skill activity within a certain period of time. The ability of each individual is also different, it depends on how the learning process, how the individual personality, and the environment around him.

Skills possessed a provision for students to improve basic techniques that are still lacking. Basic engineering skills possessed by these students become capital for students in achieving the maximum performance.

CONCLUSION

Based on data analysis, it could be concluded that long serve badminton skill's level of Physical Education male students of Universitas Islam Riau is at fair level, that is 16 students out of 40 students got percentage as much as 40%.

REFERENCES

Dinata, M., & Tarigan, H. (2004). Bulutangkis. Ciputat: Cerdas Jaya.

Nurhasan. (2001). Tes dan Pengukuran dalam Pendidikan Jasmani: Prinsip-Prinsip dan Penerapannya. Jakarta: Depdiknas.

Islahuzzaman, I. (2010). "Analisis Teknik Dasar Pukulan Bulutangkis Game 21 Pada Tunggal Putra". Jurnal Pendidikan dan Kepelatihan Olahraga, 3(1).

Ma'mun, A dan Saputra, Y.M. (2000). Perkembangan Gerak dan Belajar Gerak. Departemen Pendidikan dan Kebudayaan.

PBSI. (2001). Pedoman Praktis Bermain Bulutangkis. Jakarta: Depdiknas.

Poole, J. (2006). Belajar Bulutangkis. Bandung: Pionir Jaya.

Subarjah, H. (2010). Hasil Belajar Keterampilan Bermain Bulutangkis Studi Eksperimen Pada Siswa Diklat Bulutangkis FPOK-UPI. Jurnal Cakrawala Pendidikan, 3(3).

Sudjana, Anas. (2007). Pengantaar Evaluasi Pendidikan. Jakarta: PT. Raja Grafindo Persada.

Tohar, M. (1992). Olahraga Pilihan Bulutangkis. Departemen Pendidikan dan Kebudayaan Direktorat Jenderal Pendidikan Tinggi Proyek Pembinaan Tenaga Pendidikan.

Wicaksono, D. (2008). Permainan Bulutangkis Yang Menyenangkan. Diambil dari: Diakses pada tanggal 5 Agustus 2017. wordpress.com//sejarah-pengertian-dan-peraturan-bulu-tangkis/.

Yane, S. (2017). "Peningkatan Servis Panjang Bulutangkis Melalui Model Problem Based Learning". Jurnal Pendidikan Olahraga, 5(2), 165-174.

Table 2. Category of Long Serve Badminton Skill's Level on Male Student of Physical Education Universitas Islam Riau

Category Formula	Category	Amount	Percentage
≥42.82	Excellent	6	15%
34.33 - 42.81	Good	6	15%
25.84 - 34.32	Fair	16	40%
17.35 - 25.83	Less	12	30%
≤17.34	Poor	0	0%
Total		40	100%

19

Efforts to Improve Skills Overhand Service On Volleyball Games By Using Part and Whole

Ajib Nasir Hanifa[1] , Agus Tomi[2], Oni Bagus Januarto[3]

Universitas Negeri Malang, Indonesia[123]

Article History

Keywords:
Volleyball Game;
Overhead Service;
Part and Whole.

Abstract

The purpose of this research is to improve the overhead service techniques of volleyball related to Physical Education class in XI C Animation in SMK Negeri 4 Malang by using the method of part and whole. This research is using quantitative and qualitative descriptive approach. This research was also carried out by using two cycles and each cycle consists of four phases: (1) planning, (2) implementation, (3) observation, and (4) reflection. Subjects in this study is a 34 students of XI C class of Animation in SMK Negeri 4 Malang. The success rate of students in the first cycle is 75%, in the second cycle is 87%. Based on the results of the study is by using part and whole method can improve the ability of overhead service techniques on students of XI C class of Animation in SMK Negeri 4 Malang.

Correspondence address :
Jl. Semarang No.5, Sumbersari, Kec. Lowokwaru, Kota Malang, Jawa Timur 65145
E-mail: ajibnasirhanifa17@gmail.com

INTRODUCTION

Physical Education and Sport is a long-term investment for efforts to improve the quality of Indonesian human resources, the expected results will be achieved in a long time. Physical education according to UNESCO (in Mu'arifin, 2009) "Physical education is a process of education of a person, as an individual or as a member of society that is done consciously and systematically through various physical activities in order to obtain improvement in the ability of physical appearance, - the plant of intelligence, and the formation of character ".

Physical education learning taught in schools, especially in vocational schools, is not much different from other schools such as volleyball games, basketball games, badminton games, athletics, gymnastics, and so forth. In the sport bolavoli game already in the latest curriculum is the Curriculum 2013 SMK Class XI. A teacher of physical education and health to achieve mastery in learning the game bolavoli must know the characteristics, developments, preferences of the students so that the learning can be achieved. The top service is one of the basic techniques often used by players bolavoli to start the game which is also used as a means of attack to gain points. According to Suhadi (2009) states that "in the service there are several ways or models, namely: under serve, overhead serve, and jump serve".

Based on the results of initial observation of volleyball service technique by doing each participant perform service alternately in the service area using the net, this is done by students of class XI Animation C in SMK Negeri 4 Malang, amounting to 34 students consisting of 20 male students and 14 female student.

Description of the service above is as follows: N1 is the attitude of the body with the indicator that is: Body position The body stands straight to the ball, weight rests on the soles of the feet, and Position of the straight body facing the playing field. N2 is the attitude of the foot with the indicator that is: Legs opened shoulder width apart, One foot is in front and not parallel to the other foot, The distance of both legs arranged so that the fulcrum or balance between the middle between the legs. N3 is the position of the hand with the indicator that is: One hand holding the ball, Keep the hand outstretched in a state straight forward, Then the hand is ready to hit the ball. N4 is the ball with the indicator that is: Lambungkan ball up to the back a little ± 1 meter using the left hand, the body slightly bounced back and weight on the hind legs, Swing one hand together with the forward movement and hit the ball assisted with wiping the wrist. N5 is coordination with indicators namely: views, initial attitudes, and follow-up motion. N6 is the result. N7 is the maximum score.

From the results of preliminary observations on overhand service techniques on the N1 indicator is the score of results 64, average 1.88, the highest score 3, the lowest score 1, 63% completeness percentage. N2 score of results 64, average 1.88, highest score 3, lowest score 1, 63% completeness percentage. N3 score results 65, average 1.91, highest score 2, lowest score 1, percentage mastery 64%. N4 score result 66, average 1.94, highest score 2, lowest score 1, percentage mastery 66%. N5 score of 67 results, average 1.97, highest score 3, lowest score 1, percentage mastery 66%. N6 results score of 326, average 9.59, highest score 14, lowest score 6. N7 maximum score 510. percentage of overall mastery on overhand service technique is 64%.

Based on these observations it is important that there is a lesson focusing on the skills of volleyball game overhand service techniques, so that the technical skills of the student's game of volleyball is better and more correct.

Games used to improve overhand service skills are:

Overhand Service Without Ball

This learning is done by practicing basic service movements without using the ball. According to Baacke (1979) said "lift the ball up and touch with the wrist." Thus the researchers modify the learning overhand service without the ball. (a) Facilities and infrastructure, namely: learning field, student whistle, etc. (b) The objective of the game enhances the overhand service skills without the use of the ball by providing an example of a correct service technique movement. (c) Instruction guidance in this game some students lined up, the researcher gave an example of the technique movement of overhand service without using the ball and then followed by the students, when finished immediately replace with other students, this is done continuously until students get it right with the technique taught.

Overhand Service With Ball

This learning is almost the same as before but here already use the ball, the way is by practicing basic movements of service using the ball. According to Baacke (1979) says "lift the ball up and touch with the wrist." Broadly speaking researchers modify the service learning by using the ball. (a) Facilities and infrastructure: field for play, volleyball and students. (b) The purpose of this lesson aims to enable students to hit the volleyball that will be in service appropriately. (c) Instructional guidance In this lesson some students hold the ball, the researchers practice the overhand service movement by using the ball, followed by the students who hold the ball, after they have finished with the other students.

Overhand Service at Wall

Overhand service learning at the wall is an example of a movement in learning in a game of volleyball by pointing the ball at the target point. According to Baacke (1979) says "Throw on the point on the wall and catch".

From the above understanding the researcher uses the left right game so that students can do the passing well if the ball that came falling in front or side of the body as high as the stomach down. (a) Facilities and infrastructure, namely: students, volleyball, whistles, walls for learning, service goals. (b) The purpose of this lesson aims to increase students' accuracy of overhand service. (c) Implementation instructions For this lesson some students hold the ball. According to Budiwanto (2006) says "every testi performs a overhand service test of 10 times." So the researcher here applies to students doing overhand service to the wall, each performing alternately for 10 times the blow and done alternately with other students.

Overhand Service Using Net with 4 Meter Distance

This learning is done by practicing movement service by using media net. According to Baacke (1979) says "bait facing (bait on the head) a distance of 9m, each 30x. Distance of 6m, each 30x. Distance of 4m, each 30x ". (a) Facilities and infrastructure, namely: field, volleyball and students, whistles. (b) The purpose of this Lesson is to train students to do overhand service with the media net which is 4m away. (c) Instructional guidance in this learning some students stand in front of the net facing each other and doing service with friends who are in front. With the notes of female and male students separated because of different net height, for female students 2.24m while the male 2.43m. According to Budiwanto (2006) said "service ball must pass between the net and the rope as high as 4m. Each testi performs a overhand service test of 10x. "So the researcher here implements the above overhand service distance with the net is 4m, this is done for 10x the punch and done alternately with the other students.

Overhand Service Using Net with 6 Meter Distance

This learning is still the same as before, done by practicing service movements using the net media. According to Baacke (1979) says "bait facing (bait on the head) a distance of 9m, each 30x. Distance 6m, each 30x. Distance of 4m, each 30x ". (a) Field facilities and infrastructure, volleyball and students, whistles. (b) Objectives In this lesson, it is done to train students in the overhand service with a net medium that uses a little distance back with a distance of 6m. (c) In the implementation of this study According to Budiwanto (2006) said "every testi doing service test of 10x." So the researcher here implements the distance of this service with net a little far is 6 meters, this is done for 10x punch and done alternating with other students. With the notes of female and male students separated because of different net height, for female students 2.24m while the male 2.43m.

Overhand Service Using Net with 9 Meter Distance

This learning is a development from the previous way by practicing service movements using net media. According to Baacke (1979: 49) says "bait facing (bait on the head) a distance of 9m, each 30x. Distance 6m, each 30 x. Distance of 4m, each 30x ". (a) Field facilities and infrastructure, volleyball and students, whistles. (b) The purpose of this study is to train the students in the overhand service with the net medium that uses the rearmost distance with a distance of 9m (the back line volleyball game). (c) Implementation Instructions.

This learning is still the same as before, some students stand in front of the net facing each other and do service with friends who are in front. With the notes of female and male students separated because of different net height, for female students 2.24m while the male 2.43m. According to Budiwanto (2006) says "every testi conducts 10x overhand service tests." So the researcher here implements the service distance above this with a net of 9m (the back line of a volleyball game), performed for 10x blows and performed alternately with other students .

Edy Suyanto, (2014) entitled "Improving the Effectiveness of Learning Passing Under Volleyball Using Part and All Methods In Students of Class XI IPA 1 SMAN 2 Batu Town". The game on the research are: (1) Students do foot and knee exercises without spherical shaped sphere. (2) Students do arm exercises using the ball with a soccer catch. (3) Students perform the ball practice. (4) Students perform the overall movement exercises passing down the volleyball. The result of this research is that using part and whole method can improve the basic passing technique skill in class XI IPA 1 SMAN 2 Batu Town. Kharisma Wahyu Atmaja, (2015) entitled "Improving Quick Smash Bolavian Skills With Part and Whole Methods On Club Binayuda Club Women's Volley Ball Team Rowokangkung Lumajang District". The game on the research are: (1) Players perform shadow movements quick smash start from prefix, repulsion, jumping, perenaan ball, and landed. (2) Players make quick shash movements of bolavoli as a whole by using the ball and done starting from prefix, repulsion, jumping perenaan ball, and landing. The result of the research is that using the part and whole method can improve the technique skill of Quick Smash Volley Princess Binayuda Rowokangkung Club of Lumajang Regency. Vilan Argo Pinatas, (2014) entitled "Improving the Effectiveness of Teaching Learning by Using Part and Whole Methods In Class X Students RPL-1 SMK Negeri 5 Malang". The game on the research are: (1) Students do learning meroda with part method and Model 1 learning is a handstand that starts from the position of the body bent and both hands resting on the floor. (2) The learning model 2 is handstand starting from the initial stand attitude. (3) Models of Exercise 3 which are seduced in the sloped field. (4) Models of Exercise 4, which are flat-to-air dimatras by controlling the position of the feet and hands. (5) Students do learning merda using whole method of students doing series of gymnastics floor. The result of this research that using part and whole method can improve effectiveness of learning meroda on class X student RPL-1 SMK Negeri 5 Malang.

From some of these studies have been done on learning activities, but have not focused on basic service skills of the top techniques taught in physical education and health education.

Learning outcomes and exercises using the part and whole method are experiencing problems in the low level of quality of learning so that the interest of students for learning is still lacking, the results of this study entered in PTK (Research Action Class) that leads to aspects of overhand service skills.

Based on the problems that have been described, researchers are interested to provide learning action and overhand service techniques. Treatment to students because the learning process is less varied. So researchers will conduct research with the title " Efforts To Improve Skills Overhand Service On Volleyball Games By Using Part And Whole In Students of Class XI Animation C SMK Negeri 4 Malang."

The purpose of this study is the researcher wanted to know how after the application of part and whole method in learning overhand service can improve the skills of volleyball service on students of class XI Animasi C SMK Negeri 4 Malang.

METHODS

The approach used in this research is a qualitative research approach. Because it shows the characteristics of qualitative research is strong enough, especially on the meaning of what happens in the learning process, either in school or outside school hours, both related to the initial conditions of learning and that occur after the action is applied. Judging from the purpose of research, then this research is classroom action research. Basically a classroom action research that researchers do aims to improve learning outcomes of overhand service skills on the students of class XI Animation C SMK Negeri 4 Malang by using the part and whole method.

Classroom action research is expected in the learning process is able to learn optimally. The presence of researchers as colleagues for teachers in working together to prepare the concept of action that will be done. This classroom action research is conducted every Tuesday at 12.45 WIB until 15.00 WIB, in multipurpose field of SMK Negeri 4 Malang. The subjects of this study are students of class XI Animation C SMK Negeri 4 Malang with the number of male students 20 students and 14 female students.

Collecting techniques by researchers using (1) observation, This stage is used to obtain preliminary data for research. (2) questionnaire, this stage is used to obtain the initial needs of research in the form of quantitative and qualitative data. (3) interview, at this stage is used to obtain data that strengthen the result of questionnaire responder. (4) documentation, this stage is used to prove to have done research. In the data collection also use the following stages: (1) Preparation stage, This stage is done by: (a) the researcher made a preliminary observation in the learning process in SMK Negeri 4 Malang. (b) formulate problems that arise at the time of learning. (c) submit a class action research (PTK) and (d) prepare a research proposal. (e) the study permit (2) the stage of implementation, the next step with the implementation stage, at this stage will be done:

(a) planning to make learning overhand service on using the part and whole method (b) prepare tools to support learning (c) division of each learning game (d) explain the learning schedule to be done (e) make observations of students of class XI Animasi C SMK Negeri 4 Malang. (3) documentation. In taking the documentation of the researcher doing the shooting or photo when the students do the overhand service learning activity by using part and whole method. During the observation when learning overhand service on volleyball in SMK Negeri 4 Malang researchers assisted a teacher.

Data analysis to be used is qualitative and quantitative data analysis. Where in this qualitative data analysis technique has 3 step in doing data analysis. Sugiyono (2011) describes the steps of qualitative data analysis as follows: 1) Data reduction, ie sensitive thinking processes that require high intelligence, breadth, and depth of insight. For the new researcher, to do data reduction can discuss to the friend or others that are considered by the expert, 2) presentation of data, in qualitative research presentation of data in the form of brief description, chart, relationship between categories, flowchart, and the like, 3) ferivikasi data, the conclusions are still transient, and will still change if there is no strong evidence to support the next stage of data collection. But the conclusions raised in the initial taunt, supported by valid and consistent evidence, then the conclusion put forward is a credible conclusion.

After getting the result of observation when the implementation took place in the field then the result is calculated then included in the analysis of the following percentage **table 1**.

Tabel 1. Percentage of Succeaa Stages

Percentage	Classification
81-100%	Very Good
61-80%	God
41-60%	Enough
21%-40%	Less
<21%	Less than one

Source: Arikunto (2008)

RESULTS AND DISCUSSION

In the results of this study will be presented some data obtained results of researchers from the beginning of the research until the process of research implementation and analysis of the results of the research volleyball game in one game in class XI Animasi C SMK Negeri 4 Malang, amounting to 34 students. Then also will be presented result of observation cycle of 1 meeting 1 until meeting 3, then result of cycle 2 for 3 meeting. After getting the results then analyzed and get the results of the percentage of overall mastery of overhand service skills for students of class XI Animation C in SMK Negeri 4 Malang.

Results of Needs Analysis

From the results of observations the researchers concluded that the effectiveness of overhand passing techniques of students of class VIII B is still lacking. This can be seen from the overhand passing completeness of the students of class XI Animation C at the game of the game volley ball is 23.5%. The result of the initial observation for the overhand service of 34 students, 21 students (63%) did the right attitude, 21 students (63%) students did leg attitude correctly, 22 students (64%) students did hand attitude correctly, 23 students (65%) students did the ball spell correctly, 24 students (66%) students coordinated correctly.

Preliminary Observations

From the results of preliminary observations on service techniques on the N1 indicator is the score of results 64, average 1.88, the highest score 3, the lowest score 1, 63% completeness percentage. N2 score of results 64, average 1.88, highest score 3, lowest score 1, 63% completeness percentage. N3 score results 65, average 1.91, highest score 2, lowest score 1, percentage mastery 64%. N4 score result 66, average 1.94, highest score 2, lowest score 1, percentage mastery 66%. N5 score of 67 results, average 1.97, highest score 3, lowest score 1, percentage mastery 66%. N6 results score of 326, average 9.59, highest score 14, lowest score 6. N7 maximum score 510. percentage of overall mastery on top service technique is 64%.

Results Cycle 1 And Cycle 2

Based on the result of the research of the overhand service technique at meeting 1 cycle 1 the percentage of overall overhand service completeness up that is 67%. From that percentage it can be seen that the results have increased but not yet in accordance with existing targets, so the researchers and teachers reflect in the first meeting and continue the second meeting of cycle 1.

Based on the results of the overhand service engineering research at the 2nd cycle meeting 1 percentage of the overall completeness of the overhand service above that is 71%. From that percentage it can be seen that the result has been increased but not yet in accordance with the target, so that the researcher and teacher do reflection in the second meeting and continue the third meeting of cycle 1.

Based on the results of research overhand service technology at the meeting 3 cycles 1 percentage overall completeness of overhand service that is 75%. From that percentage it can be seen that the results have increased but not yet in accordance with existing targets, so the researchers and teachers reflect on the third meeting and continue the first meeting of cycle 2.

Based on the results of the top service engineering research at the meeting 1 cycle 2 percentage overall completeness of overhand service that is 79%. From that percentage it can be seen that the results have increased but not yet in accordance with the existing targets, so that the researchers and teachers do reflection in the first meeting and continue the second meeting of cycle 2.

Based on the results of the overhand service research techniques at the 2nd cycle 2nd percentage overall overhand service completeness over 83%. From that percentage it can be seen that the results have increased but not yet in accordance with the existing targets, so the researchers and teachers reflect on the second meeting and continue the third meeting of cycle 2.

Based on the overhand service engineering research at the 3rd cycle 2nd meeting the percentage of overall overhand service completeness over 87%. From the percentage it is seen that the results have increased so no need to continue the next cycle.

The results of the assessment of overhand service techniques on the game of volleyball in the class XI Animation C students of SMK Negeri 4 Malang can be seen from the overhand service technique indicators, the level of service success over obtained as follows: students do the right attitude of 76%, at the attitude of the foot of 75 %, hand attitude by 76%, perenaan ball by 73%, and coordination with success of 72%. In cycle 2, the result of the assessment of overhand service technique on the game of volleyball on the students of class XI Animation C of SMK Negeri 4 Malang in cycle 2 can be seen from the overhand service technique indicator, the service success rate above is obtained as follows: the students do the right attitude of 88 %, in the attitude of the foot by 86%, hand attitude by 87%, perenaan ball by 86%, and co-ordination of 85%.

DISCUSSION

From the above results can be concluded in performing overhand service techniques above there are several indicators that must be mastered, to be able to master the overhand service techniques necessary stages to be done include the treatment and intensity of meetings in learning to achieve mastery of the desired technique.

According Husdarta (2011) "physical education is the process of education that utilizes physical activity and health to produce a holistic change in the quality of individuals, both in terms of physical, mental, and emotional". Harsuki (2003) states that, "Physical education is a process of interaction between learners with the environment, through physical activity that is managed systematically to the full human". It is also revealed by Rosdiani (2012) that: "In the process of learning physical education teachers are expected to teach a variety of basic motion skills, techniques and strategies games, sports, internalization of values (sportsmanship, honest, cooperation, etc.) and healthy lifestyle habits. Implementation is not through conventional teaching in the classroom that is theoretical study, but involving physical, mental, intellectual, emotional and social elements ". From some opinions of experts can be concluded that Physical education is a process of education of a person, as individuals and members of society are done consciously and systematically through physical activity in order to obtain improved ability of physical appearance, growth of intelligence, and the formation of character.

According to Law No. 20 of 2003 on National Education System article 1 item 20 states that: "learning is a process of interaction of learners with educators with educators of learning resources in a learning environment". In addition, according to Smith in Setyosari (2001) explains that, "learning is-ah an activity that focused on the specific things learned by the learning". Meanwhile, according to Sudjana in Rusman (2013) states that "learning can be interpreted as any systematic and deliberate effort to create an activity of educational interaction between two parties, ie between learners (learners) and educators (learning resources) learning activities ". From the statement can be drawn the conclusion of learning is a process undertaken by teachers to learners to assist in the learning process with the aim to facilitate learners to improve the knowledge it possessed with facilities that support the learning process.

According to Sanchez Moreno, Miguel (2014) says "volleyball is a sport characterized by common movements such as jumping, blowing and short displacement. Attacks and blocking are very important in the bolavoli game to achieve victory in high level competition ". According to Viera (2000) "a volleyball game is played by two teams where each team consists of 6 people in a field measuring 9m for each team and the two teams are separated by a net." "For the net height of the son is 2.43m while for the net daughter is 2.24m (Ahmadi, 2007)". From that opinion it can be concluded that volleyball is a game performed by two opposing teams, each team consisting of 6 players who are separated by a net and each trying to touch the ball over the net to win the game. In this case both teams are allowed to touch the ball with all the limbs that have been determined but still by using the principle of a sportive game and not harm one of them. In this case for the net height of 2.43m son, while for the net of 2.24m.

Basically in a volleyball game there are several basic techniques that can be taught in learning. According to Del Coso, Juan (2014) says: "Volleyball is a complex team sport with certain athletic techniques, tactics, and movements. Volleyball players perform short displays, prefixes interspersed with speed and leaps in defensive or attacking positions. This game is played with a field divided by the net with a height of 2.43 m (for men), the height in the jump is the most important variable for the volleyball player ". Another case with Suhadi (2009) says "basic technique is a basic motion that must be possessed by a volleyball player both in the foot movement and also the rattle of his body. Individuals will not be the same in each of these basic movements, depending on the posture and the motion of the multilaterals of each person. "Whereas according to Ahmadi (2007) said" in the game of volleyball there are some basic techniques that must be mastered. Techniques in volleyball consist of service, passing down, passing over, block and smash ". From some statements can be concluded that there are some basic techniques that must be owned by each player, in this case the players do not have the same skills because it has different characteristics. The game of volleyball has been set so that the game is fun and interesting and not boring.

Service is a basic technique of bolavoli game that is considered trivial, but in this service has its own characteristics that are different from others. According to Parisi, Fabio (2013) says: "In volleyball there are individual skills, just like service, this is a small part of coaching technique, but service is a basic technique for volleyball skills, especially for young athletes. Service is a skill technique in which a rally is the beginning of a game of volleyball, and this can be done with top service, using a high float blow or a drive blow with a high jump. " According toSuhadi (2009) states that: "Service is also the beginning of a game of bolavoli. In the service there are several ways or models, namely: under serve, overhand serve, and jump serve. Meanwhile, according to the results of the resulting ball after the service then there is service: spin or spin, floating. From the rotation type of service ball result then there is service: topspin, backspin, sidespin ". From this understanding it can be concluded that service is part of a basic technique consisting of parts whose purpose is used to start a game of volleyball and also used for weapons in obtaining points or attacking.

According to Mahendra (2007) "part and whole method in the implementation using several steps that must be passed that is 1) Preview, 2) Experiment, 3) Review, 4) train part, 5) Synthesis, 6) Stabilization". Similarly, learning game overhand service on volleyball. This method can be spelled out and used in several steps that must be done are: 1) preview; meaning that this learning stage introduces the service material on volleyball that is studied and given a clear picture of the material being studied or practiced; 2) experiment; at this stage the student performs service accordingly in the previous stage as well as practicing; 3) review; is a repetition of student problems encountered during volleyball overhand service practice; 4) train section; for this stage the student is notified of the unknown parts 5) synthesis; this stage students perform part-by-piece overhand service volleyball repeatedly, after students understand about this technique then students try to do as a whole; 6) consolidation; in the last stage, the students re-do the previous parts of the technique to be studied and put together thoroughly.

There are so many methods or models in learning that are used in learning. According to Adisuyanto (2009) said that: "Method part is a form of learning the breaking of one part smaller. The breaking of the motion into the smallest part, has the purpose of eliminating or minimizing the possibility of making a mistake. A thorough method is a way of teaching the joining of fractions of the smallest part of a movement into a complete movement ". Based on these statements can be concluded that part and whole is a method of teaching begins by teaching from the easiest or smallest parts of the skills of motion and then the parts are combined into one whole movement. In the end, students can easily accept the learning method because it is broken down from the difficult section to become easy and simple.

Previous research conducted by Edy Suyanto, (2014) entitled "Improving the Effectiveness of Learning Passing Under Volleyball Using Part and Whole In Students of Grade XI IPA 1 SMAN 2 Batu Town" in study under passing students of SMAN 2 Batu Town, that the results of this study indicate that there is a significant increase in under passing learning by using part and whole on students of grade XI IPA 1 SMAN 2 Batu City. Kharisma Wahyu Atmaja, (2015: 6) entitled "Improving Quick Smash Bolavian Skills With Part and Whole Methods On Club Binayuda Club Women's Volley Ball Team Rowokangkung Lumajang District". In the results of this study there is an increase in the skills of quick smash bolavoli. Based on these results it can be concluded that there is an increase of part and whole to the ability of quick smash volleyball skills in SMK Negeri 1 Rasau Jaya players Team Princess Volleyball Club Binayuda Rowokangkung Lumajang District. While Vilan Argo Pinatas, (2014: 6) entitled "Improving the Effectiveness of Learning Merda By Using Part and whole In Class X Students RPL-1 SMK Negeri 5 Malang". Based on the results of the analysis. This research has effect of part and all method to learning meroda in SMK Negeri 5 Malang. From previous research findings by Edy Suyanto, Kharisma Wahyu Atmaja and Vilan Argo Pinatas, that with the use of part and whole method can improve learning and exercise in sports activities.

Cycle 1

Action Planning 1

After learning difficulties of students from the observation, researchers and teachers prepare RPP for three meetings in cycle 1. To solve the problem, researchers do variations of learning overhand service game above. (2) overhand service by using the ball, (3) overhand service on the wall, (4) overhand service using net with a distance of 4 meters, (5) overhand service using the net with a distance of 6 meters, and (6) overhand service using the net with a distance of 9 meters.

Action Implementation 1

In the implementation of the first meeting game with variations of game learning are: (1) overhand service without using the ball, and (2) overhand service by using the ball. The two students meeting the variations of game learning are: (1) the overhand service on the wall, and (2) the overhand service using the net with a distance of 4 meters. The third meeting of the students to learn the variations of the game are: (1) the overhand service using the net with a distance of 6 meters, and (2) the overhand service using the net with a distance of 9 meters.

Action Observation 1

From the observation in cycle 1, the overhand service success rate of 34 students was obtained as follows: 26 students (76%) did the correct posture, 26 students (75%) did leg attitude correctly, 26 students (76%) right hand, 25 students (73%) did the ball spell correctly, and 24 students (72%) coordinated correctly.

Cycle 2

Action Planning 2

The result of reflection on the 1st cycle conducted by the researchers and, it is done improving the learning overhand service techniques on the game volleyball done on cycle 2. Researchers and teachers prepare RPP with service engineering materials on the game volleyball for cycle 2 with 3 times meeting with variations of game learning overhand service. The researchers also prepared observation sheets for observers and field notes that aimed to record events during the lesson. The form of game variation given in cycle 2 is almost the same as in cycle 1 consisting of: (1) overhand service without using ball, and (2) overhand service on wall, (3) overhand service by using ball, (4) overhand service using net with a distance of 4 meters, (5) overhand service over using the net with a distance of 6 meters, and (6) overhand service over using the net with a distance of 9 meters.

Implementation of Action 2

Implementation of these 2 actions there are 3 meetings, in the implementation of each meeting consists of two games. Implementation of the first meeting game with a variety of games are: (1) overhand service without using the ball, and (2) overhand service on the wall. The two students meeting the variations of game learning are: (1) overhand service by using the ball, and (2) the overhand service using the net with a distance of 4 meters. The third meeting of the students to learn the variations of the game are: (1) the overhand service using the net with a distance of 6 meters, and (2) the overhand service using the net with a distance of 9 meters.

Action Observation 2

From the observation in cycle 2, the overhand service success rate of 34 students was obtained as follows: 30 students (88%) did the correct posture, 29 students (86%) did leg attitude correctly, 30 students (87%) did attitude right hand, 29 students (86%) did the ball spell correctly, and 29 students (85%) coordinated correctly.

Final Reflection

Based on the data obtained, there is an increase in overhand service techniques on the game of volleyball on the students of class XI Animasi C SMK Negeri 4 Malang, it can be seen from the percentage of overall completeness of the overhand service techniques.

Thus the aim of the researcher to improve the overhand service technique on the game of volleyball by doing variation of learning using part and whole method succeed and supported overall mastery of service technique above. The result of overhand service technique skill is obtained from observation sheet and observer which then processed by the researcher.

With the comparison of cycle 1 and cycle 2 obtained, it can be concluded that by the method of part and whole in students of class XI Animasi C SMK Negeri 4 Malang can improve the basic techniques of students in the overhand service of volleyball and has been said successful. Thus learning by applying the method of part and whole can be used for improvement of learning in order to improve the results of overhand service skills for Animation C grade students SMK Negeri 4 Malang.

CONCLUSION

The result of overhand service skill test on volleyball game after the application of part and whole method can improve the overhand service technique for grade XI Animation C students of SMK Negeri 4 Malang, completeness in overhand service technique of 87%.

Cycle 1 and 2, the conclusion by using variation of game learning are: (1) overhand service without using ball, (2) overhand service by using ball, (3) overhand service on wall, (4) top service using net with distance of 4 meter , (5) top service using the net with a distance of 6 meters, and (6) overhand service using the net with a distance of 9 meters. Some variations of this game's learning can improve the overhand service techniques on the game of volleyball in the students of class XI Animasi C SMK Negeri 4 Malang. The types of variations of this learning can improve the overhand service techniques of the game bolavoli on students of class XI Animasi C SMK Negeri 4 Malang.

REFERENCES

Adisuyanto. 2009. Cerdas dan Bugar dengan Senam Lantai. Jakarta: PT.Gramedia Widiasarana Indonesia.Ahmadi. 2007. Panduan Olahraga Bolavoli. Solo: Pustaka Utama

Ahmadi. 2007. Panduan Olahraga Voli. Surakarta: Era Pustaka Utama.

Arikunto. 2010. Prosedur Penelitian: Suatu Pendekatan Praktik. Jakarta: Rineka Cipta.

Baacke & Yatsutuka. Pedoman Melatih Bola Volley. 1979. Jakarta: Proyek Pembinaan Olahraga Bagi Seluruh Anggota Mayarakat.

Budiwanto & Mu'arifin. 2006. Evaluasi Dalam Pembelajaran Pendidikan Jasmani. Malang: Fakultas Ilmu Pendidikan Univesitas Negeri Malang.

Juan, dkk. 2014. International Journal of Sports Physiology and Performance. Enhancing Physical Performance in Male Volleyball Players With a Caffeine-Containing Energy Drink, (Online) (https://scholar.google.co.id/scholar?q=Enhancing+Physical+Performance+in+Male+Volleyball+Players+With+a+Caffeine-Containing+Energy+Drink&btnG=&hl=id&as_sdt=0%2C5), diakses 21 April 2016.

Harsuki. 2003. Perkembangan Olahraga Terkini. Jakarta. PT Raja Grafindo Persada.

Husdarta. 2011. Sejarah Dan Filsafat Olahraga. Bandung. Alfabeta.

Mahendra. 2007. Modul Teori Belajar Mengajar Motorik. FPOK UPI Bandung.

Mu'arifin. 2009. Dasar-Dasar Pendidikan Jasmani dan Olahraga. Malang: Universitas Negeri Malang (UM Press).

Parisi. 2013. INSHS International Christmas Sport Scientific Conference, 5-7 December 2013. International Network of Sport and Health. The serve in under 12-13 Italian volleyball team. (Online), (https://scholar.google.co.id/scholar?q=The+serve+in+under+12-13+Italian+volleyball+team&btnG=&hl=id&as_sdt=0%2C5), di akses 21 April 2016.

Rosdiani. 2012. Model Pembelajaran Langsung dalam Pendidikan Jasmani dan Kesehatan. Bandung: Alfabeta.

Rusman. 2013. Belajar dan Pembelajaran Berbasis Komputer. Bandung Alfabeta.

Sanchez, dkk. 2014. Federación Española de Asociaciones de Docentes de Educación Física (FEADEF). The effects of short-term resistance program on vertical jump ability in elite male volleyball players during the competition season. (Online), (https://scholar.google.co.id/scholar?hl=id&q=The+effects+of+short-term+resistance+program+on+vertical+jump+ability+in+elite+male+volleyball+players+during+the+competition+season&btnG=), di akses 21 April 2016.

Setyosari. 2001. Rancangan Pembelajaran Teori dan Praktek. Malang : Elang Mas.

Sugiyono. 2011. Metode Penelitian Kuantitatif Kualitatif dan R&D. Bandung: Alfabeta.

Suhadi & Sujarwo. 2009. VolleyBall For All. Yogyakarta: Fakultas Ilmu Keolahragaan Universitas Negeri Yogyakarta.

Viera. Bonnie Jill Ferguson,MS. 2000. Bolavoli Tingkat Pemula. Jakarta: PT Raja Grafindo Persada.

Fundamental Movement Skills and Moods as Predictors of Games Performance in Primary School Students

Ricky Wibowo[1✉], Eka Nugraha[2], Kuston Sultoni[3]

Universitas Pendidikan Indonesia, Indonesia[123]

Article History

Keywords:
Fundamental Movement Skill; Mood; Games Performance; Invasion Games.

Abstract

The purpose of this study was to determine how far FMS and mood contribute toward games performance on elementray school student through invasion games activities (modified soccer and handball games). This research uses a correlational explanatory and regression . Third grade elementary school students (n=40) were enrolled in this study consisting of 21 male students and 19 female students. To determine the games perfromance using The Games Performance Assessment Instrument (GPAI) and Brief Mood Introspection Scale (BMIS) to measure the mood of the students. The increase in FMS of 0.005 units will predict the increase in the variable SB by 0.005, then the increase in the positive mood of 0.43 will predict the increase in the variable of 0.43 units, while the increase in negative mood variable of 0.030 will predict a decline in the SB variable of 0.030. The result showed that FMS and positive moods contributed toward games performance on both games.

✉ Correspondence address :
Jl. Setiabudhi No.229, Isola, Sukasari, Isola, Sukasari, Kota Bandung, Jawa Barat 40154
E-mail: ricky_wibowo@upi.edu

INTRODUCTION

Fundamental movement skills are seen as 'the basic foundation' for lifelong physical activity. Previous studies have indicated a positive relationship between fundamental movement skills and the regular participation of children in physical activity (Vandorpe et al., 2012). The study proves that the attractiveness of displaying fundamental movement skills at the primary school level tends to contribute in improving the habit of physical activity and participating in regular physical activity, thereby being able to prevent obesity of children and adolescents (Mitchell et al., 2013). This counteracts the misconception that the fundamental movement skills of children are acquired naturally as growth into adulthood (Mitchell et al., 2013).

Therefore, children should be given the opportunity to have the widest possible physical activity in order to develop fundamental movement skills. In other words, the learning of motion skills should be given and practiced since elementary school. One strategy for developing fundamental movement skills is through play, which can facilitate the ability of a child's motor skills as this is one of the gates of the child's world. Children play with the ultimate goal of learning to recognize their body and learn to move.

Among the important factors that play a role in improving the opportunity to learn motion skills and the concept of motion is through physical activities and games. The play approach evolved from the dissatisfaction of the approach-the technique approach applied to children (Kenneth and Ronglan, 2012). Charisticistic elementary school students who love to play require elementary school teachers to carry out educational activities that charge more games for lower classes. Elementary school teachers should design learning that allows for the element of the game in it. The game in fundamental movement teaching emphasizes the aspect of how to teach students to understand the concept of fundamental movement in the context of play. Implementation of the game activity is very appropriately applied to elementary school students lower class because it is in accordance with the characteristics of students who are still in play.

Recently a lot of research has developed games to improve bafundamental movement skills, one of them is with games console (Barnett 2015a; Papastergiou 2015; Akbari et al. 2009; Johnson et al. 2016; Barnett 2015b) as well as simple motor skills games or programs - the game's physical activity game (Brian et al., 2016) (Bryant & Duncan 2016). Game-focused learning emerges to promote climate-oriented mastery of motivation to create child motivation in physical education learning (Gray et al. 2009) and also enables increased learning outcomes in school (Ericsson & Karlsson 2012).

In the game of teacher invasion provide simple games in order to adjust to the child's developmental level. But the limited research that describes what factors affect the performance of children in play, especially in the game of invasion become one of the motivations to try to dig deeper.

In the context of learning, especially physical education, the state of mood students certainly has a role in the learning process. Whereas in physical education requires physical activity and physical performance in the context of education. In implementing game activity in elementary school age children, physical education teachers need to know the various factors that influence the child to be passionate about the activities of the movement and increase the passion of the child through the activity of motion.

Previous studies have suggested that a person's mood influences play or play performance (Jani, & Amer, 2017; Russell & Newton, 2008) and sample cognitive performance (Shukitt-Hale et al., 1991; Crowley et al., 1992). When viewed from the positive mood Hansen et al. (2001) showed that moderate intensity exercise duration of 10 minutes can increase the production of positive psychological benefit. From some previous research literature, it has been able to explain how mood increases due to physical exercise (Weinberg & Gould, 2007) and how moods affect the performance of an athlete in a race. But the authors have not found a study that explores the influence of moods on learning settings of school movements, especially in primary schools.

There are several instruments to know the state of one's mood. One of them uses the Brief Mood Introspection Scale (BMIS).

As previously explained that fundamental movement skills can be developed through games. However, whether the performance of fundamental movement skills contribute to student performance in play can not be ascertained empirically. So does the student's mood when playing, does it also contribute to the performance of the child in play? It seems to need to be explored more deeply as a basis for developing children's movement skills especially in the game of invasion. The purpose of this study is to determine the contribution of fundamental movement skills and moods to play skills.

METHODS

The research method used in this research is correlational experimental method. This study used correlational design and prediction with regression analysis. This research will involve lecturers, students and elementary school students in Bandung. Subjects of students who will be involved are third grade students of elementary school (21 girls, 19 men). The sample characteristics (mean ± standard deviation) are: age = 9.1 ± 0.54 years; height = 1.25 ± 0.3; and weight = 27.4 ± 0.3). All samples are healthy without physical disability.

Analysis and data processing used in this research are: Statistical Product and Service Solution (SPSS) 22. Data analysis which researcher do in this research is, to analyze FMS contribution data and mood to play skill using correlational analysis and linear regression.

Research Procedure

The first test conducted was The Test of Gross Motor Development (TGMD-2) to measure fundamental movement skills (FMS) that can be used to measure FMS of children aged 3- 10 years (Mazzardo et al. 2008; Bardid, Huyben, et al. 2016). The fundamental motion skills test (FMS) consists of two test domains, namely the locomotor test domain and the object test control domain. Each test domain consists of six tests, the total test totaling 12 test items. Adapted from Ulrich and Wouter, (De Meester et al., 2016; Barnett, Ridgers, Zask, et al., 2015) each student was given two occasions for each test. The test results are then incorporated in accordance with the scoring criteria guidelines / converted to a percentile score according to the age and sex of the student.

A week later, students fill out the BMIS moods questionnaire and perform simple invasion activities. Filling out the moods questionnaire was done before the invasion game. Researchers help students fill out the questionnaire of each item. Then proceed to game session. The game consists of the dominant arms invasion game that is in the form of modification of handball and the dominant leg game in the form of football modification game. Both games are modified in terms of rules, wide field and goal adjusted to the student's ability. Both games are done in the same time randomly. The game is adapted from (del Campo et al. 2011; Gutiérrez et al. 2014) in the form of small-side games 4 vs 4 without the goalkeeper. Before the game students do standard heating for 10 minutes consisting of jugling, passing and passing-intercepting. Game is divided into two rounds and each round for 8 minutes. During the game, all events are recorded using Sony HDR CX405- 9.2 MP video camera. Video recordings are used to assess students' playing skills during the game. Play skills are evaluated using GPAI.

RESULTS AND DISCUSSION

From the test result on the research subjects (n = 40), first use the correlation test between skill of playing game invasion game modification (BT) and soccer (SB) to fundamental movement skill (FMS) and student Mood is shown in **table 1**. Correlation among variables variables were tested using Pearson's correlation coefficients (for parametric data), and Spearman's correlation coefficients (for non-parametric data). SPSS software (version 22.0, IBM) is used to compute all variables. While the normality test using Kolmogorov-Smirnov on each correlational test .

Table 1. Mean (± SD) Research Variable

Variable	Mean ± SD
BT	0.64 ± 0.014
SB	0.633 ± 0.005
FMS	14.22 ± 13.2
Pos Mood	2.9 ± 0.66
Neg Mood	2.7 ± 0.76

Table 2. Correlation between BT playing skills, SB against FMS, Moods Positive and negative

	FMS	Pos Mood	Neg Mood
BT Correlatio Coefficient	.337*	.336*	.170
Sig. (2-tailed)	.033	.034	.294
N	40	40	40
SB Correlation Coefficient	316*	.484**	.195
Sig. (2-tailed)	.047	.002	.228
N	40	40	40

**. Correlation is significant at the 0.01 level (2-tailed).
*. Correlation is significant at the 0.05 level (2-tailed).

Table 2 shows the results of Spearman's Rho correlations, the correlation between modified handball (BT) skills, fundamental movement skills (FMS) and Mood (positive and negative). Correlations between BT and FMS showed significant coral ($P < .05$; $r = .337$). BT correlation with positive mood also showed significant correlation ($P < .05$; $r = .336$), in contrast to negative mood showed very low correlation ($P < .05$; $r = .170$). In the modified soccer ball (SB) skill, the correlations between SB and FMS show significant coral ($P < .05$; $r = .316$). BT correlation with positive mood also showed significant correlation ($P < .01$; $r = .484$), in contrast to negative mood showed very low correlation ($P < .05$; $r = .195$).

Table 3. Linear Regression Test
Playing skill modification handball invasion

Coefficients[a]					
Model	Unstandardized Coefficients		Standardized Coefficients	t	Sig.
	B	Std. Error	Beta		
(Constant)	.371	.079		4.673	.000
FMS	.007	.006	.220	1.268	.213
Pos_Moods	.105	.040	.588	2.622	.013
Neg_Moods	-.051	.031	-.328	-1.642	.109
a. Dependent Variable: BT					
Regression Formula Y= a + b (X1) + b (X2) + c (X3)					

Based on the above linear regression test obtained equation of regression model as follows :

$$BT = 0{,}371 + 0{,}007\ (FMS) + 0{,}205\ (Pos\_Moods) - 0{,}051\ (Neg\_Moods)$$

Seen from the above regression equation it can be interpreted that the increase in fms of 0.007 units will predict the increase in the bt variable of 0.007, then the increase in the positive mood of 0.205 will predict the increase in the variable of 0.205 units, while the increase in negative mood variable of 0.051 will predict decline of bt variable of 0.051.

Based on the above regression equation it can be concluded that any increase of bt variable will be predicted by the increase of fms variable and positive mood, and every increase in bt variable will be predicted by decrease in negative mood variable.

Table 4. Linear regression test skills play invasion football modification
Skill play invasion modification handball

Coefficients[a]					
Model	Unstandardized Coefficients		Standardized Coefficients	t	Sig.
	B	Std. Error	Beta		
(Constant)	.524	.057		9.240	.000
FMS	.005	.004	.217	1.129	.266
Pos_Moods	.043	.029	.375	1.509	.140
Neg_Moods	-.030	.022	-.299	-1.350	.185
a. Dependent Variable: S_GP_1					
Regression Formula Y= a + b (X1) + b (X2) + c (X3)					

Based on the above linear regression test obtained equation of regression model as follows:

$$SB = 0{,}524 + 0{,}005\ (FMS) + 0{,}43\ (Pos\_Moods) - 0{,}030\ (Neg\_Moods)$$

Seen from the above regression equation it can be interpreted that the increase in FMS of 0.005 units will predict the increase in the variable SB by 0.005, then the increase in the positive mood of 0.43 will predict the increase in the variable of 0.43 units, while the increase in negative mood variable of 0.030 will predict a decline in the SB variable of 0.030.

Based on the above regression equation it can be concluded that any increase of SB variable will be predicted by the increase of FMS variable and positive mood, and every increase in SB variable will be predicted by decrease in negative mood variable.

Based on the results of the above research, mastery of fundamental movement skills is important for elementary school students. Students with improved motor skills will have higher physical activity (Okely, 2009). But fundamental movementskills need to be provided with attractive packaging so that students interested in physical activity. The invasion game which is one of manipulative skills can develop a child's understanding through motion in physical education (Mazzardo et al., 2008). Based on the results of this study proves that the fundamental movement skills correlated significantly with the performance of students in performing the game invasion activity. Both game invasion modification handball and football.

Similarly, the mood variable, positive mood juaga strongly correlated to the appearance of children in the game of invasion. Not unlike previous research that moods states positively correlated to play performance (Beedie et al., 2000; Lane & Chappell, 2001). But this study is a game setting in the context of learning motion instead of sports competition. The results of the study of 9-year-old elementary school students showed that mood state influences the playing skills.

Posotive moods have a positive correlation to child play skills in simple invasion games in line with previous research (Terry et al. 2000; Lane and Terry, 2005; Jani, & Amer, 2017). Therefore it is important to create a fun atmosphere in teaching the game of invasion. Previous research has shown some strategies to improve the mood of children in order to improve performance such as individual communication strategies (Stevens & Lane, 2001). Instead of engaging in the game, enthusiastic play and get the fun of playing (Aggerholm & Ronglan, 2012).

Based on the analysis of the regression equation it can be concluded that any increase in BT variables will be predicted by the increase of FMS and positive mood variables, and any increase in the BT variable will be predicted by a decrease in negative mood variables. Similarly, the SB variable will be predicted by an increase in the FMS variable and positive mood, and any increase in the SB variable will be predicted by a decrease in the negative mood variable.

CONCLUSION

Fundamental movement skills (FMS) and moods make a significant contribution to the invasion-playing skill of game modification and football. That is, any increase in the FMS and moods variables is predicted to be followed by an increase in the variable playing skills.

REFERENCES

Aggerholm, Kenneth, and Lars Tore Ronglan. 2012. "Having The Last Laugh: The Value of Humour in Invasion Games." Sport, Ethics and Philosophy 6(3): 336–52. http://www.tandfonline.com/doi/abs/10.1080/17511321.2012.689321.

Akbari, Hakimeh, Abehroz Bdoli, Mohsen Shafizadeh, and Hasan Khalaji. 2009. "The Effect of Traditional Games in Fundamental Motor Skill Development in 7 9 Year Old Boys." Iran J Pediatr 19(2): 123–29.

Bardid, Farid, Floris Huyben, et al. 2016. "Assessing Fundamental Motor Skills in Belgian Children Aged 3 – 8 Years Highlights Differences to US Reference Sample." : 281–90.

Bardid, Farid, An De Meester, et al. 2016. "Human Movement Science Configurations of Actual and Perceived Motor Competence among Children : Associations with Motivation for Sports and Global Self-Worth." Human Movement Science 50: 1–9. http://dx.doi.org/10.1016/j.humov.2016.09.001.

Barnett, Lisa M. 2015a. "Active Gaming as a Mechanism to Promote Physical Activity and Fundamental Movement Skill in Children Available from Deakin Research Online :" (February 2017)

Barnett, Lisa M., Nicola D. Ridgers, and Jo Salmon. 2015. "Associations between Young Children's Perceived and Actual Ball Skill Competence and Physical Activity." Journal of Science and Medicine in Sport 18(2): 167–71. http://dx.doi.org/10.1016/j.jsams.2014.03.001.

Barnett, Lisa M., Nicola D. Ridgers, Avigdor Zask, and Jo Salmon. 2015. "Face Validity and Reliability of a Pictorial Instrument for Assessing Fundamental Movement Skill Perceived Competence in Young Children." Journal of Science and Medicine in Sport 18(1): 98–102. http://dx.doi.org/10.1016/j.jsams.2013.12.004.

Beedie, C. J., Terry, P. C., & Lane, A. M. (2000). The Profile of Mood States and Athletic

Performance: Two meta-analyses. Journal of Applied Sport Psychology, 12, 49-68. Brawley,

Brian, Ali, Jacqueline D. Goodway, Jessica A. Logan, and Sue Sutherland. 2016. "SKIPing with Teachers: An Early Years Motor Skill Intervention." Physical Education and Sport Pedagogy (April): 1–13. http://www.tandfonline.com/doi/full/10.1080/17408989.2016.1176133.

del Campo, David Gutierrez Diaz, Sixto Gonzalez Villora, Luis M. Garcia Lopez, and Stephen Mitchell. 2011. "Differences in Decision-Making Development between Expert and Novice Invasion Game Players." Perceptual and Motor Skills 112(3): 871–88. http://journals.sagepub.com/doi/10.2466/05.10.11.25. PMS.112.3.871-888.

Crowley, J.S., Wesensten, N., Kamimori, G. and Devine, J. (1992) Effect of high terrestrial altitude and supplemental oxygen on human performance and mood. Aviation Space and Environmental Medicine 63, 696-701

Ericsson, I, and M K Karlsson. 2012. "Motor Skills and School Performance in Children with Daily Physical Education in School – a 9-Year Intervention Study." : 1–6.

García López LM, González S, Gutiérrez D, Serra J. Development and validation of the Game Performance Evaluation Tool (GPET) in soccer. SportTK. Revista Euroamericana de Ciencias del Deporte, 2013; 2: 111 129

Gray, Shirley, Shirley Gray, and John Sproule. 2017. "Developing Pupils â€TM Performance in Team Invasion Games." (January 2011).

Gray, Shirley, and John Sproule. 2011. "Developing Pupils' Performance in Team Invasion Games." Physical Education & Sport Pedagogy 16(1): 15–32.

Gray, Shirley, John Sproule, and Kevin Morgan. 2009. "Teaching Team Invasion Games and Motivational Climate." European Physical Education Review 15(1): 65–89. http://search.proquest.com/docview/810358281?accountid=9851%5Cnhttp://tf5lu9ym5n.search.serialssolutions.com/?ctx_ver=Z39.88-2004&ctx_enc=info:ofi/enc:UTF-8&rfr_id=info:sid/ProQ:ericshell&rft_val_fmt=info:ofi/fmt:kev:mtx:journal&rft.genre=article&rft.jtit.

Gutiérrez, D, J Fisette, L M García-López, and O Contreras. 2014. "Assessment of Secondary School Students' Game Performance Related to Tactical Contexts." Journal of Human Kinetics 42(1): 223–34.http://www.scopus.com/inward/record.url?eid=2-s2.0-84908136555&partnerID=40&md5=13a3043641ba03d620591a6762f455b3.

Hansen, C.J., Stevens, L.C., & Coast, J.R. (2001). Exercise duration and mood state: How much is enough to feel better? Health Psychology, 20, 267-275.

., Jani, H., & Amer, A. (2017). Mood Differences between the Winning and Losing Team during the Final Match of Razak Cup Hockey Competition 2016 Mood Differences between the Winning and Losing Team during the Final Match of Razak Cup Hockey Competition 2016, 7(January), 15–17. http://doi.org/10.5923/j.sports.20170701.04

Johnson, Tara M. et al. 2016. "Does Playing a Sports Active Video Game Improve Young Children's Ball Skill Competence?" Journal of Science and Medicine in Sport 19(5): 432–36. http://dx.doi.org/10.1016/j.jsams.2015.05.002.

Lane, A. M., & Terry, P. C. (2005). Test of a conceptual model of mood-performance relationships with a focus on depression: A review and synthesis five years on. In T. Morris, P. Terry et al. (Eds.), Promoting Health and Performance for Life: Proceedings of the ISSP 11th World Congress of Sport Psychology. Sydney: International Society of Sport Psychology.

Mazzardo, Oldemar et al. 2008. "The Relationship of Fundamental Movement Skills and Level of Physical Activity in Second Grade Children." Australian Association for Research in Education (AARE) International Conference 26(1): 71–79. http://etd.library.pitt.edu/ETD/available/etd-04302008-144205/.

Meester, An De et al. 2016. "Associations among Elementary School Children ' S Actual Motor Competence , Perceived Motor Competence , Physical Activity and BMI : A Cross-Sectional Study." : 1–14.

Mitchell SA, Oslin JL, Griffin LL. Sport Fundations for Elementary Physical Education. A Tactical Games Approach. Champaign, IL: Human Kinetics; 2003

Mitchell, S.A., Oslin, J.L., & Griffin, L.L. (2006). Teaching sport concepts and skills: A tactical games approach (2nd ed.). Champaign, IL: Human Kinetics.

Okely, D. 2012. "Prevalence and Correlates of Low Fundamental Movement Skill Competency in." (July).

Papastergiou, Marina. 2015. "The Impact of an Exergame-Based Intervention on Children â€TM S Fundamental Motor Skills Fundamental Motor Skills." Computers & Education 83(January): 90–102. http://dx.doi.org/10.1016/j.compedu.2015.01.001.

Russell, W. D., & Newton, M. (2008). Short-term psychological effects of interactive video game technology exercise on mood and attention. Educational Technology and Society, 11(2), 294–308. http://doi.org/citeulike-article-id:7693606

Shukitt-Hale, B., Banderet, L.E. and Lieberman, H.R. (1991) Relationships between symptoms, moods, performance, and acute mountain sickness at 4700 metres. Aviation Space and Environmental Medicine 62, 865-869.

Stevens, M. J., & Lane, A. M. (2001). Mood-regulating strategies used by athletes. Athletic Insight, 3. www.athleticinsight.com/vol3lss/copingissue.htm.

Ulrich DA (2000) Test of Gross Motor Development—Second Edition. Austin, TX: Prod-Ed Publishers

Weinberg, R.S., & Gould, D. (2007). Foundations of Sport and Exercise Psychology (4th Ed.), Champaign, IL: Human Kinetics.

Wouter, C., Kristine, D.M., Christiane, S., and Caroline, A. (2008). Movement Skill assessment of typically developing preschool children: A review of seven movement Skill assessment tools. Journal of sports science and Medicine 8, 154-168.

Vandorpe, Barbara et al. 2012. "Relationship between Sports Participation and the Level of Motor Coordination in Childhood: A Longitudinal Approach." Journal of Science and Medicine in Sport 15(3): 220–25. http://dx.doi.org/10.1016/j.jsams.2011.09.006.

21

The Good Governance Level's Profile of Sport Organization in Central Java

Tri Rustiadi[1], **Billy Castyana**[2], **Dwi Gansar Santi Wijayanti**[3]

Jurusan Pendidikan Jasmani Kesehatan dan Rekreasi, Fakultas Ilmu Keolahragaan, Universitas Negeri Semarang, Indonesia[123]

Article History

Keywords:
Good Governance; Sport Organization; Central Java.

Abstract

The aim of this research is to get the level of good governance of Sports Organization in Central Java. This quantitative descriptive research conducted at sports organization in 29 cities throughout Central Java. The questionnaire used was the Action for Good Governance in the International Sports Organization (AGGIS) Sports Governance Observer developed by the Danish Institute of Sports Studies, Denmark and data analysis used the Sports Governance Observer (SGO) Index to generate the average percentage score of four dimensions. From the analysis result, Kota Salatiga and Kota Pekalongan have the highest level of good governance with 60%. However, Kabupaten Tegal becomes the lowest level of good governance, 21.88%, and overall, the average level of good governance of sports organizations in Central Java is only 38.62%. The low average score has affected by the transparency rate, only 37%, because the organization does not have a website or social media so the community to monitor the use of budget and activities. Later this initial data could be a basis for determining the policy in improving the good governance and similar research can be done every one period.

Correspondence address :
Jalan Kutilang Barat No.1 Cilacap 53215
E-mail: billycastyana@mail.unnes.ac.id

INTRODUCTION

Indonesia is home to many talented athletes. So many athletes in Indonesia are triumphing at the international level, such as Susi Susanti, Alan Budikusuma, and many more. However, this country is also a place for sports problems that, might be, never end.

The problems that arise are very closely related to the Sports Organization in Indonesia and how the Sports Organization is running. It happened because the Sports Organization, now, has become an organization that has its own governance system. The organizational governance system is a system that directs, controls, and regulates organizational elements. This system not only provides a framework for the direction of the Sports Organization but also helps increase the level of public confidence in the institution (Hoye & Cuskelly, 2007). However, not all Sports Organizations have good governance systems, whereas governance or governance systems are an important component of managing sports organizations because they relate to the policy issues and performance directions of a sports organization (Ferkins, Shilbury, & McDonald, 2005, Hoye, 2006; Hoye & Auld, 2001).

Since the beginning of the 21st century, corruption, doping, and scoring in sports competitions, as well as mismanagement and lack of efficiency in the Sports Organization. This has resulted in the emergence of the term Good Governance. In the corporate world, Good Governance, commonly referred to as corporate governance or good corporate governance, is related to the various ways companies, whether private or public, are run in an accountable manner to stakeholders (OECD, 2004; Jordan, 2008). With Good Governance, the activities of sports institutions can be monitored so that the institution can provide benefits to the institution itself, members, and society (Hoye, 2006). Due to the failure to have a good governance system to control and monitor the Sports Organization may result in loss of interest from sponsors to work together, the decline in membership and participation, and intervention from external agencies.

The importance of good governance systems in the Sports Organization cannot be underestimated. If analogous to the business world, good economic management can ensure that the Sports Organization can achieve their long-term goals, so that the Sports Organization can continue to operate in the long term (Bonollo De Zwart & Gilligan, 2009). That way, sports organizations have proven that he is able to steer the sport forward.

In addition to improving public health through physical activity, sports have the potential to communicate sports values, contribute to social-economic integration and integration, and to provide entertainment for society (European Commission, 2007). However, many studies have shown that socio-cultural values derived from sports, today, have been corrupted by corruption. It is also related to the commercialization of sports significantly, especially over the last two decades, which has resulted in problems facing the Sports Organization as well (Katwala, 2000).

The statement reflects that the lack of a good governance system in the Sports Organization has the potential to have a significant negative impact on society. Finally, since the Sports Organization has a burden on society, it is very important for them to take care of sport responsibly and transparently (Katwala, 2000; Henry & Lee, 2004).

METHODS

This research is quantitative descriptive research with questionnaire method. The population in this study were all sports organizations in Central Java in accordance with Act No.3 of 2005 on National Sports System article 1. The sampling method used was total sampling involving all sports organizations in Central Java.

Questionnaires will be based on the AGO Governance Observer developed by Danish Institute of Sports Studies, Copenhagen - Denmark. This instrument is divided into four dimensions: Transparency, Democratic Process, Check and Balance, and Solidarity.

Each dimension consists of 10-14 indicators, with a total of 48 indicators, and each indicator is classified as a core or additional indicator. If the indicator is categorized as a core indicator and the answer from the questionnaire is "yes", then the indicator is assigned a value of 4.

After all the data is obtained, the researcher will analyze data using Sports Governance Observer (SGO) Index. This analysis technique will be used for each sports organization, so can know the level of good governance of each organization.

RESULTS AND DISCUSSION

Participants of this study are all sports organizations in Central Java in accordance with Law No.3 of 2005 on National Sports System article 1, which is a group of people who work together to form an organization for the organization of sports in accordance with the provisions of legislation, invitation. In this study, researchers conducted data collection at the District Board of National Sports Committee of Indonesia (KONI) throughout Central Java, which is as many as 35 districts and there were only 29 districts were willing to be surveyed.

After conducting the research process in the Sports Organization of Central Java, researchers used descriptive analysis to get an overview of each assessment points in each region. From each rating point the average score is taken which can finally show the region with the lowest average score in each rating point. The data shows that there are eleven regions with the average value of "Transparency" M=x<1, namely Semarang, Kendal, Demak, Tegal, Tegal, Klaten, Prworejo, Kudus, Rembang, Sukoharjo, and Kebumen.

In addition to transparency, there are three other important points that form the basis of the assessment in this study. For the average value of the "Democracy Process" point, there are three regions that have M = x <2.5, namely Tegal, Kudus and Surakarta, while the average value of "Checks and Balances" points, six regions have the lowest value M = x <2.5, namely Semarang City, Tegal District, Pemalang, Grobogan, Klaten, and Purworejo. The last assessment point of this research is "Community" and there are eight districts that have M = x <2.5, namely Tegal, Pekalongan, Kudus, Grobogan, Blora, Surakarta, Magelang, and Temanggung.

From the analysis, the researcher found that Kota Salatiga and Kota Pekalongan have the highest level of good governance with 60%. However, Kabupaten Tegal becomes the region with the lowest level of good governance, which is 21.88%. Based on these results, researchers can convey that, overall, the average level of good governance of sports organizations in Central Java is only 38.62%.

According to the results of data analysis conducted earlier, the research can show that the average level of good governance in Central Java is still low because the level of transparency is only 37%. In some areas, the transparency is very low and not even transparent at all, this can occur as a result of the lack of attention of the board of sports organizations to be open to the public about the activities of the organization, list of boards, and the budget. Transparency, in essence, provides information that enables external stakeholders, whether sports enthusiasts, media, sponsors, government, athletes, and the public, to monitor internal work and organizational performance. The key to transparency is accurate information.

Lack of transparency can also occur because the organization does not have a website or social media that can be used by the community to access and monitor the extent of budget use, list of managers, and what activities are undertaken.

For your information that in organizations, the system used is an open system where the organization gets a very big influence from the external environment, one of which is the community. Since sports organizations in Indonesia still rely on revenues from National Budget / Regional Budget derived from public taxes, so transparency not only reports activities and budgetary usage to fellow management but must also be reported to the public.

In addition to transparency, the democratic process of an organization is also highlighted in measuring the level of good governance. The process of democracy is done in various decision-making situations, either to choose the chairman or in the making of the work program, so that all activities can be run jointly by all administrators. In this study, research results show that sports organizations in Central Java already have a good level of the democratic process with 82%, this is seen from the total percentage of the average value obtained by the entire organization.

On the third point of a good governance level assessment are checks and balances. This point focuses more on the accountability of sports organizations because from an organizational point of view, accountability is an obligation to explain what they do and why they take action, but also about accountability reports. Successful organizations understand accountability and they understand that they need to manage their relationships with their key stakeholder groups and that is a herb in their success. If we look at the results obtained in this study, the accountability of sports organizations in Central Java is 84%.

As has been previously stated that the system used in sports organizations is an open system because society has a very strong influence to run the organization. Therefore, a good sports organization should have a responsibility to help develop sports in the community or at the very bottom. In addition, sports organizations should also take into account operational standards in running the organization, where proposals should be submitted funds and how the process should be clear so that the board of sports can also understand well. In addition, a good organization should also pay attention to the board and its members in improving the ability and capability to support organizational performance. The organization also has responsibility for gender representation in the stewardship and must apply anti-discrimination in running the organization. In this study, we can see firsthand the involvement and role of sports organizations for the community. If we look at the data obtained, sports organizations in Central Java already have a good level of the community by reaching 77% from the total percentage of the average value received.

CONCLUSION

This research is expected to be an initial data about the extent of good governance level owned by sports organizations in Central Java. Later this preliminary data could be a basis for determining policies in improving the level of good governance and similar research can be done every one period of stewardship to measure whether there is an increase in the level of good governance of the sports organization or not. Keep in mind that this study only provides value and percentage only, but it does not cover the deeper issues that each sports organization has. Further research is necessary to find out and find the problems that make the level of good governance in sports organizations get a bad score.

REFERENCES

Bonollo De Zwart, F. and Gilligan, G. (2009) Sustainable governance in sporting organisations. In: P. Rodriguez, S. Késenne and H. Dietl, eds. Social responsibilityand sustainability in sports, Oviedo, Universitat de Oviedo, 165-227.

European Commission. (2007) White Paper on Sport, COM (2007) 391 final.

Ferkins, L., Shilbury, D. and McDonald, G. (2009) Board involvement in strategy: Advancing the governance of sport organizations, Journal of Sport Management, 23, 245–277.

Henry, I. and Lee, P.C.,(2004) Governance and ethics in sport. In: S. Chadwick and J. Beech, eds. The business of sport management, Harlow, Pearson Education, 25-42.

Hoye, R., & Auld, C. (2001) Measuring board performance in non-profit sport organisations, Australian Journal of Volunteering, 6(2), 109–116.

Hoye, R. (2006) Leadership within voluntary sport organization boards, Nonprofit Management and Leadership, 16(3), 297–313.

Hoye, R. and Cuskelly, G. (2007) Sport Governance, Sydney, NSW, Elsevier.

Katwala, S. (2000) Democratising global sport, London, The foreign policy centre.

Jordan, A. (2008) The governance of sustainable development: taking stock and looking forwards, Environment and planning C: Government and policy, 26, 17-33.

OECD. (2004) Principles of corporate governance 2004, Paris, OECD publications.

22

The Physical Education Learning in Municipal Yongkang Junior High School Taiwan

Sri Febriyani[1], **Cheng Yun-Wen**[2]

Jurusan Pendidikan Jasmani Kesehatan dan Rekreasi, Fakultas Ilmu Keolahragaan, Universitas Negeri Semarang, Indonesia[1]
Department of Physical Education Master, National Kaohsiung Normal University, Taiwan[2]

Article History

Keywords:
Learning; Curriculum; Taiwan; Junior High School; Physical Education.

Abstract

The objective of this research is to know the descriptive result of curriculum, process learning, infrastructure and facilities, educators, and learners in Tainan Municipal Yongkang Junior High School Taiwan. The method research is used descriptive qualitative. The data collection techniques were observation, interview, data searches and documentation. The data analysis used data reduction, data serve, and result conclusion. The results showed the used curriculum is the curriculum-based school. The learning process is carried out with the stage of planning and execution. The availability of sufficient infrastructure and facilities both in quantity as well as quality. Educators have met the qualification standards, competency standards, and test the feasibility of a teacher. Learners are required to pay for the operational cost and other unit adapted to the economic level of the family.

Correspondence address :
E-mail: srifebriyani0@gmail.com

INTRODUCTION

The curriculum is one of the guidelines is important in planning the process of formal education. Efforts are being made to achieve the goal of education is to serve as catalysts for the curriculum guidelines and reference in planning, and implementing a learning. (Prastowo, 2017). According to Ralp Tyler (1949), defines the curriculum is all lessons pupils who planned and carried out by the school to achieve educational goals (Jihad, 2008:1). Indonesia itself always doing curriculum development, and currently Indonesia enacted curriculum 2013 nationally, but in some areas they still use a curriculum unit level education (KTSP). In addition to the curriculum that serve as reference in national education, there is also a learning component which cannot be separated from the education system i.e., a component of the learning process and infrastructure, educators and learners. Based on ministerial regulation Number 32 year 2013 explained that learning process in Indonesia namely teachers are required to make the learning design of the implementation will be done with the basic competencies and based on core competencies that available in the curriculum, education in Indonesia and the allocation of hours of face-to-face learning middle school 40 minutes x 3 meetings and pembelajarn approach in Indonesia using a scientific approach where learners as Center in learning. Educators in Indonesia, especially for teachers of physical education should be a graduate of an educational institution. Facilities and infrastructure in Indonesia have been regulated in the regulation of the Minister of education and culture Number 24 year 2007 concerning minimum standards sarpras owned by the school. This depends on your opinion of Edward f. Melcer, (2017) that good physical education Planning will correlate success in his education. Different theories advanced by (Sun, Li, Shen, & 2017) that profiles students will mempresepsikan the nature of the learning environment that supports the-autonomous or control, need for satisfaction, and motivation as determined by themselves. This is called the theory of self-determination.

Difference theory challenging the observer and Regent education policies for to continue to develop the system in accordance with the national environment. The curriculum development of research and evaluation through cross-regional comparison of curriculum in the country even. Comparative study of the curriculum and its implementation of one, two or more countries is one of the businesses complement deficiencies in the Organization of national education. (Hans, 2012).

The author through his research seeks mempelajarisistem education in Taiwan, education reform over the past decade in Taiwan has provided new challenges to teachers at the school, since teachers are not only required to provide pengetahunan and skills to the students but also the teacher is required to develop their capacity in developing existing curriculum in all schools. Responsibility for planning specific curriculum has been given to the school and identified as "school-based curriculum development" (Tomas & Luyi Lien, 2005:177).

Physical education is one of the subjects of the national curriculum in taiwan for primary and secondary school education first in Taiwan. The curriculum known as the "1-9 Grade Curriculum" (Tomas & Luyi Lien, 2005), which consists of the following subjects: Civics and Ethics, Health Education, Mandarin Chinese), English, Mathematics, Social Sciences, History, Geography, Natural Science, Physical Education, Home Economics, Music and Computers (Li, 2005; nuffic, 2015; Who, 2002).

Based on the preliminary studies researchers conducted on 20 September-31 October 2016 related learning physical education in Tainan Yongkang Municipal Junior High School in Taiwan, found some phenomena in the implementation of education physical learners are required to have a good kesehataan first, if sick or having health problems then the learners are allowed to break wait until the study is completed. The methods used by teachers in teaching is centered on the teacher or teacher centric. In planning the learning teacher learning implementation plan does not make or RPP. Adequate facilities and infrastructure in physical education learning good indor pools as well as support the success of the learning objectives. Topics that will be developed in this paper is the implementation of physical education kurikullum Yongkang Municipal Junior High School in Taiwan.

The purpose of this research is to study the implementation of physical education curriculum in the Yongkang Municipal Junior High School Taiwan.

METHODS

The qualitative approach is undertaken in this research to describe the phenomenon of Learning of physical education in Tainan Yongkang Municipal Junior High School in Taiwan.

Qualitative research is the attempt to understand the subject's experience of the phenomenon by researchers such as behavior, perceptions, motivations, actions and others, in holistolik, and descriptive manner in the form of words and language, in a context of special natural and by utilizing various methods of natural (Moleong, 2014). The subject in this study is the head of school, physical education teacher, student field employees, parents of learners and learners class VIII with the object of study of physical education activities in the year 2016. Location of implementation research in Tainan Yongkang Municipal Junior High School, Chung Shan Road No. 43, 71089 Tainan City, Taiwan. Data retrieval method using interviews, observation, data searches and documentation. According to Sugiyono (2013:244) data analysis is the process of finding and compiling systematic data obtained from the results of the interview, cacatan field and the other ingredients, so it is easy to understand and everything can be communicated to others. Plot data collected as it looks in the picture below:

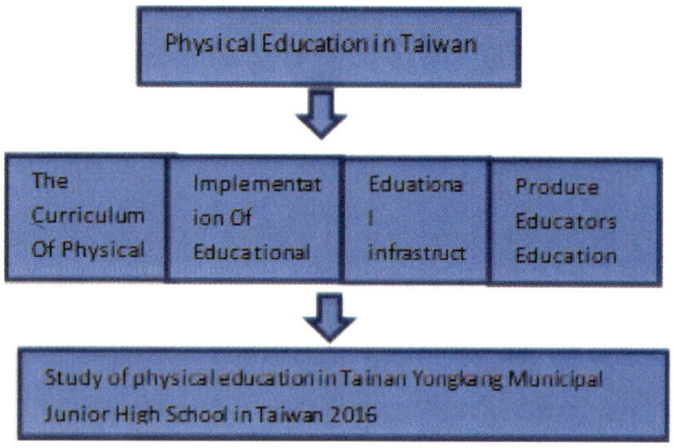

Figure 1 data Flow Research

The analysis of the data to be used in this study is the analysis of qualitative data such as expressed by Arikunto (2002) that includes the components of data research results collected and reduced data, data presentation, and a false assertion results

RESULTS AND DISCUSSION

Results of the study explained that in Tainan Municipal Yongkang Junior High School in Taiwan to use the school-based curriculum, namely the curriculum specified by Board meeting teachers and school administrators are tailored to the needs in the region around the school. In the curriculum used by the Tainan Yongkang Muncipal Junior High School Taiwan contains learning objectives i.e. through learning activities students could learn to live appreciated each other and can protect yourself, learn to avoid free sex behaviour, illegal drugs and have a healthy life patterns, learners can understand the relationship between food, nutrition, hygiene and health, learning and practicing special motion skills to develop the ability of self, reaching the goal of improving health through recreational activities. The curriculum contains about implementation time learning starting from the months, weeks and days, exams and test the working ability of the indicators, indicators, ability and learning activities of the unit name, learning objectives, barriers or major problems, indicators other capabilities, the number of parts, the measurement or assessment methods and records.

The process of implementation of the learning of physical education in Tainan Yongkang Municipal Junior High Schoool Taiwan explained that the study was done with the stage of planning and execution. In the introduction, the core activities and activities cover. Teachers are based on a syllabus that has been created based on the results of the meeting of the Board of teachers of physical education with school administrators about the title which contains the syllabus, date of execution, allocation of time, and the material being taught. Teachers don't make the execution plan of learning but the teacher make learning each end of the evaluation report, the teacher prepares the media learning and tools/equipment to support the success of learning. Teachers do not do modifications and infrastructure because teachers feel in quantity and quality to meet the needs already support the teaching and learning process. Allocation of time hour face-to-face learning physical education in Tainan Yongkang Municipal Junior High School in Taiwan is a 45-minute face-to-face 2 x each week

The available facilities and infrastructure in support of physical education learning success is very adequate in quantity as well as quality. Physical education teachers have entrances and are not joined with teachers of other subjects, with supporting facilities such as a television, table and chairs, armchair, serious air conditioner, document storage space, and a bulletin board. In order to achieve the learning objectives of physical education is to be expected, the school has facilities in the form of 3 basketball court equipped with mast ring and cement floor is smooth so that it does not hurt if the fall. Two volleyball courts are equipped with poles and nets net. Athletic fields in the form of a running track, Javelin, discus throwing area, decline of deciduous, high jump and skip away in the form of sandbox. Indor swimming pool with a depth of 150 cm, with supporting facilities, a pond keeper rinse, dressing room, hairdryer, clothes lockers, floats, and one bathroom for student disability. Hall/Hall,

3 badminton courts indor, warehouse equipment and supplies, 1 indor room table tennis, fitness room with well-maintained condition. Teachers do not do modifications to the infrastructure and facilities in the study because it was available with either. In addition the learners are given a textbook lesson for each semester with a display of colorful, illustrated and exciting.

The results of the research on educators or teachers of physical education in Tainan Yongkang Municipal Junior High School in Taiwan meet the qualification standards of teachers. Academic qualifications possessed by teachers of physical education, teacher in Yongkang have undergraduate education even have attended Graduate studies physical education course from one of the universities in Taiwan. Before teaching in schools teachers are required to follow the practice of teaching 6 months and through the test of eligibility and competence of teachers to obtain a certificate to teach.

The number of teachers of physical education is a teacher with a total of 11 hours of teaching that is tailored to the varying length of teaching as a teacher. Average hours of teaching physical education every teacher is 21 x 45 min/week-24 x 45 min/week. Teachers can memamahami characterisitics of learners who come from different backgrounds and mastering the material being taught, it is visible in the implementation process of learning teachers explain the material in a way that is easily understood by learners and provide examples of everyday dalamkegiatan. The teacher be objective in giving judgment in the aspect of the attitude, knowledge and skills.

Learners in Tainan Yongkang Muncipal Junior High School in Taiwan is the citizens who live in the area near the school. Learners should pay a little over 3,644 NTD for Class VII, 5,714 NTD for class VIII, and 7.941 for class IX. The payment covers books, uniforms, lunch for one month, insurance, extracurricular, and an additional disore class today.

Learners are required to create their own sports uniform design, so each class has a different uniform. Students are obligated to follow any rules that existed in schools. Based on search results document the number of learners in Tainan Yongkang Municipal Junior High School in Taiwan is 1746 learners with details of 1729 regular learners, and 17 students in need. Based on the results of observation, interview and search data that learners are classified in the three classes i.e., exercise classes, art classes and regular classes. Sports class is a class that contains an active learner and have the potential in the field of sports as athletes. However the sport in education referring to four types of physical activity i.e. Olympic competition sports, games and recreation outside the room, the fitness sports, music and movement (Rahayu, 2013; Samsudin, 2008; Malobulu dkk, 2011). Art class is a class that contains the learners who have the skills and interest in the art of good dance, fine arts and other arts. Regular class is a class that contains the learners who want formal education without specialization skills. But physical education is one unit within the framework of the education are inseparable and have an important role in the formation of character in learners so that the purpose of education can be achieved with either. Physical education is an important part and cannot off in the overall education system that has been widely realized by many circles both in Indonesia, Asia, and the world (Hardman, 2014). This is due to physical education is an educational process that utilizes the physical activity that is planned systematically aims to develop and enhance the entire realm, physical, cognitive, psychomotor or affective each learners with the material presented is about sports, fitness and recreation outside the room. If the purpose of physical education is associated with educational purposes in Indonesia in line and synergistic i.e. develop potential learners in order to become a man of faith and piety to God Almighty, precious, healthy, have learned, accomplished, creative, self-sufficient, and become citizens of a democratic and accountable. (Gerald Crawford, 2017; Noddings, 2018)

CONCLUSION

Based on the results of analysis and discussion, then the conclusions that can be drawn from this research is the study of physical education in Tainan Yongkang Municipal Junior High School in Taiwan the year 2016 are:

1. The curriculum used by the Tainan Yongkang Municipal Junior High School is a school-based curriculum.

2. The process of implementation of the learning consists of planning, and the implementation of learning.

3. Facilities and infrastructure in a very adequate in supporting the successful achievement of the learning objectives of physical education.

4. Physical education educators in Tainan Yongkang Municipal Junior High School in Taiwan have met the qualification standards of good teachers in the academic eligibility, exams teachers and teacher competence sesai with subjects that diampu.

5. Learners in Tainan Yongkang Municipal Junior High School in Taiwan are required to

pay in accordance with the classification of economic families, learners are distinguished into three classes i.e., exercise classes, art classes and regular classes.

REFERENCES

Arikunto, S. (2002). Metode penelitian. Jakarta: Rineka Cipta, 89-71

Eka Trikanthi Agustina. 2013. Survei Kelayakan Sarana dan Prasarana Pelaksanaan Belajar Mengajar Penjasorkes SLB B DON BOSCO Kabupaten Wonosobo tahun 2013. Diambil dari ACTIVE: Journal of Physical Education, Sport, Health and Recreations

Creswell, J. W., & Plano Clark, V. L, 2007. Designing and conducting mixed methode research. Thousand Oaks, CA : Sage Publications, Inc.

Hans, N. (2012). Comparative education: A study of educational factors and traditions. Routledge.

Hardman Ken. 2008. Physical Education In Schools : A Global Perspective. UK : University of Worcester. Diambil dari: https://hrcak.srce.hr/index.php?show=clanak&id_clanak_jezik=39135

Hardman,Ken. 2014. Final report. Diambil dari: https://core.ac.uk/download/pdf/132614193.pdf

Kardman, Ken. 2008. situation and sustainability of physical education in scghools: a Global Perspective. Diambil dari: https://www.researchgate.net/profile/Ken_Hardman/publication/228680229_Physical_education_in_schools_A_global_perspective/links/00b49529dc5d5b83a4000000/Physical-education-in-schools-A-global-perspective.pdf

Li, L. (2005). Quiet revolution in the classroom: The nine-year integrated curriculum. (R. Taylor, Trans.). SINORAMA Magazine. Diambil dari: http://www.sinorama.com.tw/en/print_issue.php3?id=200229102016e.txt&mag=past

Moleong, J. (2014). Lexy, Metodologi Penelitian kualitatif, Penerbit PT. Remaja Rosdakarya bandung.

Nuffic. (2015). Education System Taiwan : The Taiwanese education system described and compared with the Dutch system. Diambil dari https://www.nuffic.nl/en/publications/find-a-publication/education-system-taiwan.pdf.

Prastowo, A. (2017). Menyusun Rencana Pelaksanaan Pembelajaran (RPP) Tematik Terpadu. Kencana.

Rahayu, Ega Trisna. 2013. Strategi Pembelajaran Pendidikan Jasmani. Bandung : Alfabeta.

Salinan Peraturan Menteri Pendidikan Nasional Republik Indonesia Nomor 24 Tahun 2007 Tentang Standar Sarana dan Prasarana Untuk Sekolah Dasar, Menengah Pertama, dan Menengah Atas.

Salinan Peraturan Menteri Republik Indonesia Nomor 32 Tahun 2013 Tentang Perubahan Atas Peraturan Pemerintah Nomor 19 Tahun 2005 Tentang Standar Nasional Pendidikan.

Salinan Undang-Undang Nomor 20 Tahun 2003 Tentang Sistem Pendidikan Nasional.

Samsudin. 2008. Pembelajaran Pendidikan Jasmani, Olahraga dan Kesehatan. Jakarta : Prenada Media Group.

Malobulu. S, Abdi Rahmat, and Taga Radja Gah, 2011. Olahraga dan Pendidikan Jasmani dalam Wajah Keutuhan NKRI. Jakarta : Ardadizya Jaya.

Thomas Ruth and Luyi Lien. 2005. Alternative Curriculum perspectives : Implications for Teachers' Curriculum Developments in Taiwan. . Journal of Educational Research and Development.

Malik, A. A. (2013). "Ular Tangga Olahraga" Media Permainan Edukatif Untuk Olahraga Dengan Menggunakan Sistem Sirkuit Training Bagi Siswa Kelas X Sma Negeri Ajibarang Tahun 2013. Active: Journal of Physical Education, Sport, Health and Recreation, 2(10).

Ramdhani, M. A. (2017). Lingkungan Pendidikan dalam Implementasi Pendidikan Karakter. Jurnal Pendidikan UNIGA, 8(1), 28-37.

Noddings, N. (2018). Philosophy of education. Routledge.

Jihad, A. (2008). Pengembangan kurikulum matematika. Multi Pressindo.

Edward F. Melcer (2017). Exploring the Effects of Physical Embodiment in a Puzzle-Based Educational Programming Game, Proceedings of the 2017 ACM SIGCHI Conference on Creativity and Cognition, June 27-30 Singapore, Singapore

Sun, H., Li, W., & Shen, B. (2017). Learning in physical education: A self-determination theory perspective. Journal of Teaching in Physical Education, 36(3), 277–291. https://doi.org/10.1123/jtpe.2017-0067.

23

Development of Outbound Activities to Embed The Values of Character Education Through Interactive Multimedia

Muhammad Virga Gustifajar[1], Wasis D. Dwiyogo[2], Febrita Paulina H.[3]

Universitas Negeri Malang, Indonesia[123]

Article History

Keywords:
Interactive Multimedia; Character Education; Outbound; Extracurricular.

Abstract

The purpose of this research and development is to generate outbound activities to instill the values of character education through interactive multimedia for participants of nature lovers extracurricular. The design of this study uses a research and development model from Lee and Owens. The results of research and development of large group trials on 45 participants resulted in 86.18% percentage of product validation and 90% results from product effectiveness.The conclusion of this research and development is the product is valid with very good category and well used as training media.

Correspondence address :
Kampus Universitas Negeri Malang, Jalan Semarang No.5 Malang
E-mail: virgagusti48@gmail.com

INTRODUCTION

Character education is a term used for any effort that can be done to influence a student's character. According Zubaedi, (2011) people who are character are those who have good morals, morals, good manners. At this time, Indonesia is experiencing a crisis of character values of the nation, which is marked by the increasingly widespread crime and other acts that do not reflect the values of national character, conducted by educated people in the work environment and society. Therefore, character education in Indonesia today is highly emphasized in both formal and non-formal education in the community. Character education is a very important thing to be instilled in every learner. Individuals with good character and superior will try to do the best thing to God Almighty, herself, environment, fellow and always have motivation to do goodness (Aqib, 2011) Permendikbud number 23 year 2015 states that character education should be able to be a joint movement involving government, local government, community and parents. Recognized or not recognized today there is a real crisis in the nation of Indonesia that involves the generation of the nation, especially teenagers where many crimes against friends, cheating, pornography, bullying in schools and brawl.

The purpose of character education is basically to encourage the birth of a good child by growing and having a good character that encourages learners to grow with the capacity and commitment to do the best things and do everything right and have a purpose in life. In the scope of school there are extracurricular activities that become a container for learners who have the talent of interest and ability.

According to Permendikbud no. 62 year 2014, extracurricular activities are activities undertaken by learners outside the hours of learning intrakurikuler activities, under the guidance and supervision of educational units. One of the most popular extracurricular activities today is nature lovers. Andri (2016) nature lovers is an organization or a forum for students who want to develop themselves in this regard. So this nature lovers means very wide, love forests, sea and so on. Nature lovers are related to the outdoors. Outbound activities can be enjoyed and studied, one of them as a medium.

According to Dwiyogo (2008) the word "media" comes from the "medius", which means "middle". Media selection aims to motivate and attract interest in message recipients and can take place optimally. One form of media that he considers capable of attracting students' attention is interactive multimedia. Interactive multimedia is a multimedia that can be used Autoplay Media Studio which is a software that can be used to create a professional presentation is considered to attract and bring huge benefits to participants. Autoplay media studio allows users to be able to create interactive multimedia even though the user is not from a programmer. In reality practice at the time of training conducted in extracurricular nature lovers are still a lot of students who are not active and time is not effective and this incident is exacerbated by the absence of media that can attract the interest of participants such as interactive multimedia so that the material is running less than the maximum and boring.

Based on observations from 3 high schools of SMAN 1 Situbondo, SMAN 2 Situbondo, and SMAN 1 Panji, extracurricular nature coach lovers stated that rarely deliver material by using interactive multimedia. All coaches extracurricular nature lovers in the four schools agreed if developed interactive multimedia planting the values of character education through outbound. From result of requirement analysis for student obtained result among others 88,3% participant interested with development of interactive multimedia planting character value through outbound.

From the results of a study conducted by Indri (2011) on his thesis that the results of 95% effectiveness and 100% attractiveness in small group trial and 98% effectiveness and 100% appeal in large group trials after being given the product of intermediate multimedia development results, and the results of Wijanarko's (2010) research on his thesis that there is a significant influence on student leadership after being given treatment through outbound method. From the above description is expected through the development of interactive multimedia of the values of character education through outbound can attract students because this multimedia is a collection of various media such as text, images, sound, video and others where the material contains outbound activities can be a fun medium and designed with the themes of character education, extracurricular participants of high school nature lovers are expected to understand, emulate and apply nilia-value character education as a capital to become a good and dignified nation.

Character education is a system of inculcating character values to the citizens of the school which includes the components of knowledge, awareness or willingness, and actions to implement those virtues (aqib, 2011). The purpose of character education is basically to encourage the birth of a good child by growing and having good character so as to encourage learners to grow with the capacity and commitment to do the best things and do everything right and have the purpose of life. Character education should begin with a process of cultivating knowledge and intelligence on the individual about good things worth doing and not and existing knowledge can be applied to the attitude form (Dianti, 2014). The values of the characters that are embedded and developed in schools in Indonesia and their descriptions (Kemendiknas, 2010: 9) are as follows: (a) religious,, (b) honest, (c) tolerance, (d) discipline, (e) hard work, (f) creative, (g) independent, (h) democratic, (i) curiosity, (j) (m) friendly / communicative, (n) peace loving, (o) reading, (p) caring about the environment, (q) social care, always sharing , (r) responsibility.

Understanding the media leads to something that delivers information between the giver and the recipient of the message. If the media carries instructional or instructional information then it is called learning media (arsyad, 2014). Daryanto (2011) stated that instructional media is a means of intermediary in the learning process. The use of media has the purpose of providing motivation to learners. Good media will also enable learners to respond, feedback and also encourage learners to practice properly.

Multimedia that is a technology to optimize the role of computers as a means of displaying and manipulating text, graphics, and sound in an integrated view (Rusman, 2013). While interactive multimedia is a multimedia equipped with a controller that can be operated by the user (Wijaya, 2010). When users get the flexibility in controlling the multimedia, then it is interactive multimedia. As information technology grows rapidly, interactive multimedia enables users to get richer output from conventional media. Users can view three-dimensional images, photos, moving videos, or animations, and hear sound, or music (Dwiyogo, 2008).

Interactive multimedia always use supporting software for display media software, supporting software that is Autoplay Media studio. Autoplay Media studio is a vector-based two-dimensional animation software with professional capabilities. The software is to create a multimedia device by integrating various types of media such as pictures, text, sound, and vidio into presentations made (Hernawati, 2010).

Outbound is the delivery of material to students through outdoor activities to stimulate self-development and character. Activities provided will be able to stimulate the ability to beroganisasi, physical challenges and adventure. Susanta (2010) states Outbound is a method of development through a combination of sequences of psychomotor, cognitive, and affective activities in the learning approach through experience. In outbound there are games that involve motion, thinking, emotional, and social activities as part of the formation of character and character for a person (Jatmiko, 2015).

Skills gained through outbound is more daring to take risks. An open-ended experience enables one to be bolder and confident in facing obstacles. Characters are formed by repetitive behaviors that become habitual. In line with this, it needs to be embedded values from childhood so that human characters can be formed. According to Asti (in, Wijanarko, 2011) in many studies the outbound method was effective in building an understanding of a concept and building behavior.

Here are some games that will be given to extracurricular participants of nature lovers for high school: (1) chain messages, (2) spinning together, (3) throwing a ball, (4) guessing motions, (5) mystery hats, (6) rotating, (7) glass balls, (8) life obstacles, (9) magical ball bales, (10) pretty retreat.

Based on the above problems, then conducted a research entitled "Development of Outbound Activities To Embed the Values of Character Education through Interactive Multimedia For Esktrakulikuler Participants Lovers Nature High School".

METHODS

The design of this research using research and development of outbound activities through interactive multimedia using autoplay software which is packaged in CD form to instill the values of character education as a learning media which refers to multimedia research development model. This development model has a full flow from the analysis and assessment phase, the design phase, the development stage, the implementation stage, and the evaluation phase. Interactive multimedia development steps or procedures used by the developer in this study.

Here are the steps of this research and development: (1) analysis, this stage is the initial stage for the development which includes two steps of activity, the first step is the need assessment. Need Assessment is a systematic step to determine the gap between the actual state and the desired state. In this research, the initial needs analysis is done directly by the researcher by spreading the questionnaire to the extracurricular coach of nature lovers of High School in Four schools, namely SMAN 1 Situbondo, SMAN 2 Situbondo, SMAN 1 Panji, and SMAN 1 Panarukan, (2) design at this stage the planning stage of the product to be developed. There are several activities that need to be done in this phase, that is activity schedule, media specification, (3) development, after design is made then the next step is development step. Basic principles of computer-based media development, (4) implementation, at this stage media products have been declared ready uutuk used and if at evaluation stage found deficiencies will be revised again with the aim of collecting data as the basis of establishing the feasibility of products produced from the media so support the achievement the. (5) evaluation, evaluation aims to determine whether the product developed has achieved the established goals.

The test subjects in this research and development are: (1) experts, using two experts outbound material experts and media experts who have characteristics and competent in the field. (2) field trials conducted on students extracurricular nature lovers from four high schools SMAN 1 Situbondo which has a population of 35 students, SMAN 2 Situbondo which has a population of 37 students, and SMAN 1 Panji with a population of 28 students, then used the technique Simple Random Sampling technique is stated simple because sampling of population members is done randomly without regard to strata

The instrument used in this study is a questionnaire.

Data analysis techniques used are qualitative and descriptive analysis techniques in the form of percentages.

RESULTS AND DISCUSSION

Outbound activity products that have been developed to instill the values of character education through interactive multimedia as a medium of learning or training extracurricular participants of nature lovers in high school. Developers of interactive multimedia products can be run or operated through computers and laptops. This interactive multimedia using autoplay media studio software that can integrate various media in it such as text, images, music, video and the exit button is very interactive so that it can connect as per the desire of the user. A good product is a product that meets the criteria of validity.

In this study, the researchers conducted a needs analysis that was done in the form of initial observation of extracurricular nature lovers in three high schools, namely SMAN 1 Situbondo, SMAN 2 Situbondo, and SMAN 1 Panji by giving questionnaires or questionnaires to 15 participants in each school and at the same time coach or pembinaekstrakurikuler nature lovers. The next step to obtain expert evaluation data in the process of development of product in the form of outbound activities to instill the values of character education through interactive multimedia on the extracurricular nature lovers, researchers use the method of data collection of instruments presented in the form questionnaire and accompanied by suggestions or inputs. Expert evaluation consists of 2 experts namely Outbound experts and media experts. While for the test is presented in the form of a questionnaire (1) small group test of 9 extracurricular participants, (2) large group test of 45 participants of natural nature extracurricular in three high schools.

From the result of requirement analysis for trainer that 100% outbound can be used as method to inculcate character value, 100% trainer has never used interactive multimedia, 100% agree if developed interactive multimedia.

From the result of requirement analysis for student, the result is 98,47% of participants say the importance of character education, 82.9% of participants have never done outbound educational activities, 88.3% of participants are happy and interested in the development of interactive multimedia planting the character's value through outbound.

From the validation of 2 outbound experts after the average obtained the results of 83.33%, so the material outbound in interactive multimedia is very feasible. From this expert outbound obtained input that the game sorted from easy to difficult, the music is replaced with traditional music and added score on evaluation.

From media expert validation obtained 77% results, so the product from development feasible to use with a small revision.From the media expert obtained input that onfinishing needs to be optimized, the type of music needs to be replaced and added.

From the results of small group testing on the validity of the product obtained a score of 476 results, a maximum score of 540 and the percentage obtained 88.14%, so that interactive multimedia development products is very decent-digunakan.Dari small group test results on the effectiveness of the product obtained score of 42 results, a maximum score of 45 and a percentage of 93%, so that interactive multimedia development products is very feasible use.

From the results of large group trials of product validity obtained by 2327 result score, maximal score 2700 and percentage obtained 86.18%, so that interactive multimedia development products is very feasible use. From the results of large group trials to the effectiveness obtained 203 results score, a maximum score of 203 and 90% percentage, so that interactive multimedia development products is very feasible use.

DISCUSSION

The product of the development of outbound activities inculcates the values of character education through interactive multimedia that has been produced is used for extracurricular participants of high school nature lovers as a medium of learning or media training.Suatu media that brings an information that aims instructional or contains the purpose of teaching then the media called learning media (arsyad, 2014).

At the time of implementation of learning or training must occur interaction between messenger to the recipient of the message, therefore it takes the media in the form of interactive multimedia. Interactive multimedia is a multimedia equipped with controller that can be operated directly by the user. According to Wijaya (2010) if users get the flexibility in controlling the multimedia, then it is interactive multimedia.

One form of interactive multimedia is autoplay media studio. It is software to create an interactive multimedia software by integrating various types of media such as pictures, text, sound, and vidio into presentations made (Hernawati, 2010).

The values of the characters contained in this medium (Kemendiknas, 2010) are as follows: (a) religious, (b) honest, (c) tolerance, (d) discipline, (e) hard work, (f) creative, (i) curiosity, (j) the spirit of nationalism, (k) love of the homeland, (l) respect for achievement, (m) friendly / communicative, (n) peace loving, o) reading, (p) care about the environment, (q) social care, and (r) responsibility. There are 10 kinds of outbound activities: (1) chain messages, (2) rotating together, (3) throwing balls, (4) guessing motions, (5) mystery hats, (6) bolabergergir, (7) glass balls, (8)) obstacles of life, (9) magical ball ball, (10) pretty retreat.

Products that will be produced through this research process in the form of development of outbound activities to instill the values pendididkan characters through interactive multimedia. Darmawan (2014) explains that multimedia learning is basically a learning that is expected to empower all learning activities.

A small revision was made after receiving input and suggestions from material experts and media experts. The following inputs and suggestions as a whole from the experts used as a benchmark by researchers to revise the product are as follows (1) The concept is good, (2) finishing media needs to be optimized, (3) selection of musical instruments more attention (4) for CD cover yet (8) the value of the character needs to be added to the explanation (9) the outbound activity is sorted by the difficulty level and given the number.

CONCLUSION

The results of research and development can be summarized as follows: (1) based on the results of the evaluation of the experts that the product development from the development of outbound activities inculcate the values of character education through interactive multimedia for extracurricular participants of nature lovers SMA valid otherwise used on students extracurricular activities lovers nature in high school. (2) based on the results of the evaluation of large-scale product test on the subject try as a candidate from product users that product development outbound activities inculcate the values of character education through interactive multimedia is declared valid and has the attractiveness, ease, clarity to be trained in the students extracurricular nature lovers in high school.

REFERENCES

Arsyad A. 2014. Media Pembelajaran. Jakarta: Raja Grafindo Persada

Aqib,Z. & Sujak. 2011. Panduan dan Aplikasi Pendidikan Karakter. Bandung: Yrama Widya.

Darmawan,D. 2011. Teknologi Pembelajaran. Bandung: PT Remaja Rosdakarya.

Darmawan,D. 2012. Inovasi Pendidikan. Bandung: PT Remaja Rosdakarya Offset.

Daryanto. 2011. Media Pembelajaran. Bandung: PT. sarana Tutorial Nurani Sejahtera

Dianti P. 2014. Integerasi Pendidikan Karakter Dalam Pembelajaran Pendidikan Kewarganegaraan Untuk Mengembangkan Karkater Siswa. Jurnal Pendidikan. (Online) 23 (1), (http://www.ejournal.upi.edu) diakses 23 Desember 2016

Dwiyogo,W. 2008. Aplikasi Teknologi Pembelajaran: Pengembangan Media Pembelajaran Pendidikan Jasmani dan Olahrga. Malang: Fakultas Ilmu Pendidikan Universitas Negeri Malang.

Hernawati, Kuswari. 2009. Modul Pelatihan AutoPlay Media Studio, (Online).

(http://staffnew.uny.ac.id) diakses tanggal 5 Februari 2017.

Jatmiko T. 2015. Pendidikan jasmani melalui outbound, (online). (http://ejournal.unesa.ac.id)

diakses tanggal 12 Januari 2017.

Kemendiknas. 2010. Pengembangan Pendidikan Budaya Dan Karakter Bangsa. Jakarta: Kemetrian Pendidikan Nasional

Permendikbud No 23 Tahun 2015. (online), (http://www.kemendikbud.go.id), diakses 26 Desember 2016

Permendikbud No 62 Tahun 2014. (online), (http://www.kemendikbud.go.id), diakses 26 Desember 2016

Rusman. 2013. Belajar dan Pembelajaran Berbasis Komputer. Bandung: Alfabeta.

Susanta,A. 2010. Outbound Profesional. Jogjakarta: Andi Offset.

Wijanarko, W. 2011 . Pengaruh Metode Outbound Terhadap Pendidikan Karakter Kepemimpinan Seklah Alam Indonesia. (online). (http://repository.uinjkt.ac.id/dspace/bitstream/123456789/4835/1/WAHYU%20WIJANARKO-FPS.PDF), diakses 15 Desember 2016

Wijaya E. 2010. Pengembangan Bahan Ajar Berbasis Multimedia Interaktif Untuk Meningkatkan Hasil Belajar Siswa. Skripsi Tidak Diterbitkan. Malang : UIN

Zubaedi. 2011. Desain Pendidikan Karakter: Konsepsi dan Aplikasinya dalam Lembaga Pendidikan. Jakarta: Rencana Renada Media Grup

24

Motivation to Community for Following Aerobic Sports

Dhian Kusmiyanti[1], Agus Kristiyanto[2], Tri Aprilijanto Utomo[3], Hartini[4]

Program Studi Ilmu Keolahragaan, Program Pascasarjana Universitas Sebelas Maret, Surakarta, Jawa Tengah, Indonesia[123]
Pendidikan Kepelatihan Olahraga, Fakultas Keguruan Dan Ilmu Pendidikan, Universitas Tunas Pembangunan, Surakarta, Jawa Tengah, Indonesia[4]

Article History

Keywords:
Aerobic Gymnastic; Community; Descriptive Qualiative Methods .

Abstract

The purpose of this study is to determine the role of motivation what is the basis of the community following aerobic gymnastics. The method used in this research is using qualitative descriptive. Data collection techniques used are using survey techniques. The research results show that the role of motivation for the public to participate in aerobic exercise is very important. People who follow this aerobic gymnastics come from different backgrounds that is from the educational environment both teachers and students, teenagers, housewives, and elderly. The results of five aerobic gymnastics workshops namely Yoyok Fans Community amounted to 18 people, Maria Center amounted to 63 people, Lotte Mart Morning Gymnastic Community, 82 people, Ira Gymnastic Studio numbered 12 people and Dee Dee Gymnastic Studio numbered 11 people. Of the five gymnastics studios studied then the total amounted to 186 people. The motivation of society is so that body become healthy and fit 108 people then get 58,06%, recreation 30 people then get 16,13%, add friend 21 people then get 11,29%, want to channel knowledge to other people equal to 14 people then obtained 7.53%, and became the champion when following the race 13 people then obtained 6.98%.

Correspondence address :
E-mail: kusmiyanti1993@gmail.com

INTRODUCTION

Physical fitness is a primary requirement of all levels of society, through fitness then any performance will increase. A study conducted by Dian Windarwati (2014) on public fitness exercise conducted at the time of government car free day policy in Semarang City showed that 77% of participants have high motivation on relevance factor requirement ie body desire to be healthy and fit. In addition to awareness of the needs of the public, there needs to be a high motivation both from within and from outside to push toward the fit through exercise and sports. Hamzah B. Uno (2016) says that "motivation as an inner strength of the individual, which affects to do something. Sardiman, (2012) says "motivation is a business under certain conditions to do something. While the opinion of Sary, I(2015) understanding of motivation is the power (energy) of an individual individual either sourced from within and from outside a person.

Improved physical fitness requires a regular, planned, periodic physical activity and has a beneficial effect on physical and mental health. One form of physical activity that is cheap and fun and cause a fit effect is gymnastics. In line with the opinion Wardani, (2012) states that Gymnastics is a physical exercise that is planned and systematic to form and develop personally in harmony. Aerobic aerobics is a sport that has been known by the public, fun and provide a fit effect. In the opinion of Chrisly M. Palar & Djon Wongkar ., (2015) says that aerobic exercise is a sport that has a category of physical activity from low intensity to moderate intensity in a certain time one of them is Aerobic Gymnastics is also associated with the utilization of oxygen. It was also conveyed by Fajar et al. (2014) that aerobics need extra oxygen because this sport lasts a long time. This sport is very good for health if in the execution done with regular and regular. While understanding aerobic exercise by Adi Trisnawan (2010) is a series of movements and music created intentionally to achieve certain goals. Aerobic aerobics have received positive responses and high interest for the community. It is seen in every public place on the morning of a gymnastic event along with always attended by many people.

So here can be seen that the role of society is very important. Syahrial Syarbaini and Fatkhuri (2016) said that "society is a group of people interact and stay together for a long time". While "Participation is the involvement of the community in the activities and implementation in its environment". (Remiswal, 2013; Fadil, 2013).

Surakarta is one of the big cities in Central Java with a population of about 514171 people spread in 5 districts of Laweaan, Serengan, Pasar Kliwon, Jebres and Banjar sari. It appears that growth is increasing, this requires handling of various things, especially in the health section as shown in **table 1** below.

Table 1. The rate of growth and population of Surakarta City.

Growth Population	2012	2013	2014	2015	2016
Total Population	505413	507825	510077	512226	514171
Population Increase From The Previos Time	2547	2412	2252	2121	1945
Growth Population	0.08	0.08	0.08	0.47	0.46

https://surakartakota.bps.go.id/dynamictable/2018/03/14/43/pertumbuhan-penduduk-pertahun-kota-surakarta.html

Awareness of participating in aerobic fitness gymnastics led to the emergence of gymnastics centers began to grow and develop in the city of Surakarta. Recorded 5 (five) gymnastics regularly and growing in serving aerobic gymnastic activity Surakarta City Community is Yoyok Fans Community, Maria Center, Lotte Mart Morning Gymastic Community, Ira Gymnastic Studio, and Dee Dee Gymanstic Studio. In addition, the notion of community participation is not seen from the participation of the community to perform gymnastics only. In the opinion of Permana & Sastaman (2015) community participation involves the planning and development of gymnastics activities. People who follow aerobic exercise are not only followed by women, but aerobic exercise is also followed by men. Similarly aerobic exercise is not only done for adults only, but done by children, adolescents, and elderly. However, the level of community participation in gymnastes varies depending on the participants' motivation. The author feels the need to know what motivation underlies the participation of participants in aerobic gymnastics at gymnasium. It aims to improve the service of aerobic gymnastics activities at studios in Kota Surakarta.

Based on the above background the focus of the problem you want to know is how the motivation of participants who joined aerobic gymnastics at gymnasium in the city of Surakarta. The purpose of this research is to know the motivation of aerobic gymnastics participants in Surakarta gymnastics gigs.

METHODS

This study used descriptive qualitative. Where in taking data using survey technique. For the results of the study indicated by the percentage. Implementation of this research was conducted in September 2017 until December 2017. The location of this research is in five gymnasium namely Yoyok Fans Community, Maria Center, Lotte Mart Morning Gymastic Community, Ira Gymnastic Studio, and Dee Dee Gymanstic Studio. Instrument data collection is carried out based on the opinion of Sugiyono (2013) namely interviews, observation and questionnaire (questionnaire).

The data collection technique is done in three ways, namely as follows:

a. Interviews were conducted by asking the gym instructors and the people who follow aerobic exercise. Where it is very important to be interviewed is related to the role of motivation for the community and the actual motivation of what is the basis of the community to follow aerobic gymnastics in the city of Surakarta.

b. Observations made is observing aerobic exercise activities that have been running in the community of Surakarta.

c. Questionnaire distribution (questionnaire) done after the community finished doing aerobic exercise. So in the questionnaire the researchers should be helped, because the community after aerobic exercise is usually in a hurry to go home, although previously it has been told there will be a questionnaire. Filling in the questionnaire (questionnaire) takes about five to ten minutes, because the answer type is a multiple choice.

This data analysis technique uses descriptive percentages (%) based on opinions from (Sudjana, 1990). With the formula below:

$$P = \frac{f}{N} x\, 100\ \%$$

Keterangan
P = Percentage result
f = the number of acquisition data
N = Total data

RESULTS AND DISCUSSION

Surakarta city is a densely populated city of 512 thousand inhabitants. The second most populous city after the city of Semarang which amounted to 1700 thousand inhabitants. Public awareness of health and cultivate physical activity to maintain body fitness increases with the proliferation of fitness centers in Surakarta. In table 1 below will first be shown the number of people who follow aerobic gymnastics in each aerobic gymnastics.

Table 2. Number of Communities Following Aerobic Gymnastics.

Studios Name	Amount
Yoyok Fans Community	18
Maria Center	63
Lotte Mart Morning Gymnastic Community	82
Ira Gymnastic Studio	12
Dee Dee Gymnastic Studio	11
Total	**186**

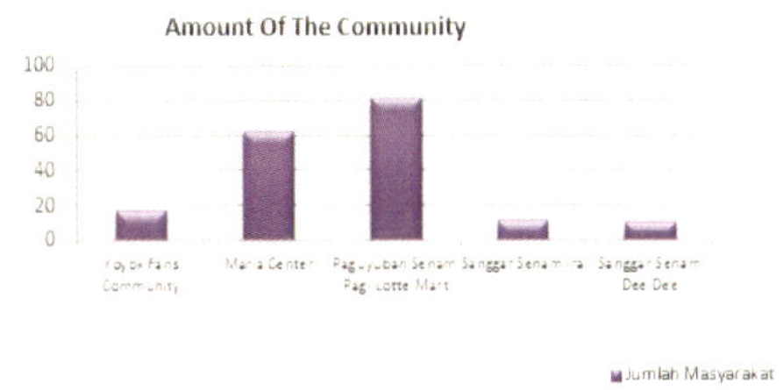

Picture 1. The Number of Participants in Aerobic Gymnastics

The number of participants in gymnastics enthusiastically follow the course of aerobic gymnastics must be based on certain motivations both extrinsic and encouragement from within.

Picture 2. Spirit and enthusiasm of Aerobic Gymnastics at Lotte Mart Morning Gymnastic Community

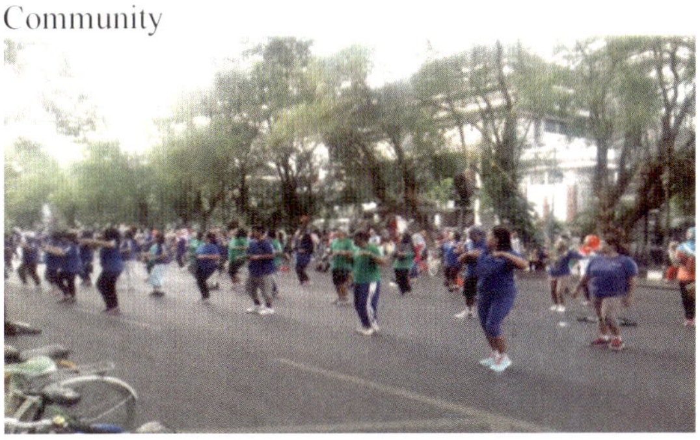

Every aerobic gymnast in the community has an underlying motivation so they are willing to participate in aerobic exercise. Data collected through the results Questionnaire, interview on gymnastics participants, then analyzed using descriptive percentage. The results are illustrated and found what

underlies the motivated people to follow aerobic gymnastics. Table 2 below shows the percentage of aerobic exercise motivation participants:

Table 3. The Underlying Motivation of People Following Aerobic Gymnastics

Motivation	Participants	Results (%)
HealHealthy Body	108	58.06
Recreation	30	16.13
Adding Friends	21	11.29
Channel knowledge	14	7.53
Being a winner in Competition	13	6.98

Picture 3. Underlying Motivation of People Following Aerobic Gymnastics

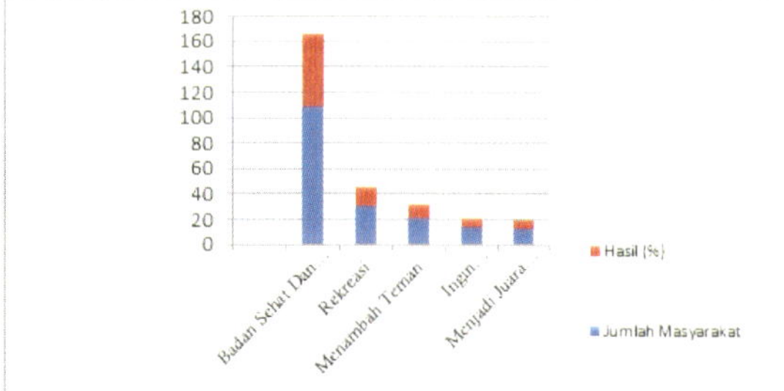

DISCUSSION

The role of motivation of what is the basis of society following aerobic exercise is very important. People who follow this aerobic gymnastics come from different backgrounds that is from the educational environment both teachers and students, teenagers, housewives, and elderly. The motivation that becomes the basis of society following aerobic exercise is to want the body to be healthy and fit, recreate, add friends, distribute knowledge to others, and become the champion while following the race. According to research results, the greatest motivation comes from within a person or intrinsic motivation. Intrinsic motivation will spur someone to get good results because the activity is done with cheerfulness and without coercion (Zuraida & Ifwandi, 2016).

The greatest motivation of people following aerobic exercise is to want the body to be healthy and fit. The results showed that of the 186 people who followed aerobic gymnastics, 108 people stated that the motivation is the basis for the body to be healthy and fit. This result is also supported by research from (Ircham Nur Majid, 2015) which takes issue with the theme of "Motivation of aerobic gymnastics participants in Eristy Management Semarang City in 2013. The results show the motivation of people following aerobic exercise is because to maintain body health and fitness. In addition according Utomo et al., (2012) Aerobic gymnastics has also been proven to maintain the elasticity and health of the skin so it does not quickly wrinkles and looks ageless. There are other discoveries about aerobic exercise with high intensity category its function can burn approximately 100 calories in the body (Dawn & Permana, 2014).

Motivation to follow aerobic exercise is for recreation. Recreation is needed to eliminate saturation and tension for the body. Recreation is also entertainment. Recreation can be done anywhere, anytime and by anyone. Recreational sports is a sport that is done in his spare time so as to obtain physical satisfaction (Retnoningsih & Subyono, 2015).

Motivation to follow aerobic exercise is to add friends. Goal here because basically we live can not own and always need other people to social interaction. Ssocial interaction occurs because of contact and communication with other people (Nismawati, n.d., 2014) Because in society we encounter different characteristics, then we must be careful in choosing friends. Do not let us get carried away to negative things. Because the motivation to follow aerobic exercise to add friends, then usually in following the gymnastics movement is not maximal and many jokes.

Motivation to follow aerobic exercise is to channel knowledge to others, especially about gymnastics. This is usually done by a gym instructor, teacher and student. Each has a different background according to the field. The goal is to increase knowledge so that in the delivery of science is not monotonous because it has a lot of uptake of new science and make those who receive knowledge is not bored and saturated. In addition, the community also needs a place or a container to always be able to exercise regularly and regularly there must be sports facilities (Prasetyo, 2013).

Motivation to follow aerobic gymnastics is to become a champion when following the race is usually done by athletes and ordinary people. The purpose of following this aerobics gymnastics is to prepare yourself if one day there is aerobic gymnastics body condition is ready. Because the preparation of the race can not be sudden and must follow step by stage so that the body condition becomes ready. To follow the race required a high motivation for maximum results. Motivation will affect performance (Mediawati, 2010).

CONCLUSION

Based on the results of research conducted it can be concluded that the role of motivation in following aerobic exercise is very important. People who follow this aerobic gymnastics come from different backgrounds that is from the educational environment both teachers and students, teenagers, housewives, and elderly. The results of five aerobic gymnastics workshops namely Yoyok Fans Community amounted to 18 people, Maria Center amounted to 63 people, Lotte Mart Morning Gymnastic Community, 82 people, Ira Gymnastic Studio numbered 12 people and Dee Dee Gymnastic Studio numbered 11 people. Of the five gymnastics studios studied then the total amounted to 186 people. The motivation of society is so that body become healthy and fit 108 people then get 58,06%, recreation 30 people then get 16,13%, add friend 21 people then get 11,29%, want to channel knowledge to other people equal to 14 people then obtained 7.53%, and became the champion when following the race 13 people then obtained 6.98%. The results of this survey can be the basis for action in serving aerobic exercise participants.

REFERENCES

Adi Trisnawan. (2010). Senam Aerobik. Semarang: Aneka Ilmu.

Chrisly M. Palar & Djon Wongkar, D. S. H. . T. (2015). Manfaat Latihan Olahraga Aerobik Terhadap Kebugaran Fisik Manusia. Jurnal E-Biomedik (Ebm) Volume 3 Nomor 1, Januari-April 2015, 3(April).

Fadil, F. (2013). Partisipasi Masyarakat Dalam Musyawarah Perencanaan Pembangunan Di Kelurahan Kotabaru Tengah. Jurnal Ilmu Politik Dan Pemerintahan Lokal, Ii(8), 287–294.

Fajar, D., & Permana, W. (2014). Pengaruh Latihan Aerobic Class Dan Body Language Terhadap Penurunan Persentase Lemak Tubuh. Jurnal Media Ilmu Keolahragaan Indonesia, 4.

Galih Tri Utomo , Said Junaidi, S. R. (2012). Latihan Senam Aerobik Untuk Menurunkan Berat Badan, Lemak, Dan Kolesterol. Journal Of Sport Sciences And Fitness, 1(1).

Hamzah B. Uno. (2016). Teori Motivasi Dan Pengukurannya. Jakarta: Pt. Bumi Aksara.

Ircham Nur Majid. (2015). Motivasi Peserta Senam Aerobik Di Eristy Management Kota Semarang Tahun 2013. Journal Of Physical Education, Sport, Health And Recreations Http://Journal.Unnes.Ac.Id/Sju/Index.Php/Peshr, 4(2), 1590–1595.

Mediawati, E. (2010). Pengaruh Motivasi Belajar Mahasiswa Dan Kompetensi Dosen Terhadap Belajar. Jurnal Pendidikan Ekonomi Dinamika Pendidikan, V(2), 134–146.

Zuraida , M & Ifwandi, A. (2016). Motivasi Intrinsik Masyarakat Dalam Mengikuti Senam Aerobik Di Stadion Harapan Bangsa Banda Aceh Tahun 2015 Meiria. Jurnal Ilmiah Mahasiswa Pendidikan Jasmani, Kesehatan Dan Rekreasi, 2(2), 73–81.

Nismawati. (N.D.). Jurnal Sosialisasi Pendidikan Sosiologi-Fis Unm Pengaruh Syarat Interaksi Sosial Guru Terhadap Motivasi Nismawati Pendidikan Sosiologi Fis-Unm Pendahuluan Manusia Merupakan Makhluk Sosial Yang Tidak Dapat Hidup Tanpa Bantuan Orang Lain . Oleh Karena Itu ,. Jurnal Sosialisasi Pendidikan Sosiologi- Fis Unm, (C), 86–90.

Permana, A., & Sastaman, P. (2015). Sdm Keolahragaan Kota Pontianak Provinsi Kalimantan Barat Ditinjau Dari Sport Development Index (Sdi) Yang Menganalog Konsep Human Development Index Atau Hdi , Dalam Konsep Hanya Kepada Proses Pelaksanaan Kegiatan Saja , Tetapi Juga Melibatkan Masyaraka. Jurnal Pendidikan Olahraga, 4(1), 9–19.

Prasetyo, Y. (2013). Kesadaran Masyarakat Berolahraga Untuk Peningkatan Kesehatan Dan Pembangunan Nasional. Jurnal Medikora, Vol.Xi, 219–228.

Pribadi, A. (2015). Pelatihan Aerobik Untuk Kebugaran Paru Jantung Bagi Lansia, Ii(2), 64–76.

Remiswal. (2013). Menggugah Partisipasi Gender Di Lingkungan Komunitas Local. Yogyakarta: Graha Ilmu.

Retnoningsih, T., & Subyono, H. S. (2015). Journal Of Sport Sciences And Fitness, 4(2), 49–53.

Sardiman. (2012). Interaksi Dan Motivasi Belajar Mengajar. Jakarta: Rajawali Pers.

Sary, I (2015). Buku Mata Ajar Evaluasi Pendidikan. Deepublish.

Sudjana. (1990). Teknik Analisis Data Kualitatif. Bandung: Tarsito.

Sugiyono. (2013). Metode Penelitian Pendidikan (Pendekatan Kuantitatif, Kualitatif, dan R&D). Bandung: CV. Alfabeta.

Syahrial Syarbaini dan Fatkhuri. (2016). Teori Sosiologi Suatu Pengantar. Bogor: Ghalia Indonesia.

Wardani, A. A. K. (2013). Meningkatkan Hasil Belajar Roll Depan melalui Pemanfaatan Alat Bantu Bidang Miring pada Siswa Kelas VII C SMP Negeri 1 Purwodadi Tahun Pelajaran 2011/2012. Jurnal Phederal Penjas, 1(1).

Utomo, G. T., Junaidi, S., & Rahayu, S. (2012). Latihan senam aerobik untuk menurunkan berat badan, lemak, dan kolesterol. Journal of sport Sciences and Fitness, 1(1).

The Influence of Imagery on The Improvement of Three Point Shoot Ability in Basketball Games

Yogha Tri Pamungkas[1], Aris Mulyono[2], Uen Hartiwan[3]

Department of Physical Education, Faculty of Sport Science, Universitas Negeri Semarang, Indonesia[123]

Article History

Keywords:
Imagery; Basketball; Three Point Shoot.

Abstract

The purpose of this study was to determine the effect of imagery on improving the three point shoot ability. The population of this study are extracurricular participants of men's basketball SMK Negeri 1 Gombong with twenty number of students and the sampling technique used is total sampling. The research method using True Experimental method, that is Pretest-Posttest Control Group Design. The control and experimental group was divided by matched by subject (M-S) method. The data analysis used are normality test, homogeneity test and hypothesis test. The results showed that the exercise of imagery has a significant effect on the improvement of basketball three point shoot skills. The average of pretest is 14,3 and the average of posttest is 17,7, therefore the influence of imagery to improve three point shoot ability is 19,5%. The conclusion of this research that there is significant influence from imagery exercise to increase basketball three point shoot ability of SMK Negeri 1 Gombong's extracurricular participants.

Correspondence address :
E-mail: javanesemoiro@gmail.com

INTRODUCTION

Basketball is one of the many extracurricular activities carried out by secondary schools. By participating in basketball extracurricular activities, it is expected that the participants can improve the basic skills and techniques of playing basketball, becoming the school's core team that represents basketball matches, and is expected to gain achievement in basketball.

One of the main goals in basketball games is the creation of scores, namely by shooting. (Abdul Rohim, 2008) One type of shot in a basketball game is a three-point shot. (Kosasih,2008; Ambler, 2008 ; Oliver, 2007)

In accordance Hopla(2012) with the relevant basketball game style. That is simple basketball, three-point shots today are used as the main weapon for scoring numbers. At a sports analysis conference in the United States held in 2017, Seth Partnov, one of the speakers who is the Research Director of Milwauke Bucks, stated that in the present era the fundamental defense in basketball games that is applied is to protect the paint area. Therefore, the three-point shot is now increasing in frequency. In one team there can be four shooter players. This is shown by the role of power foward which now concludes as a three-point shooter.).

Even statistics show that this year the center position scored 1479 three-point shots. More than the previous four seasons combined. In the present era almost all basketball teams apply a simple philosophy of basketball. Drives and lay-up shots are now rarely used. While the medium shot from the perimeter area and the three point shoot has a larger portion. This is marked by the increase in the three point shoot trend since 2011 until now. And inversely, the portion of two-digit shots has decreased.

Cooper (1975) said the results of the analysis of the three-point shots show that the movement in this shot is more difficult than other shots because of the longer distance, making it more difficult to adjust the coordination and rhythm of the shot. There is a form of training that is still not well known among the basketball team, namely the exercise of imagery.

Seikh & Korn (1994) stated that Imagery exercises occur in the brain and muscles. When an athlete imagines a particular exercise skill, the muscle will contract, this is the same condition as the athlete displays a range of skills in the actual context. It's just that the magnitude is smaller so it doesn't cause any physical movement. Imagery training is one of the effective training methods to be given to anyone, including basketball players who want to improve their three point shoot skills. Because in practice imagery someone will imagine and put each movement according to the limbs that work, so that the nerves that move the body members will be used to a technique that is being studied in his mind. Neuromuscular stimulation associated with the brain in our body will make it easier for the person concerned to transform something imagined into actual physical action or movement. And in the end the movements that have been stored in the minds of players can become easier to do while practicing actual techniques in the field. (Fauzee , 2009; Abdin, 2010, Kosslyn et al, 2001)

Three-point shoot skills of extracurricular participants at SMK 1 Gombong are still not consistent and need to be improved. Based on the observations that the authors did, at the 2016 AOS Cup basketball event the average for three point shooting attemps was a lot in each match, but the comparison between the three point shoot made and the three point shoot attemp was still very small at around 5%. Therefore imagery training is expected to be applied to facilitate basketball extracurricular participants in SMK Negeri 1 Gombong in an effort to increase the ability of three-point shots.

METHODS

This study uses a quantitative approach or numbers because the research conducted is a type of experimental research. So the analysis is based on numbers using statistical analysis. That is a research activity that begins with an initial test then gives treatment or exercises to the subject and ends with a test to be tested for the truth. The experimental method is the most appropriate method to investigate the causal relationship (causal relationship) between two factors that are deliberately generated by researchers by reducing or eliminating other factors that can interfere (Suharsimi Arikunto, 2006: 12).

This experimental research design uses the Pretest-Postest Control Group Design. In this design there are two groups selected through ordinal pairing. Previously the pretest was carried out to find out the initial state. After going through a certain treatment, posttest was carried out to find out the condition after the treatment. And in the end the results are to find out the difference between the experimental group and the control group.

The population in this study were all male students who took basketball extracurricular activities at SMK Negeri 1 Gombong, amounting to 20 students. In this study the sampling technique used is saturated sampling. According to Soegiyono (2010: 61) saturated sampling is a sample determination technique if all members of the population are used as samples. This is often done if the population is relatively small, less than 30 people. Another term saturated sample is a census, where all members of the population are sampled. Then the sample used in this study is all male students of SMK Negeri 1 Gombong who take basketball extracurricular activities. The number of students consists of 20 students consisting of tenth grade students and eleventh grade students.

The research instrument used in this study was a three-point shot with an angle of 0, 90 and 135 degrees. This instrument is taken from previous research conducted by M. Dzul Fikri in 2013. Assessment is the number of scores obtained during the three point shoots as much as 15 times, and each ball gets a score of one. Here you will see more scores, the results will be better. The test was started with a warm up and continued by trying to do a three-point shot several times, then carried out a three-point shot test 15 times.

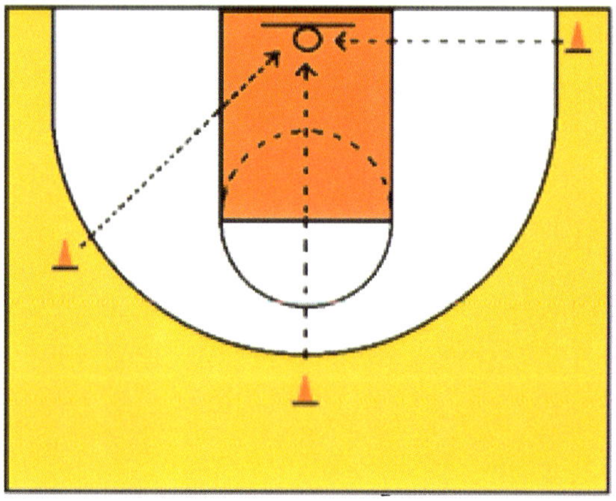

Picture 1. Test position for three point pada sudut 0°, 90° and 135°

Instrument testing tests were carried out on the members of the Gombong Basketball Enthusiast community to find the validity and reliability of the instruments that will be used in this skill test. The amount of validity in the trial of this instrument is 0.731 and the reliability in the trial of this instrument is 0.813, with r-table at 5% significance is 0.444. Because r-count is greater than r-table, the instrument is said to be valid and reliable. So that it can be used for research.

RESULTS AND DISCUSSION

From the results of data analysis can be known, the results of the control group normality and experimental groups are normally distributed. This is shown from the test value of the significance of normality of the control group 0.968 and the experimental group 0.505. The homogeneity test serves to test the similarity of the sample, namely the uniformity of the sample variants taken from the population. The results of this test provide information that the p value (Sig.) Is 0.840, because p (Sig.)> 0.05, it is said that a variant of two or more data population groups is the same or homogeneous, so data analysis can be continued with parametric statistics.

The t-test in the analysis of this study was conducted twice. Based on the results of the t-test it is known that the mean (mean) pre-test of the experimental class is 14.3 and the average pre-test value of the control class is 14.0. The t-count value obtained is 0.213. The value of t-table at a significance level of a = 0.05 is 2.101. From this description it can be seen that t-count is smaller than the t-table, this means there is no significant difference between the experimental group and the control group, both have the same level of ability before the experimental group is given imagery training treatment. This means that if there is an increase in value after treatment, it is assumed that the increase in value is due to the treatment given.

Furthermore, based on the results of the t-test it is known that the average post-test experimental class is 17.7, while the average post-test of the control class is 14.6 and the t-count value is 2.798 with a significance of 0.012. The value of t table with df = 18 at a significance level of a = 0.05 is 2.101. From the explanation above it is known that the t-count value is greater than the t-table value of 2.798> 2.101. If the t-count value is greater than the t-table value, then there is a difference in significance. Thus the null hypothesis (Ho) which states "The absence of the influence of imagery training on increasing the three-point skills of basketball basketball shoots for male extracurricular participants of SMK Negeri 1 Gombong" was rejected. The results showed that the average value of the post-test experimental class was 17.7 greater than the average (mean) post test in the control class which was 14.6. This means that imagery training has a significant effect on increasing the three-point shoot results of male extracurricular participants of SMK Negeri 1 Gombong.

Aiming to find out how much skill improvement is in the form of percentages, a percentage analysis of influence is needed. The results of the analysis can be seen in the table below.

Table 1. The Influence of the Control and Experiment Group

Group	Mean Pre test	Different Post test-Pre test	Influence (%)
Control	14,0	0,6	4,2%
Experiment	14,3	3,4	23,7%

From the **Table 1** above it can be seen that

the use of imagery training in three-point basketball ball training increased 23.7%. Whereas in the control group who did the three point shoot exercise without imagery exercise also experienced an increase of 4.2%. The difference in the percentage of the process between the experimental group and the control group was 19.5%. So it can be concluded that imagery training has an effect of an increase of 19.5% on increasing the three point shoot skills of male basketball extracurricular members of SMK Negeri 1 Gombong in 2017.

Discussions

This study aims to determine the effect of imagery training on improving the three-point shoot skills of the extracurricular participants of SMK Negeri 1 Gombong. Treatment for 16 meetings with frequency of 2 to 3 times a week for 90 minutes per session. The analysis was carried out using the t-test to determine the effect of imagery training on increasing the three point shoot skill. Based on the results of the analysis that has been obtained, it can be seen that the three-point shoot exercise accompanied by imagery training has a significant effect on the results of the three-point shoot basketball basket for extracurricular participants at SMK Negeri 1 Gombong. The results of the t test showed that there were an increase in the three point shoot results of the extracurricular participants of SMK Negeri 1 Gombong. This is indicated by the value of t-count = 2.789> t-table = 2.101, meaning that there is a significant influence. Thus the null hypothesis (Ho) which reads "There is no influence of imagery on the increase in the ability of three points of basketball shoots for extracurricular participants in SMK Negeri 1 Gombong" was rejected. This means that imagery training has a significant effect on increasing the three-point shoot results of extracurricular participants at SMK Negeri 1 Gombong.

The group that did the basketball three-point shoot exercise which was accompanied by imagery training increased 23.7%. Whereas in the control group who did the three point shoot exercise without imagery exercise also experienced an increase of 4.2%. The difference in the percentage of the process between the experimental group and the control group was 19.5%. So it can be concluded that imagery training gives an effect of an increase of 19.5% on the increase of three point shoots for male basketball extracurricular members of SMK Negeri 1 Gombong in 2017.

Imagery training itself is one way to help improve the skills of a player or athlete in the process of mastering difficult techniques in the sport he is practicing. According to Komarudin (2013: 85) imagery exercises proved to provide benefits for athletes / students to re-create the motion experience in their brains, so that the athlete made it possible to display the motion patterns well. Furthermore Hopla (2012) states that a basketball player can improve their overall skills through mental imagery. For example, players who want to improve their shooting skills can take a few minutes and imagine becoming a successful shooter. Each step in the shooting process is visualized and felt in the imagery exercise.

According to Wissel (2000) today some practitioners basketball have used mental imagery exercises that describe structured mental training techniques to create an optimal exercise performance. Based on research that has been conducted on students of basketball extracurricular participants at SMK Negeri 1 Gombong, it is known that imagery exercises can improve the three point shoot skills. This is because imagery exercises provide a deeper experience not only in the experience of physical motion, but also the experience of motion in students' cognitive. So that students will find it easier to master difficult and complex movements. However, students must be really serious when doing this exercise if they want to get maximum results, because imagery training requires good concentration in the process.

The study of the effect of imagery training on the improvement of three-point bolabket basketball technique for extracurricular participants at SMK Negeri 1 Gombong provides an opportunity for students to be able to master and improve the three-point shoot skill well. Besides intu students also get knowledge about what is imagery training and its uses related to efforts to improve mastery of techniques that exist in basketball. The results of this study also inform that the treatment of imagery exercises can be used as an effective way to improve the mastery of the three point shoot skills of basketball extracurricular participants.

From the discussion above, it can be concluded that imagery training has an effect on increasing the three-point skills of basketball extracurricular participants in SMK Negeri 1 Gombong. Thus this imagery exercise can be a solution for students of basketball extracurricular participants in an effort to improve the ability of the three point shoot. This was indicated by the results of the study which showed that there were differences in the improvement of three point shoot technique skills between students who were given imagery exercise and students who were not given imagery exercise treatment.

DISCUSSION

In accordance with the result findings elaborated in the previous part, some aspects related to this research implementation are presented as follows.

First, the aspect of social behavior is categorized as good. Human is a growing being that always thrive on living. Children's growth and development are rapid and fundamental in their early age. The children's development depends greatly on the stimulation given in the early age. It is in line with Singh (2016: 282) opinion stating that

"... the important part of social development is on how children interact in their environment to serve the children's need on developing their social skill and mental."

This opinion supports the research findings in which respondents learn to provide curriculum which enables children to learn to interact and exercise and then develop their emotional and social skills. The environment this study took place enables children to interact with each other, so it can develop good social and emotional skills. On the contrary, Su et al. (2016: 159-160) argues that the inability to interact in physical activities through sports causes inadequacy of social behavior including the lack of self-conception. The argument concludes that the high level of self-conception will improve children motivation to be actively participate in physical activities and exercise.

The development of human resources who are physically, psychologically, mentally, and emotionally healthy depends on the growth and development processes. The development involves physical, cognitive, emotional, and psychological growth of children at the age of infancy and toddlerhood (0-3 years old), early childhood (3-6 years old), and middle childhood (6-11 years old). A study done by Güçlü (2016: 2) proves that the social skill level and the personality of an athlete enhance as his/her physical and sport abilities are improving. It proves that movement development is closely related to children's social and character development. Moreover, it is supported by a research finding revealed by Vlahov (2014: 289) that early age children's movement development can predict their physical fitness and health when they are in senior high school.

Second, regarding the aspect of fine motor skill, it can be concluded based on the obtained mean score that the children's motor skills are categorized as good. It indicates that children of early age get opportunities to develop fine motor skill in a good education. Early childhood is the golden age of individual development span. At this period, children have the greatest motor skills, emotional, cognitive, and psychological growth. Children's development is a holistic process. Thus, stimulation should be provided in holistic activities. Perceptual motor skill can be used to develop fine motor skill as Hong (2010: 77) says that activities, such as arranging blocks, building Legos, drawing, or playing games requiring fingers usage are essential in improving children's fine motor skill.

Third, based on the research findings, it is concluded that the children's language skill aspect is categorized as good. 61.91% of the children have good vocabulary mastery. Besides, in relation with children's cognitive and language skills, Santrock(2017) said its (50) states that language skill is influenced by other developmental aspects especially physical and intelligence aspects. Children who interact using different languages show significant language skill development. As it is shown from the research findings, each child's development has different physical development as in language skill development. There are children who grow rapidly or slowly. Fourth, in accordance with the children's gross motor skill, the respondents of the study (4-6 years old) have well-coordinated gross motor skill. Their movements are in accordance with their need and desire. This period is shown with hyperactive and movements. The children tend to perform plenty agile and energetic gross motor skill movements. Hence, the age range (4-6 year old) is the ideal period to learn motor skills in some activities such as: writing, drawing, painting, swimming, playing football, and doing athletics activities. Kelly (2010: 20) states that in that period children have mastered locomotors skills in order to participate in various games, sport, and physical fitness activities.

The understanding of children growth and development pattern is really needed by parents and teachers in order to take care of the environments where children are stimulated to learn. Children's growth and development are rapid processes. Every process leads to the skills. However, there is no sufficient evidence in relation to benefits of children's physical activities and sports. Vella (2014; 6) states maintaining information on children's development on report cards can help parents and teachers in optimizing children's movement development.

Children's motor skills development, social and emotional development, and abilities to acquire and use language are very essential in developing new skills needed for their growth in every stage of development to become the pinnacle of future generation. Parents and teachers can enhance children's exploration and curiosity by improving their growth and development holistically. Jarani (2015: 11) states that there needs to be an intervention on physical education program and curriculum to improve children's physical abilities. It is in line with the research done with children in Albania. Based on the explanation, children's motor skills development will become a good potential when supported with sufficient preparation on a good physical education program and a curriculum that is developed based on children's movement development.

Based on the previous discussion, it can be inferred that children's motor skills development is an important part in the human life span. On the other hand the more important thing is how children innate motor skills can be optimized in a program suitable with children needs, so they can benefit from doing appropriate physical activities. Veldman et al. (2017:53) states that children's physical and sports inactivities should be noticed; especially when they are incapable in most everyday life skills. This indicates that motor skills development is an aspect people should focus on in order to make sure that children will grow as qualified and competitive human resources.

CONCLUSION

Based on the research results obtained with the data analysis and hypothesis testing, it can be concluded that there is a positive and significant effect of treatment of imagery exercises to increase the ability of three point shoot the basketball game participants extracurricular student of SMK Negeri 1 Deal. Basketball extracurricular student participants who obtain additional imagery exercises on an exercise program three point shoot, was found to increase the ability of the more significant when compared with students in extracurricular basketball participants who do not obtain additional imagery exercises on an exercise program three point shoot .

REFERENCES

Allen, K.E. & Marotz, L. R. (2010). Developmental profiles: pre-- birth through twelve, 6th edition. Belmont, CA: Wadsworth, Cengage Learning.

Berg, L. E. (2002). Infants, children and adolescents, 4th edition. Boston, MA: Allyn and Bacon.

Bergen, Doris. 2008. "Stages of Play Development," Play as a Medium for Learning and Development. Doris Bergen,ed.,Portsmouth, NH: Heinemann.

Biechler, RF & Snowman, J. (2003) Psychology Applied Teaching. Toronto: Houghton Mifflin Company.

Bowlby, J and Ainsworth, M. 1992. The Origins Of Attachment Theory. Developmental Psychology, 28, 759-- 775; available at: http://www.psychology.sunysb.edu/attachment/online/inge_origins.pdf

Bremner, J. G. (2017). An introduction to developmental psychology. John Wiley & Sons.

Güçlü, Mehmet et. al. 2016. An Examination On The Personal And Social Adjustment Levels Of The Athletes According To The Gender, Age And Branch Variables. The Online Journal of Recreation and Sport – January 2016 Volume 5, Issue 1

Hong, Chia Swee.; Gabriel, Helen.; St. John. 2010. Sensory Motor Activities for Early Development. Specchmark Publisher Ltd.

Indrawati, Maya dan Nugroho, Wido. 2006. Mendidik dan Membesarkan Anak Usia Pra-Sekolah. Jakarta: Prestasi Pustaka Publisher.

Jarani et. al. 2015. Effects of two physical education programmes on health- and skill-related physical fitness of Albanian children. Journal Of Sport Sciences. Routledge Taylor & Francis. http://dx.doi.org/10.1080/02640414.2015.1031161

Jürimäe, Toivo & Jürimäe, Jaak. 2000. Growth, physical activity, and motor development in prepubertal children. Washington DC: CRC Press.

Kelly, Luke E. et. All. 2010. Everyone Can: Skill Development and Assessment in Elementary Pysica Education. Champaign IL.: Human Kinetics.

Kurtz And Lisa A. 2007. Understanding Motor Skills in Children with Dyspepsia, ADHAM, Autism, and Other Learning Disabilities: A Guide to Improving Coordination (KP Essentials Series) (KP Essentials). Jessica Kingsley Pub. ISBN 1-84310-865-8.

Logan, S. W., Barnett, L. M., Goodway, J. D., & Stodden, D. F. (2017). Comparison of performance on process-and product-oriented assessments of fundamental motor skills across childhood. Journal of sports sciences, 35(7), 634-641

Lowery, S. E., Kurpius, S. E. R., Befort, C., Blanks, E. H., Sollenberger, S., Nicpon, M. F., & Huser, L. (2005). Body image, self-esteem, and health-related behaviors among male and female first year college students. Journal of College Student Development, 46(6), 612-623.

Marta, C. C., Marinho, D. A., Barbosa, T. M., Izquierdo, M., & Marques, M. C. (2012). Physical fitness differences between prepubescent boys and girls. The Journal of Strength & Conditioning Research, 26(7), 1756-1766.

O'Regan, J. Kevin & Noe, Alva. 2000. What it is like to see: A sensorimotor theory of perceptual experience http://nivea.psycho.univparis5.fr/Synthese/MyinFinal.-html

Payne, V. Gregory & Isaacs, Larry D. 2017. Human Motor Development A lifespan Approach. Nineth Edition. Routledge.

Riduwan. 2012. Belajar Mudah Penelitian Untuk Guru, Karyawan, Peneliti Pemula. Bandung: Alfabeta

Singh, Kuldeep. 2016. Role of physical education and sports in Indian prospective: An over view. IJPESH. P-ISSN: 2394-1685, E-ISSN: 2394-1693

Su, Xiaoxia et. al. 2016. At-Risk Boys' Social Self-Efficacy and Physical Activity Self-Efficacy in a Summer Sports Camp. Journal of Teaching in Physical Education, 2016, Vol 35, 159 -168. Human Kinetic Inc.

Sudjana. 2003. Metoda Statistika. Bandung: Tarsito Press.

Supartini. Y. 2004. Buku Ajar Konsep Dasar Keperawatan Anak. Jakarta: EGC

Tientje, Nurlaila N.Q. Mei dan Iskandar, Yul. 2004. Pendidikan Anak Dini Usia Untuk Mengembangkan Multipel Inteligensi. Jakarta: Dharma Graha Group.

Thelen, E., & Bates, E. (2003). Connectionism and dynamic systems: Are they really different? Developmental Science, 6, 378–391

Veldman, et. al. 2017. Promoting Ball Skills In Preschool-Age Girls. Journal Science and Medicine In Sport. Vol. 20(2017). 50-54.

Vella, Stewart A., et. al. 2015. The contribution of organised sports to physical activity in Australia:Results and directions from the Active Healthy Kids Australia 2014 Report Card on physical activity for children and young people. Journal of Science and Medicine in Sport, 2015

Vlahov, Eric et. al. 2014. Preschool Motor Development Predicting High School Health-Related Physical Fitness: A Prospective Study. Perceptual And Motor Skill: 2014, (Published Manuscript) 119, 1, 279-291. ISSN 0031-5125

Spencer, J. P., Perone, S., & Buss, A. T. (2011). Twenty years and going strong: A dynamic systems revolution in motor and cognitive development. Child Development Perspectives, 5(4), 260-266.

Phillips, E., Davids, K., Renshaw, I., & Portus, M. (2010). Expert performance in sport and the dynamics of talent development. Sports medicine, 40(4), 271-283.

Santrock, J. W., & Rollo, D. (2017). Psicologia dello sviluppo. McGraw-Hill Education.

26

Short Run Capability Improvement Efforts Through Varied Learning Approaches

Jasmani

Department of Sport Coaching Education, Faculty of Teacher Training and Education, Universitas Tunas Pembangunan, Indonesia

Article History

Keywords:
Class action; Run; Learning Approach

Abstract

The purpose of this research was done to upgrade the learning approach through the short run variable on the students grade 3 son SD N Krebet 3 Masaran Sragen 2015/2016 school year. This research is Class action, research was conducted with two-cycle and do the analysis it can be concluded that increased learning outcomes atltetik number of short run through the learning variable approach is characterized by an increase in the value of the average student. The average value of the students on the initial conditions of 60.56 with ketuntasan percentage of 6.67%. The condition has increased the value of the average students in cycle I, i.e. of 62.20 and ketuntasan percentage of 10.00%. However, the increase has still not reached the targets set earlier. Then after continuing to cycle II the average value of the short run capability of the students again experienced an increase of ketuntasan percentage of 74.70 with 80.00%. This indicates that the target set previously already accomplished so research stopped in cycle II. The process of learning the number of short run Athletics through learning approach markedly dynamic and fun takes place and the results of observation of the teacher when learning is also increasing in every meeting.

Correspondence address :
Jl. M Walanda Maramis no. 31 Cengklek Mojosongo, Surakarta District, 57127 Central Java
E-mail: j.jasmani9@gmail.com

INTRODUCTION

Athletics for elementary school different from adult athletics, athletics for primary emphasis on aspects of play because playing is part of children's lives. Sujiono (2009) "for a child's play is an activity that they do throughout the day due to the child's play is life, life is a game". While according to Soejadi (1981) "children's games are games that have rules simple is easy to understand, easy to implement, and will affect the child's development and growth of children". In a form of the game should give pleasure, satisfaction, joy and happiness because it is favored by children. Athletics are playing can increase motivation and attention to children and do not let go of the items contained in the Athletics itself as the basic motion run, the way, jump, and throw. Athletic games does not mean eliminating the element of seriousness, ignoring the element of dexterity or eliminate substance through an athletic staple material itself but the athletic game which contains a set of basic motion run, the way, jump, and throwing the game presented in the form of which varies in enriching the Treasury of children's basic motion.

One of the basic motion of Athletics was run. A run is a capability that is marked by the process of with moving the position of the body from one place to another quickly with the movement of the float in the air. According to S (2001), generally running movement characteristics are (a), the attitude of the body leaning slightly forward, the point is to minimize air resistance coming from the direction of the front runner and the benefit to penapakan point weight is more forward, (b) steps must be longer, make this walk along it may be possible at the beginning of the legs off from the start, so that the balance of the body stay awake then step foot should already begin shortened but with the frequency of the motion accelerated, fixed or (c) when the landing legs, landing to the ground while being exposed should always on the tip of the sole of the foot with the knee slightly skewed position so limber at the time would have made the next step, (d) the movement of the arms, fingers or dikepalkan opened the meeting and relax, swing hands must be coordinated with the movement of the legs and at a time when the left foot stepping forward as then the left hand must be behind, and vice versa at a time when the right foot stepping in the future, then the right hand must be behind.

Based on observations conducted researchers against the teachers of physical education and student son SD N Krebet 3 Masaran Sragen upon learning the basic motion run Athletics retrieved data as follows: (1) students who do not look running movement semangan and doing random, (2) at the time of short-run movements of the students focus in a race with the temennya of the truth movement in flight, (3) lack of infrastructure mejadikan students must undertake activities learning running short on the school, (4) while learning the basic of athletic motion in particular short run many students who are lazy to do.

According to Rusyan (1989) how active student learning is not intended so that the students do a variety of learning activities learning activities by origin but that take precedence are learning activities that involve mental optimally though often requires the involvement of physical activities. In addition to the lack of ability of teachers in a fun learning methods applying to result in students being excited and not lose the liveliness of the students in the process of teaching and learning. Varied learning methods to run short, namely: (1) the game run short, (2) games run across the barrier (3) games run Chase pungung, (4) short-run Game with racing, (5) games running relay pass through obstacles. With the form of the variation of learning used in the short run in the short run capabilities expected of students can be increased and the learning process more fun and children are not easily bored.

Based on the background of the problems that have been presented so researchers took the title "short run capability improvement efforts through varied learning approaches at students grade 3 son SD N Krebet 3 Masaran Sragen 2015/2016 school year". The purpose of this research was done to upgrade the learning approach through the short run variable on the students grade 3 son SD N Krebet 3 Masaran Sragen 2015/2016 school year.

METHODS

Further research done 2 cycles, each of the main activities that exist in each cycle, namely: (a) planning, (b) implementation, (c), (d) the observation of the reflection which is described in **picture 1**. In operating the research steps are as follows

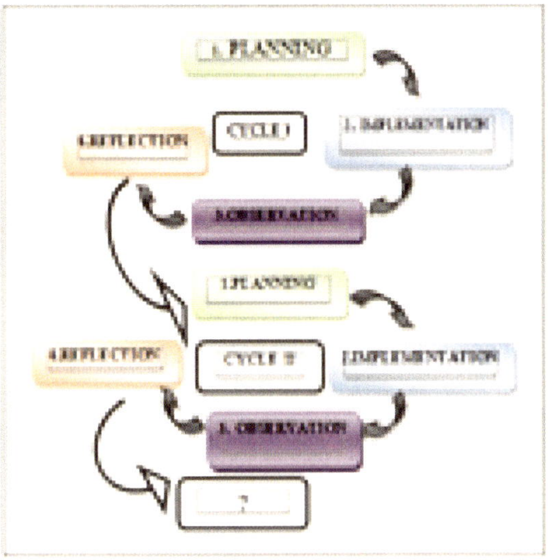

Picture 1. the flow of execution of the Research Action Class. (Source: Suharsimi Arikunto, 2008)

Population and sample in this research is the grade III elementary school ELEMENTARY SCHOOL N 3 Krebet Masaran Sragen which numbered 30 students comprise 17 students are sons and 13 daughters schoolgirl, and the entire population of class III will be in research namely sempel 30 students.

The technique of data collection has a very important role in a studies because the data used to address problems in research. Therefore activities to collect data should be based on your with the right techniques so that the retrieved data is really relevant and useful. According to Winarno (2007), "data collection is the process of identifying and collecting information that researchers do, in accordance with the purpose of research". Data collection procedure that is done in this research are as follows; observations, interview, documentation, field notes.

RESULTS AND DISCUSSION

Initial conditions

Initial conditions based on basic competency test atltetik test on the material the ability run short, it turns out that the result is still less satisfying, even though the teacher had already tried everything possible so that students understand. The results of the cognitive domain of learning results obtained average value of the mean value, 43.34 realm of affective students of 56.78, and average values for the results of a study on the psychomotor domain of 63.56. Short-run assessment of results obtained from the highest grade students is 75 and the lowest value 55. The average value of the class for a short run of only material 60.56, with the number of students who "finished" just as much as 2 students (6.67%) of the total number of students in whole 30 students. While the students are "not finished" as much as 28 students (92.33%) of the amount entirely 30 students. So it was concluded that the value of the grade 3 students in learning the material in short run Athletics first-year lessons 2015/2016 are still not in accordance with the indicators of the success of student learning. Indicators of the success of the learning of students who applied in SD N Krebet Masaran, Sragen 3 Masaran, Sragen district is a minimum of 70% of the total students in one class have reached the criteria of "mastery".

Observations of the cycle I

Observations are used to observe learning learning approach through short run variable is created using the criteria of the assessment so that it is easy to conclude the results of the observations. The results of observations of the collaborators against the teacher in the learning cycle I produce a value of 70 (category enough). Result observation of short-run floor gymnastics learning through game approach markedly on the students grade 3 son SD N Krebet 3 Masaran Sragen school year 2015/2016 on cycle I presented in **table 1-4** as follows:

Table 1. Assessment of the Psychomotor domain

Aspect	Description
Average Value	68,8
The Number Of Learners Has Been Completed	10
The Number Of Participants Who Havent Completed	20
Percentae Of Mastery	33,33%
Unfinished Percentage	66,67%

Table 2. Assessment of the Affective domain

Aspect	Description
Average Value	66,00
The Number Of Learners Has Been Completed	12
The Number Of Participants Who Havent Completed	18
Percentae Of Mastery	40,00%
Unfinished Percentage	60,00%

Table 3. Assessment of the Cognitive domain

Aspect	Description

Average Value	62,20
The Number Of Learners Has Been Completed	3
The Number Of Participants Who Havent Completed	27
Percentae Of Mastery	10,00%
Unfinished Percentage	90,00%

Table 4. Recapitulating the value cycle I

Aspect	Description
Average Value	52,33
The Number Of Learners Has Been Completed	5
The Number Of Participants Who Havent Completed	25
Percentae Of Mastery	16,67%
Unfinished Percentage	83,33%

Based on the results of the test cycle I obtained results are still less satisfying, even though the teacher had already tried everything possible so that students understand. The results of the cognitive domain of learning results obtained average value of the average values, 52.33 realm of affective students amounted to 66.00, and the mean value of the results of the study on the psychomotor domain of 68.80. Short-run assessment of results obtained from the highest grade students is 82 and the lowest value is 45. The average value of the class for a short run of only material 62.20, with the number of students who "finished" just as much as 3 students (10.00%) of the total number of students in whole 30 students. While the students are "not finished" as much as 27 students (90.00%) of the total number of students, then 30 entirely research resumed in cycle II.

Observations

Observations were used to observe the short run through the learning game approach markedly created using criteria so easily summed up the results of the observations. Observations a. Observations observations used to observe learning game approach markedly pendekmelalui a run was made using criteria so easily summed up the results of the observations. The results of observations of the collaborators against the teacher in the learning cycle I produce a value of 70 (category medium) and increased in cycle II of 90 (both categories). Result observation of short-run learning through learning approach markedly on the students grade 3 son SD N Krebet 3 Masaran Sragen school year 2015/2016 on cycle II is presented in **table 5-8** as follows:

Table 5. Assessment of the Psychomotor domain

Aspect	Description
Average Value	75,15
The Number Of Learners Has Been Completed	26
The Number Of Participants Who Havent Completed	4
Percentae Of Mastery	86,67%
Unfinished Percentage	13,33%

Table 6. Assessment of the Affective domain

Aspect	Description
Average Value	72,00
The Number Of Learners Has Been Completed	22
The Number Of Participants Who Havent Completed	8
Percentae Of Mastery	73,33%
Unfinished Percentage	26,67%

Table 7. Assessment of the Cognitive domain

Aspect	Description
Average Value	74,73
The Number Of Learners Has Been Completed	24
The Number Of Participants Who Havent Completed	6
Percentae Of Mastery	80,00%
Unfinished Percentage	20,00%

Table 8. Recapitulating the value cycle II

Aspect	Description
Average Value	73,33
The Number Of Learners Has Been Completed	21
The Number Of Participants Who Havent Completed	9
Percentae Of Mastery	70,00%
Unfinished Percentage	30,00%

Based on the results of the test cycle I obtained results still less satisfying, even though the teacher already tried everything possible so that students understand. The results of the cognitive domain of learning results obtained average value of the average values, 72.00 realm of affective students of 77.33, and average values for the results of a study on the psychomotor domain of 75.15. Short-run assessment of results obtained from the highest grade students is 90 and the lowest value is 58. The average value of the class for a short run of only material 74.70, with the number of students who "finished" as many as 24 students (80.00%) of the total number of students in whole 30 students. While the students are "not finished" as 6 pupils (20.00%) of the total number of 30 entirely students, then the research is considered successful.

CONCLUSION

After a class with two action research cycle and do the analysis it can be concluded that increased learning outcomes atltetik number of short run ahead through varied learning approaches are characterized by an increase in the value of the the average students. The average value of the students on the initial conditions of 60.56 with ketuntasan percentage of 6.67%. The condition has increased the value of the average students in cycle I, i.e. of 62.20 and ketuntasan percentage of 10.00%. However, the increase has still not reached the targets set earlier. Then after continuing to cycle II the average value of the short run capability of the students again experienced an increase of ketuntasan percentage of 74.70 with 80.00%. This indicates that the target set previously already accomplished so research stopped in cycle II. The process of learning atltetik number of short run ahead through learning approach markedly dynamic and fun takes place and the results of observation of the teacher when learning is also increasing in every meeting.

REFERENCES

BSNP. 2006. Standar Isi Sekolah Dasar (SD)/Madrasah Ibtidaiyah (MI). Jakarta: Badan Standar Nasional Indonesia.

Dwiyogo, W. D. 2010. Dimensi Teknologi Pembelajaran Pendidikan Jasmani dan Olahraga. Malang: Wineka Media.

Rusyan, T. 1989. Pendekatan Dalam Proses Belajar Mengajar. Bandung: Remaja Karya CV.

Sidik, D. Z. 2010. Mengajar dan Melatih Atletik.

Sujiono, Y.N., 2009. Konsep dasar pendidikan anak usia dini.

Winarno, B., 2007. Kebijakan Publik: Teori dan Proses. Yogyakarta: Media Pressindo.

Implementation of Physical Education Learning K-13 Class 11 Semester I in Senior High School

Angga Adi Prasetya[1], M E Winarno[2], Dona Sandy Yudasmara[3]

Universitas Negeri Malang, Malang, Indonesia[123]

Article History

Keywords:
Learning; Physical Education; Curriculum.

Abstract

The purpose of this study was to investigate the implementation of physical education learning based on the 2013 Curriculum in the 11th grade at Senior High Scholl "SMAN 8 Malang". The method used in this research was non-experimental research design in the form of descriptive survey. The subjects used were 3 physical education teachers as well as 110 students of 11th graders, and there were 10 students taken from each class. The sampling technique used was proportionate sampling. The instruments used for collecting data were observation techniques, questionnaires, interviews and documentation. Meanwhile, the technique used to analyze the data was qualitative descriptive. From the results obtained of the questionnaires, it was found that only 88% the acquisition of the physical education learning based on the 2013 Curriculum was used, while 12% were not implemented. Suggestion that could be given to the teacher was teaching physical education should be given in accordance to the 2013 Curriculum as a whole.

Correspondence address :
E-mail: dona.sandy.fik@um.ac.id

INTRODUCTION

The learning process of Physical Education, Sport and Health (PJOK) in schools in the current era has changed. This happens because the implementation of government policies that are set to be implemented in schools. One of the policies applied is about the use of the curriculum as a description of the learning content to be implemented. The curriculum used today is the 2013 curriculum.

The curriculum is a curriculum that puts forward the scientific approach in its implementation process. The scientific approach emphasizes the learning process thoroughly and gives students the opportunity to literate on the subject matter learned. Literacy will lead learners not only to read, write and perform movements (in physical education), but to enable students to study, understand, construct and analyze learning materials. Literacy can encourage students to be able to develop self potential optimally and can do learning activities holistically (Lundvall, 2015; Roetert & Mac Donald, 2015)

All subjects in the 2013 curriculum are taught by the (scientific) approach. That students are invited to observe, reason, ask and try. A total of seven study materials that must be mastered by students. Yet essentially scientific approach has also been used in KTSP, but the term used is the approach of inquiry. Thus will be realized learning atmosphere and learning process so that learners can actively develop their potential. Selection of teaching method becomes one of the factors of realizing a conducive learning atmosphere. The selection of this teaching method will depend on the classroom management, the amount of study time, and the student's activity. (Syrmpas et al., 2017). The scientific approach in Curriculum 2013 becomes an important supporting factor to create a conducive learning environment. This scientific approach also makes it possible to create group learning dynamics, unite ideas for the completion of learning tasks, learn to respect each other's opinions, provide experience in decision making, can be a motivation to always do learning activities and control group learning dynamics to be better (Leonard, 2015).

The true scientific approach is in line with the term inquiry because the sequence of the sequence of implementation of the method is the same as the scientific approach. The phase sequence in the inquiry approach is generalized to several steps.

The inquiry approach starts from the conceptualization phase of the idea in which the student frames the idea idea of matter, the investigation phase where the student will make the planning, exploration and hypothesis of the material being studied, the experimentation phase where the student will experiment as well as the discussion and reflection phase as to review the process , inputs and outcomes of the learning activities undertaken. Some of the previous research findings suggest that this inquiry approach can also increase students' learning motivation because the series of processes performed provide extrinsic stimuli for students in conducting learning activities (Pedaste et al, 2015; Bayram et al, 2013)

There are some contents in the 11th semester physical education curriculum for high school. The contents of the curriculum include: (a) Games and sports consisting of soccer games, volleyball games, basketball games, table tennis softball games, martial arts badminton games, Racewalking, bullets, long jumps. (b) Gym activities consisting of straddle jump and tuck jump. (c) Development activities consist of body composition, heart and muscle resistance, speed, agility, balance, and coordination. (d) Rhythmic activity consists of systematic exercises with music (e) water activities consisting of freestanding pools, chest pools, backstroke pools, butterfly swimming pools (f) from concepts, benefits, principles, impacts and designing physical activity, hazards, modes of transmission, and how to prevent HIV.

The purpose of physical education is to change the behavior of learners through the activity of motion. Development of potential learners can be maximized through physical education because in it allows children to learn various activities of body movement that allows residual meninkatkan potential physical, skills, knowledge, skills and social and moral aspects (Paturusi, 2012). Physical education allows students to develop personal potential because in its implementation allows students to develop a mindset, it is because the capacity of motion skills of each individual is different so that to meet the demands of the motion students must be able to find the capacity of each individual self (Balan et al, 2012). The result of initial observation on physical education learning activity found that the learning is not implemented as a whole and the learning done in SMAN 8 malang is only done based on existing facilities and infrastructure but less well optimized, whereas inSenior high scholl "SMAN 8" Malang has many field and facilities adequate to physical education learning activities. Existing sports facilities include 1 badminton court in the hall and 1 room with gymnastics floor, 1 basketball court, 2 indoor and outdoor futsal courts, 1 volleyball court, while the facilities in sma 8 are 6 soccer balls, 12 basketball, 1 table and net table tennis, 4 bolavoli, 4 wicket futsal, basketball hoop, 2 net badminton, 2 mats. Teachers play an important role as planners, managers, colleagues, physical education professionals, counselors (teacher counselors). Lutan (2002) states the effectiveness of learning which is the task of teachers consisting of several management dimensions that include, (1) management of teaching tasks, (2) behavior management, (3) time management, equipment. Teachers are expected to be able to translate well the content of the study written in the curriculum document. The success of one learning activity will be determined by the suitability of the content of the teaching materials taught with the curriculum documents that serve as the basic reference. The findings of previous research mentioned that the learning of K-13 physical education for high school students in Bondowoso city level 2 is less in accordance with the 2013 curriculum as reference. This study aims to determine learning physical education and health Curriculum 2013 class 11 semester I in high school " SMAN 8 Malang".

METHODS

Based on the research problem, then in this research using non experimental research design in the form of Descriptive Survey, because in this research do not give treatment. Judging from the purpose of research is to know the implementation of physical education education K-13 class 11 semester 1 in SMA 8 Malang, then this research includes the type of descriptive research The method used in this research is descriptive qualitative research with qualitative approach. Subjects used in this study were physical and sports education teachers at SMAN 8 Malang, and 11th graders . The data about the number of physical education teachers of sports and health teaching in SMAN 8 Malang amounted to 3 teachers, and 110 students of the total 11 students of grade 11 which amounted to 346 students and each class will be taken 10 students. The sampling technique used in this research is the technique of proportional sampling. The instrument used in this research is non test instrument in the form of questionnaire which will be filled by physical education teacher of sport and health, and 11th graders in SMAN 8 Malang. Questionnaire is a data collection technique that is done by giving a set of questions or written statement to the respondent to be answered. (Sugiyono, 2009).

Data collection techniques in this study is to use observation techniques, questionnaires / questionnaires, interviews and documentation. Data analysis technique used is qualitative descriptive analysis technique. The results of the research will be described as qualitative research results, while data processing in this study using Miles and Huberman model analysis. There are three stages in doing the analysis with data reduction (summarizing, choosing the main points, then focusing on the things that are important, searched for the theme and pattern, display data (display data in the form of tables, graphics and the like) and conclusion or verivication, and data deduction will be grouped into nine sections based on research variables (Sugiyono, 2009) .Then the results will be presented in the form of quantitative research with percentage, after which the results are quantitative in the form of calculated figures search percentage, then be interpreted with a quantitative sentence.

RESULTS AND DISCUSSION

The availability of facilities and infrastructure supporting physical education learning activities at SMAN 8 Malang is sufficient. Based on the findings of research conducted SMAN 8 Malang has facilities and infrastructure supporting physical education as follows:

Table 1. Infrastructure Supporting Learning Activities Physical Education at SMAN 8 Malang

Type Of Infrastructure	Acount	Discription
badminton court	1	-
Floor Gymnastics Room	1	-
Basket court	1	-
Indoor Futsal Field	1	-
Outdoor Futsal Field	1	-
Volleyball field	1	-
Total	**6**	

Table 2. Supporting Facilities of Learning Activities Physical Education at SMAN 8 Malang

Type of Facilities	Acount	Discription
Football Balls	6	-
Basketball Balls	12	-
Table Tennis and Net	1	-

Volleyball Balls	4	-
Basketball hoop	4	-
Net Badminton	2	-
Floor Gymnastics Mat	2	-
Total	**31**	

The amount of facilities and infrastructure of learning physical education in SMAN 8 Malang can be served to provide learning materials listed in the Curriculum 2013 (K-13). It can be seen from several types of facilities and existing infrastructure that allows to be used, both for materials in accordance with the function of facilities and infrastructure or for other materials that are not in accordance with the functions of facilities and infrastructure. Several types of existing facilities can be used for other materials that require space availability that can utilize some existing field, so that learning can still be implemented.The results of observations made on learning activities carried out on materials physical education, sports and health in SMAN 8 Malang obtained data as follows:

Table 3. Design of Learning Process on PJOK subjects for games and sports activities, Athletics, Ritmik and Gymnastics at SMAN 8 Malang

Elements Supporting Learning Activities	Physical fitness			Aqua-tik	Health
		Blnc	Agl	crawl	Health
Availability of learning devices	The Benefits of Physical Activity	1	1	1	1
Number of meetings	1	1	1	1	1

Sp: Speed; Blnc: Balance; Agl: Agility

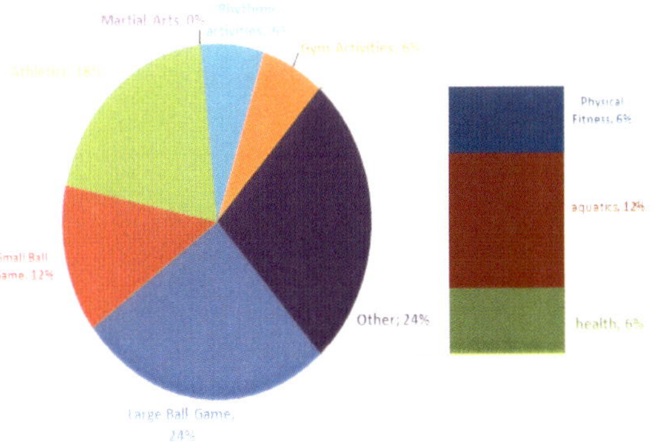

Figure 1. Percentage of instructional materials taught in 1 semester.

Table 4. Design of Learning Process on PJOK subjects for Physical Fitness, Aquatics, and Health at SMAN 8 Malang

Elements Supporting Learning Activities	P. Big Balls			P. Small Balls		Athletics		Rit-mic	Gym-nastic
	FB	VB	BB	SfB	BT	RB	Sp	Arb	Arg
Availability of learning devices	1	1	0	0	0	0	0	0	0
Number of meetings	1	2	1	1	1	2	1	1	1

Informasi :

FB : Football SfB: Softball Sp: Sprint

VB: Volleyball BT: Badminton Arb: Aerobik

BB: Basketball RW: Racewalking Sn.Kt: Artistic gymnastic

Based on the results of research conducted, the implementation of physical education education Curriculum 2013 (K-13) class 11 semester I in SMA Negeri 8 Malang is appropriate. The basis can be seen based on the lessons learned, but for the lesson of physical education subject with the implementation of K-13 physical education less than complete and less appropriate, the existing RPP only 5 include: (1) big ball game (football and volleyball). (2) Physical fitness (physical fitness exercise). (3) Water activities (pool freestyle) (4) Health.

K-13 physical education learning outcomes conducted at SMAN 8 Malang, physical education learning K-13 in accordance with the curriculum listed in the school described in **tebel 5** following;

Table 5. Data on Learning Result Analysis of Physical Education K-13

Material	Result Score	Percentage
Large Ball Game	4	24%
Small Ball Game	2	12%
Athletics	3	18%
Martial Arts	0	0%
Rhythmic Activities	1	6%
Gym Activities	1	6%
Physical Fitness	1	6%
Water Activities	2	12%
Health	1	6%
Total	**15**	**88%**

Based on the above description, the findings in this study are as follows: (1) Lessons and teachers of physical education are less creative in developing lesson plans and learning media of physical education that can help the implementation of physical education learning K-13, and the lack of attention of physical education teachers to certain subjects so that students can not accept the material well (2) In every lesson, physical education teacher always apply scientific study, so that in physical education education which is done not only focus on teacher and there is reciprocity between student and teacher. (3) Lesson Plan (RPP) used in learning is incomplete and not in accordance with K-13 physical education learning, so less interesting learning and does not vary. (4) Physical education education K-13, teacher never made lesson plan, so learning physical education done without any lesson plan.

Table 6. Summary of Research Findings.

Types of Learning Materials	Availability of Learning Device	Findings
Large Ball Game	There is a learning tool, but only on soccer and Volleyball material	Large ball games are presented presented four meetings covering the soccer material sub presented one time, the bolavoli is served twice, the bolabasket is served once.
Small Ball Game	There is no learning tool	mall ball game presented twice meeting encompassing softball sub subject presented once, badminton served once, small ball game.
Athletics	There is no learning tool	Athletics presented three meetings covering the material sub-street quickly presented twice, a short run distance is served once, high jump is not served at all, the bullets are not served at all.
Martial Arts	There is no learning tool	Martial arts are not presented due to lack of adequate facilities and infrastructure.
Rhythmic Activities	There is no learning tool	Rhythmic motion presented once a meeting, sub-material presented is a systematic exercise of motion with the accompaniment of rhythm.
Aquatics Activities	There is a learning tool, but only swimming material crawl style	Aquatics sub-material presented is the swim movement of the crawl style
Gym Activities	There is no learning tool	Gym Activities presented at one meeting, sub-material presented by gymnastics floor
Physical Fitness	There is a learning tool, but only on Agility, Balance and Speed	Physical fitness is presented once a meeting, sub-material presented type of physical activity and measurement of physical fitness.
Health	There is a learning tool, but only on the physical activity benefit material	Health presented 1 one meeting encompasses sub content of physical activity benefit
Out door Activities	There is no learning tool	Not present

DISCUSSION

Means of learning activities in physical education consists of classrooms, field games and the race, while the infrastructure in the form of sports equipment support games and measurable. Two things must be fulfilled due to the learning process using motion activities that are adapted from sports activities as the main media. In an effort to fulfill the facilities and infrastructure, several things are done such as adjustment of human resources condition and management of learning activities. This resource adjustment is done to avoid overloading teachers in teaching activities and maximizing the availability of learning facilities. Overly high teaching loads will result in reduced teaching practice practices will decrease as well as smaller classroom volume arrangements may allow students to have more participation to move. (Turner et al, 2017; Kirkham-King et al, 2017)

Sports activities require field or equipment supporting the game. Each school does not necessarily have an overall facility that matches the material contained in the PJOK 2013 curriculum. Teachers of physical and health education subjects are expected to make modifications and improvisation activities tailored to the availability of facilities and infrastructure in the school. Intervention to learning activities due to certain conditions (lack of condition of facilities and infrastructure) can encourage students to learn maximally (Kawabata & Harimoto, 2018). Modifications need to be done in an effort to deliver the subject matter as a whole. Planning of learning activities must be done by the teacher. Planning a good learning activity will determine the learning process that will be done. There is a positive influence between the readiness of learning devices with the learning process keselurahan done, but if the readiness of instructional devices are not well prepared then the learning process will not take place effectively, both from the aspects of the process of implementation of activities, content and assessment. Planning of learning activities will also determine the learning objectives to be achieved. (Soumokil & Zamroni, 2013; Wibawa & Kartowagiran, 2014; Wang et al, 2017). Learning planning is also the basis for program activities during the learning process takes place. Planning of learning activities can be done by teachers with various levels.

Based on previous research findings mentioned that there is no significant difference in the preparation of learning tools by teachers who have different levels of teaching experience and different levels of education (Stănescu, 2013). Activity planning is very important to be done by teachers, especially by teachers who do not have the experience to facilitate communication to students and do good class management (Wahl-alexander et al, 2017). The findings of the research obtained that the teachers Physical Education And Health in SMAN 8 Malang only set up learning tools on certain material alone so that the administrative completeness of learning activities are still declared less.

Data analysis of the implementation of learning PJOK K-13 in SMAN 8 Malang, teachers PJOK apply scientific approach, in accordance with the mandate on K-13. Learning is designed not to center on the teacher. The scientific approach involves inviting students to begin observing, reasoning, questioning and experimenting. These activities can trigger students to be more actively involved in learning activities. The learning process is emphasized on the collaboration of teachers and students and the pattern of assignment to students. The pattern allows students to have more interest in learning than when students only do the instructions given by the teacher. Collaboration between teachers and students can improve students' active learning activities. (Roure & Pacso, 2017)

Implementation of K-13 for subject of physical and health education at SMAN 8 Malang can be done although some completeness related to learning administration has not been done optimally. The scientific approach to learning process of physical education and health remains the main focus of teachers in conducting learning activities. In line with previous studies related to the implementation of the scientific approach in the learning of physical and health education it is stated that there is an increase in the average value and percentage of learning completeness after the application of scientific approach to learning physical education and health (Rangga, 2016). In contrast to other research findings stating that K-13 learning practice has not been able to give a significant impact on student learning outcomes due to the acceptability of teachers and students to the new curriculum practice has not been less than the maximum due to changes in the management process of learning and different teaching load. (Putra & Qoriah, 2016)

Optimizing the implementation of K-13 in Senior High School will be possible when all the elements involved can be open and follow the changes actively. In K-13 all written materials are expected to be taught to students. Implementation of physical education and health education K-13 in SMAN 8 Malang has not been categorized perfect because there is still material that is not presented in the learning activities. Martial material is not taught to students due to lack of facilities for martial activities. In line with other research findings mentioned that found obstacles in the provision of martial material due to inadequate infrastructure and low interest in the material martial art. (Tama & Purwono, 2017). Lesson K-13 will run optimally when all the supporting elements have been met well.

CONCLUSION

Based on the results of data exposure and discussion it can be concluded the implementation of physical learning K-13 class 11 semester 1 year 2016/2017 in SMAN 8 Malang is in accordance with the curriculum 2013, It can be seen in the implementation of learning that has been designed in the number of scheduled meetings. In relation to instructional tools (RPP) is poorly administered, it is because the lesson plans (RPP) that exist in the school are only composed of large ball games (soccer and bolavoli), physical fitness (physical fitness measurements), water activities (pool) and health (physical activity).

REFERENCES

Balan, V., Marinescu, G., Ticala, L., & Shaao, M. (2012). Physical Education–Longlife Learning

Factor. Procedia-Social and Behavioral Sciences, 46, 1328-1332.

Bayram, Z., Oskay, Ö. Ö., Erdem, E., Özgür, S. D., & en, . (2013). Effect of inquiry based learning method on students' motivation. Procedia-Social and Behavioral Sciences, 106, 988-996.

Kawabata, M., & Harimoto, F. (2015). Facilitating flow experience in physical education settings. Manuscript in preparation for publication.

Kirkham-King, M., Brusseau, T. A., Hannon, J. C., Castelli, D. M., Hilton, K., & Burns, R. D. (2017). Elementary physical education: A focus on fitness activities and smaller class sizes are associated with higher levels of physical activity. Preventive medicine reports, 8, 135-139.

Leonard, F. J. (2015). The Analysis of the Scientific Research Projects Management in the Higher System of Physical Education. Procedia-Social and Behavioral Sciences, 180, 1248-1252.

Lundvall, S. (2015). Physical literacy in the field of physical education–A challenge and a possibility. Journal of Sport and Health Science, 4(2), 113-118.

Lutan et al., 2002. Supervisi Pendidikan Jasmani. Depatermen Pendidikan Nasional, Jakarta

Paturusi, A. 2012. Manajemen Pendidikan Jasmani dan Olahraga. Jakarta: Rineka Cipta

Pedaste, M., Mäeots, M., Siiman, L. A., De Jong, T., Van Riesen, S. A., Kamp, E. T., ... & Tsourlidaki, E. (2015). Phases of inquiry-based learning: Definitions and the inquiry cycle. Educational research review, 14, 47-61.

Putra, y. S., & qoriah, a. (2016). Implementasi kurikulum 2013 mata pelajaran penjasorkes di sekolah pengembangan dan percontohan. Active: journal of physical education, sport, health and recreation, 5(3), 122-125.

Rangga, g. (2016). Peningkatan hasil belajar sepak bola melalui pendekatan scientific dalam pembelajaran penjasorkes. Active: journal of physical education, sport, health and recreation, 5(3), 158-164.

Roetert, E. P., & MacDonald, L. C. (2015). Unpacking the physical literacy concept for K-12 physical education: What should we expect the learner to master?. Journal of Sport and Health Science, 4(2), 108-112.

Roure, C., & Pasco, D. (2017). The Impact of Learning Task Design on Students' Situational Interest in Physical Education. Journal of Teaching in Physical Education, 1-29.

Soumokil, A., & Zamroni, Z. (2013). Kontribusi perangkat pengajaran, motivasi belajar, pelatihan ktsp terhadap proses pembelajaran PPKN sman kota ambon. Jurnal evaluasi pendidikan, 1(2), 103-115.

St nescu, M. (2013). Planning physical education–from theory to practice. Procedia-Social and Behavioral Sciences, 76, 790-794.

Sugiyono. (2009). Metode penelitian kuantitatif, kualitatif dan r&d. Bandung: alfabeta.

Syrmpas, I., Digelidis, N., Watt, A., & Vicars, M. (2017). Physical education teachers' experiences and beliefs of production and reproduction teaching approaches. Teaching and Teacher Education, 66, 184-194.

Tama, r. A., & purwono, e. P. (2017). Survei kendala pelaksanaan pembelajaran pjok materi pencak silat smp negeri di kabupaten semarang. Active: journal of physical education, sport, health and recreation, 6(1), 53-61.

Turner, L., Johnson, T. G., Calvert, H. G., & Chaloupka, F. J. (2017). Stretched too thin? The relationship between insufficient resource allocation and physical education instructional time and assessment practices. Teaching and Teacher Education, 68, 210-219.

Wahl-Alexander, Z., Curtner-Smith, M. D., & Sinelnikova, O. A. (2017). Influence of a Training Program on Preservice Teachers' Ability to Negotiate With Students. Journal of Teaching in Physical Education, 1-31.

Wang, J., Shen, B., Luo, X., Hu, Q., & Garn, A. C. (2017). Validation of A Teachers' Achievement Goal Instrument for Teaching Physical Education. Journal of Teaching in Physical Education, 1-27.

Wibawa, E. A., & Kartowagiran, B. (2014). Kesiapan perangkat pembelajaran pengantar akuntansi dalam rangka implementasi kurikulum 2013. Jurnal evaluasi pendidikan, 2(2), 123-134

Physical Condition as a Contribution of Shooting Accuracy with Flick Drag Technique

Kartika Septianingrum[1], Sugiyanto[2], Agus Kristiyanto[3], Nuril Lolita Hudayhana[4], Dhevana Pradika Yanda Putra[5]

Postgraduate Program, Sebelas Maret University, Surakarta, Indonesia[123]
Departement of Sport Science, Surabaya State University, Surabaya, Indonesia[4]
Project Fellow, University of Muhammadiyah Semarang, Semarang, Indonesia[5]

Article History

Keywords:
Physical Condition; Contribution; Drag Flick.

Abstract

The purpose of this study was to examine how much the contribution of grip strength, arm muscle power, flexibility togok, and eye and hand coordination to shooting accuracy with drag flick technique. This research uses correlational method. A total of 40 men's hockey players were selected as samples in this study. The data analysis technique used multiple regression and coefficient determination test (R2). It can be concluded that the grip strength variable, arm muscle power, togok flexibility, and eye and hand coordination have an effect on shooting accuracy with drag flick technique and produce significant contribution. Relationship with Flick Drag shot accuracy was power muscle arm with a result of 34.6%, then body flexibility of 20.5%, holding strength of 17.9%, and the least contribution of hand-eye coordination of 14.3%.

Correspondence address :
E-mail: kartika_septianingrum@yahoo.co.id

INTRODUCTION

Exercise is an activity that has many benefits. Sport is not only aiming to be healthy but sports can also measure the achievement of a person or team. Like the sports hockey which is a sport that much in demand. This can be seen with the many holding of hockey cleric either local, national or international level. In a hockey sport every individual or team must outperform the other both technically and strategically to win the game. Increased technique should also be supported by the increase in physical condition (Bompa, 2018). Measurement of physical conditions is important in supporting the practice of a hockey player to achieve excellence in play. A focused hockey player there is a development of physical conditions as part of their preparation in play. Currently the measurement of physical condition becomes a guide for the coach as well as the hockey player itself to create a training schedule to support hockey players in mastering the technique of playing hockey.

A good hockey player must master the basic techniques of sports hockey one of them is shooting techniques. The shooting technique becomes one of the techniques in hockey sport that needs to be mastered properly because shooting is the decisive victory of a team. The more shots are generated the greater the team's chance to win. The shot in the hockey game is the Attacker's action trying to score by playing the ball into the goal of the inner circle. "The ball may miss the mark but it is still a" shot on goal "if the player's intention is to score with a shot towards the goal. (FIH, 2016). The attacking player must be able to put his shot in an accurate position or position that is difficult to reach by the goalkeeper. The quality of the resulting shot depends on how the physical condition is owned by each player. Good physical condition is needed by players to support the success of shooting. Each player has different physical conditions that will affect motor skills, techniques, tactics. The performance of a hockey player depends on the level of motor skills, techniques and tactics during the competition. (Septianto, 2016; Elferink-Gemser et al., 2004). Drag flick is one of the most commonly used shooting techniques in hockey games. Research conducted by (Rajinikumar, 2015) says that 59% of goals occur because of direct fire, 38% occurred because of penalty corner, and 2.5% occurred due to penalty stroke. Of the three, 34.5% of the techniques used in goal scoring are the drag flick technique. (Hussain, et al 2012) explains further in recent years, the penalty corner, especially with the advent and popular hit drag flick, has gained an important part of the game as a scoring opportunity.

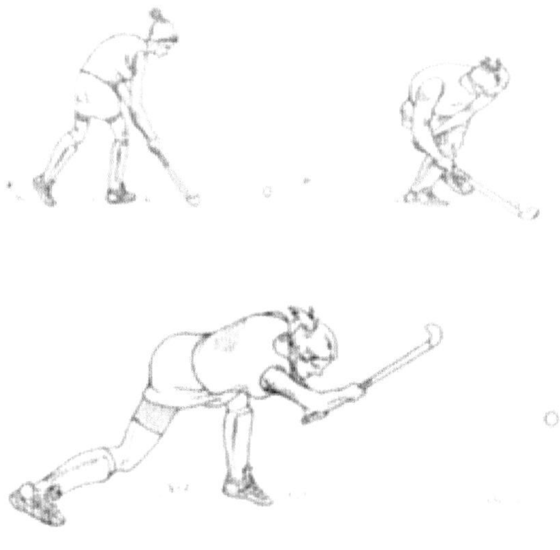

Picture 1 :Drag flick
(Anders, 1951)

The popularity of drag flick techniques became an innovation and became an important part of the team while attacking. Drag flick is an important technique, which makes the game more interesting. Drag flick is commonly used in the penalty corner, and is used as a variant to shoot. In addition to the above techniques are also required physical capabilities that support the results of shooting performance on the game hockey. Arm muscle strength, hand strength, flexibility of arms and leg strength are the physical components that support the game of Hockey (Nurhidayah et al., 2014; Lythe et al., 2011). In this tuliasan, the author will reveal what factors are related, forming the accuracy of Drag flick and punch determination. This study also aims to find out how big the contribution of physical performance relationship to the accuracy of drag flick blows.

METHODS

The method in this research is correlational research. Correlational research is a study that aims to determine the relationship between two or more variables and to detect the extent to which variables on one factor relate to variations on one or more other factors based on correlation coefficient (Siswanto, 2013). This research is a correlation research, which want to investigate whether or not correlation between independent variables with dependent variable. The independent variables in this study are the holding power (X1), arm muscle power (X2) flexibility posture (X3), and hand eye coordination (X4), while the dependent variable is shooting accuracy with drag flick (Y) technique.

Researchers used a sampling technique with cluster random sampling, where in this sampling the population is divided into several clusters or clusters. Randomly the necessary clusters are taken with the randomization process. Each of the different members in the randomly selected clusters is a necessary sample (Sudjana, 2002). In this study there are 4 research variables and researchers using random sampling technique. So the sample to be taken by researchers amounted to 40 players hockey in Central Java.

The instrument used to measure hand grip strength using handgrip dynamometer is a tool for measuring grip strength (Sri, 2009). To measure the arm muscle power is a medicine ball weighing 2 kg, with the validity of 0.77 and reliability 0.84 (Johnson, 1986). The instrument used to measure togok flexibility uses sit and reach test (Verducci, 1980). The instrument used for measuring hand eye coordination is a ball-throwing test (Maskum, 2007). The instrument used to determine the accuracy of the shot with the drag flick technique is using shooting test with the validity of 0.89 and the reliability of 0.94 (Puji, 2013)

Analytical techniques in this study using multiple regeneration anaisis because the independent variable has more than two variables. Regression equation in this research is to know how big influence of independent variable or free that is handheld strength (X1), flexibility of strike (X2), eye coordination (X3) and power of arm muscle (X4), to shooting accuracy by Drag Flick Technique Y). The mathematical formulas of the multiple regression used are:

To measure how far the whole independent variable can explain the dependent variable using the coefficient of determination (R2).

$$Y = a + b1X1 + b2\ X2 + b3X3 + b4X4 + e$$

To measure how far the whole independent variable can explain the dependent variable using the coefficient of determination (R2).

RESULTS AND DISCUSSION

Based on the results of measurements of grip strength, arm muscle power, flexibility togok, hand eye coordination, and shooting accuracy by drag flick technique in Central Java in June 2017 through a survey with test techniques. In this research get the respondent counted 40 respondents, with characteristic for first variable that is holding strength biggest result is 52 kg, smallest result is 26 kg and result of power average equal to 37,38. The second variable is the largest arm muscle power yield is 560 cm, the smallest result is 250 cm, and the average 389 cm. The third variable is flexibility of togok largest result is 23 cm, the smallest result is 0 cm, and the average value is 10.97. The fourth variable is the largest hand-eye coordination result is 18 times, the smallest result is 7 times, and the average value is 12 times the average value of throw is 12 times the throw. The fifth variable is the accuracy of the result of shooting with drag flick the greatest result is 19 points, the smallest result is 6 points, and the average value is 12 points. Here are the results of Multiple Regression Analysis shown in table 1 below :

Table 1. Results of Double Regression Hypothesis Test

Variable	Unstandardized Coefficients Beta
Constant	1,763
Gripping Power	0,064
Arm Powe	0,015
Body Flexibility	0,054
Eye and Hand Coordination	0,150

Source : Processed Data, 2017.

The regression equation is known :

Shooting Results = 1,763 + 0.0,0 KM + 0.015 POL + 0.054 FT + 0.150 KOM + e

The constant of 1.763 with positive parameters indicates that grasping power, arm muscle power, body flexibility, and hand eye coordination will improve shot accuracy by drag flick technique. Based on the above equation can be interpreted as follows:

1) Coefficient value of grip strength of 0.064. This implies that the variable holding power has a positive relationship with the result of shooting with drag flick technique which means that every increase of power holds one unit then the accuracy of firing with drag flick technique will increase by 0,064 with the assumption that the other independent variable from the regression model is fixed.

2) regression coefficient of arm muscle power equal to 0,015. This implies that the arm muscle power variable has a positive relationship with the results of shooting with drag flick technique which means any increase in arm muscle power of one unit then the accuracy of shooting with drag flick technique will rise by 0.015 with the assumption that other independent variables of the regression model is permanent.

3) The regression coefficient of posture flexibility is 0,054. This means that the variable flexibility of body has a positive relationship with the result of shooting with drag flick technique which means any increase of flexibility body one unit then the accuracy of firing with drag flick technique will rise by 0.054 with the assumption that other independent variables of the regression model is fixed.

4) Regression coefficient of hand eye coordination of 0.150. This implies that hand eye coordination variables have a positive relationship with the results of shooting with drag flick technique which means any increase of eye hand eye coordination then the accuracy of firing with drag flick technique will rise by 0.150 with the assumption that other independent variables of the regression model is permanent.

The following table 2 shows how much power the relationship with the accuracy of the drag flick technique shot

Table 2. R2 Test Determination

Equation	R	R Squared
Gripping Power	,423	,179
Arm Power	,589	,346
Body Flexibility	,453	,205
Eye and Hand Coordination	,378	,143

Source : Processed Data, 2017.

1) The Power of Grasping

The value of correlation relationship (R2) is 0,179. The effect of gripping force on firing accuracy with drag flick technique is equal to R value of 0.423 indicates that the proportion of contribution of power variable grips against shoot accuracy variable with drag flick technique of 17.9%. This means that the contribution of power gripping the shoot with drag flick technique contributes 17.9%.

2) Power Sleeve Muscles

The value of correlation relationship (R2) is 0.346. The effect of Powerotot lenganterhadap shooting with drag flick technique is equal to R value of 0.589 indicates that the proportion of variable contribution of arm muscle to shoot accuracy variable with drag flick technique of 34.6%. This means that the arm muscle power contribution to the accuracy of shooting with drag flick technique contributes 34.6%.

3) Flexibility of Strike

The value of correlation relationship (R2) is 0,205. Effect of togok flexibility on firing accuracy with drag flick technique is equal to R value of 0.453 indicates that the proportion of contribution of body flexibility variable to shoot accuracy variable with drag flick technique is 20.5%. This means that the contribution of body flexibility to shoot results with drag flick technique contributes 20.5%.

4) Speech Coordination

The value of correlation relationship (R2) is 0,143. The effect of hand eye coordination on shooting accuracy with drag flick technique is equal to R value of 0.378 indicates that the proportion of contribution of hand eye coordination variable to shoot yield variable with drag flick technique is 14,3%. This means that hand eye coordination donation to the accuracy of shooting with drag flick technique contributes 14.3%.

Multiple regression analysis of grip strength measurement, arm muscle power, body flexibility, hand eye coordination have a positive relationship to shooting accuracy with drag flick technique. The biggest contribution in the accuracy of shooting with drag flick technique is the arm muscle power with the result of 34.6%, then the flexibility of togok is 20.5%, the holding power is 17.9%, and the least contribution is hand eye coordination of 14, 3%.

The arm muscle power is required to provide the strength and speed of the ball speed while performing the ball pushing motion. (Nurhidayah, 2014). Movement of the arm by the hockey player when firing using drag flick technique causes the ball to escape from the stick and slide toward the target. While the strength of the arm muscles when carrying the stick and pushing the ball will produce accurate shots if in pelaksanannya accompanied by the speed. A hockey player with a good togok flexibility will easily make drag flick moves and produce the perfect movement, otherwise if the hockey player has the flexibility togok the less well will eat difficulty in doing drag flick movement. as it is said (Ibrahim, 2009) in his research concludes that the flexibility of body is an underlying ability of a person's motion. The low body flexibility causes rigid movement, thereby reducing flexibility and flexibility of movement, which is a critical determinant element in successful field hockey shooting. A hockey player who has high body flexibility has the ability to perform better skill moves, rather than players who have low body flexibility.

Body flexibility is required when the ball is released or loose, the stick is on the body of the stick, because when the ball is in the shape of the shot more quickly and accurately different if the ball feels at the end of the stick when it is released then the shot becomes weak and widened. (Mohd et al., 2014) states that after crossing the foot the player is forced to position his body as low as possible and advocate the stick as low as possible with the ground. In addition, in the movement to release the ball from the hip, chest, and shoulder sticks to rotate to produce the right target shot.

In addition, the strength of the grip is also influential to determine the direction of the ball, with a good grip then the stick will not be easily separated because if the stick is released during the shot then will change the position of the stick face and will change the target of the targeted shot. Verma (2014) in his research reveals that holding power helps players defend angles.

Coordinate when doing drag flick technique is on the accuracy of placement of the ball on the body of the stick so that the ball can be pushed to the maximum then gouged and placement of the shot to enter the goal in accordance with the desired target. The eye receives the first stimulus of the brain to do the motion and then the hand gives an answer in the form of the movement. Both of these tasks must be done jointly.

Seeing the usefulness of drag flick is important for any hockey player to master this technique and can be applied during the competition. Physical condition factors are needed to support success in performing this technique. In addition technical factors become supporters in doing drag flick. Increased exercise especially for body parts used to perform drag flick techniques need to be done by players and coaches to assist players in supporting success in training and in competitions that will impact on improving hockey achievement.

CONCLUSION

The conclusions in this research are (1) There is a positive relationship between grasping power to the accuracy of shooting with drag flick technique which means the stronger grip the stick the accuracy of the shot more accurate. Contribution of power variables grasping to shoot yield variable with drag flick technique equal to 17,9%. (2) There is a positive relationship between arm muscle power to shooting accuracy with drag flick technique which means bigger arm muscle power then accuracy of fire more accurate. Contribution of variables of arm muscle power to shoot yield variables with drag flick technique of 34.6%. (3) There is a positive correlation between togok flexibility to shooting accuracy with drag flick technique which means better body flexibility then accurately more accurate shot accuracy. Contribution of variable body flexibility to variable result of firing with drag flick technique equal to 20,5%. (4) There is a positive relationship between hand eye coordination to the accuracy of shooting with drag flick technique which means the better hand eye coordination then the more accurate the shots. The contribution of hand eye coordination variable to shoot yield variable with drag flick technique is 14,3%.

REFERENCES

Anders, E. (1951). field hockey step to success. USA: Human Kinetics.

Bompa, T. O. (2009). Periodization: theory and methodology of training. Orietta Calcina.

Elferink-Gemser, M., Visscher, C., Lemmink, K., & Mulder, T. (2004). Relation between multidimensional performance characteristics and level of performance in talented youth field hockey players. Journal of Sports Sciences, 22(11-12), 1053-1063.

FIH. (2016). Rule of Indoor Hockey. Switzerland: International Hockey Federation.

Hussain, I., Ahmed, S., & Khan, S. (2012). Biomechanical Study on Drag Flick in Field Hockey. INTERNATIONAL JOURNAL OF BEHAVIORAL SOCIAL AND MOVEMENT SCIENCES, 186-193.

Ibrahim. (2009). PERBEDAAN PENGARUH METODE LATIHAN DAN FLEKSIBILITAS TOGOK TERHADAP KETERAMPILAN MENEMBAK HOKI LAPANGAN. Surakarta: Universitas Sebelas Maret.

Johnson, B. L. (1986). Practical Measurements for Evaluation in Physical education (3rd ed.). New Delhi: Surjeet Publications Indian reprint.

Khan, I. H. (2012). Biomechanical Study on Drag Flick in Field Hockey. NTERNATIONAL JOURNAL OF BEHAVIORAL SOCIAL AND MOVEMENT SCIENCES, 186-193.

Lythe, J., & Kilding, A. E. (2011). Physical demands and physiological responses during elite field hockey. International Journal of Sports Medicine, 32(07), 523-528.

Maskum, A. (2007). Tes dan Pengukuran dalam Olahraga. Surabaya: Universitas Negeri Surabaya.

Mohd, A., Tel, A., & Fuzail, B. (2014). Three Dimensional Analysis of Drag-flick in The Field Hockey of University Players. Advances in Physics Theories and Applications, 87–93.

Nurhidayah, E., Rahayu, S., & Waluyo, M. (2014). Sumbangan Power Otot Lengan, Kekuatan Genggaman, Fleksibilitas Pergelangan Tangan dan Kekuatan Tungkai terhadap Kemampuan Tembakan Penalti pada Hockey. Journal of Sport Sciences and Fitness, 3(1).

Puji, R. (2013). Pengaruh Senam Otak (Brainn Gym) terhadap Pemahaman Bermain Hoki. Bandung: Universitas Pendidikan Indonesia.

Rajinikumar, P. (2015). Analysis of field goal and penalty corner in hero hockey india League - 2013. Asian Journal of Multidisciplinary Research, 7-10.

Septianto, R. (2016). Tingkat Kebugaran Jasmani Siswa Peserta Ekstrakurikuler Hoki Di Smp Negeri 1 Mlati Sleman Tahun Ajaran 2015/2016. Pendidikan Jasmani Kesehatan dan Rekreasi, 1(9).

Siswanto. (2013). Metodologi Penelitian Kesehatan dan Kedokteran. yogyakarta: Bursa Ilmu.

Sri, H. (2009). Buku Pedoman Praktek Laboratorium mata kuliah Tes dan Pengukuran Olahraga. Semarang: Sang Pencipta.

Sudjana. (2002). Metode Statistik. Bnadung: Tarsito.

Verducci, F. M. (1980). Measurement Consepts in Physical Education. London: The C. V. Mosby Company.

Verma, S. K. (2014). Assessment of physical variables of drag flick performance in field hockey. Internaional Journal of Physical Education, 78–80.

29

Long Limb Prediction, Body Mass Index, Flexibility and Speed to Long Jump Style Squatting

Abdurrachman[1], Sugiyanto[2], Mucshin Doewes[3]

Program Pascasarjana, Universitas Sebelas Maret, Surakarta, Indonesia[123]

Article History

Keywords:
Length of Limbs;
Body mass index;
Flexibility of Strike;
Running Speed.

Abstract

This study aims to determine the relationship and how much the prediction of long jump squat style achievement in terms of limb length, body mass index, body fleksibility and running speed. The objective of this research is that trained students of state senior high school in Pekalongan Regency, with a total sample of 60 students. The independent variables in this research is limb lenght, body mass index, body flexibility, and running speed whereas dependent variable was long jump with squat style achievement. This study uses multivariat correlational method. The results showed that the length of the legs, body and togok flexibility has a positive relationship, whereas the body mass index and running speed has a negative relationship with the long jump squat style achievement. Prediction value at limb length was 0.027, body mass index was -0.049, body flexibility was 0.026 and running speed was -0.234. The conclusion of this study is that there is a significant relationship and can be predicted between limb length, body mass index, body flexibility and running speed against long jump squat style achievement.

Correspondence address :
Kampus Pusat Universitas Sebelas Maret. Jalan Ir. Sutami 36 A, Surakarta (Solo), Indonesia, 57126
E-mail: mans.fisio@gmail.com

INTRODUCTION

Long jump is a form of jumping movement that begins with horizontal movement and is transformed into vertical movement by doing repulsion on one of the strongest legs to get the distance as far as possible (Wiarto, 2013). According to Aip Syarifuddin (1992) the long jump is a form of moving forward foot forward in an effort to carry weight as long as possible in the air (flying in the air) is done quickly by doing repulsive force on one foot to reach a distance as far as possible. The fundamental factor that a jumper must possess is the ability to master the technical skills and ability of the physical condition. Adequate physical condition that will support the appearance of long jump when making a leap. Thus, physical conditions become important for jumpers because of the physical condition as a foundation for learning techniques, tactics, strategies, and mental. As for some components of the physical condition that greatly support the achievement of long jump, the elements are power, strength, flexibility, speed, kelinicahan, balance, coordination and reaction (Sajoto 1998). in the opinion of Suharno HP (1993) that the factors that determine maximal achievement include: (1) indogenous factors: good physical and mental health, body shape and body proportions, physical conditions and abilities, perfect mastery of techniques, mastering the problem of tatik, having the psychological aspect and the good personality and having the maturity of soul; (2) Exogenous factors: Coach (coach), coach assistant, trainer, venue, equipment, finance, organization, environment, government participation, methods and training system.

Long jump is a form of jumping movement that begins with horizontal movement and is converted to vertical movement by performing repulsion on one of the strongest legs to obtain the greatest distance (Wiarto, 2013). Ballesteros in Ade Mardiana, et al (2009) suggests that long jumps are the result of horizontal speeds made during the prefix with the vertical power generated from the strength of the repelling leg.

According to Ade Mardiana, et al (2009) that the basic principle of long jump is to build the fastest prefix and do the strongest repulsion toward the front-up with one leg to reach the optimal height when flying so as to produce the distance leap that far - he said.

Hadi Marwanto (2007) explains that the length of the leg is the vertical distance between the feet to the groin as measured by standing upright. The legs as a member of the lower motion serves as a support for upper limb motion, as well as determinants of movement in walking, running, jumping or kicking. According to Ade Mardiana et al. (2009) that the basic principle of long jump is to build the fastest prefix and do the strongest repulsion upward with one leg to reach the optimum height when flying so as to produce a leap- away. The longer the muscle gets stronger to move. A person who has longer leg lengths with another will likely have a better jump because of the wider jump or wider step toward the front. So the longer the legs will be the further jump or run in the long jump (Syaifudin Ilham, 2016).

The ideal body porposes are very important in achieving high achievement, as each sport demands an ideal body ideal in accordance with the terms of the sport that is followed. In general, athletes especially for long jump athletes should have the ideal high body size or portion (Amirudin, 2016). Hamlin (2013) states that a large body portion of his influence on a person's ability to exercise aktvitas. This is very much for the long jumping athlete, because with a good body poseposi the athlete will be easy to do repulsion and get a longer drift time during floating phase.

The flexibility of the body is thought to play a role in the determination of the long jump achievement whereby an athlete is concerned with the body during the floating phase, because the flexibility of the flexible body makes it easier for an athlete to position his body while flying and also when it falls (Syaifudin Ilham, 2016). In this case it is explained that flexibility is the effectiveness seserang in penyusuaian himself to do all the activities of the body with stretching as far as possible, especially on the muscles, ligaments around the joints. The higher the body flexibility the angle of body movement in the swing is also greater so that the power generated is also greater (M. Sajoto, 1995).

Running speed or prefix speed is one component of basic physical conditions that may affect jumping performance in long jump numbers, students will get good long jump performance. Due to the speed of a jumper run a jumper can increase the power of a forward impulse and when doing repulsion or take off (Jess Jarver, 2005). Running speed is defined simply, the step length of step frequency, is the determinant of running speed. To determine the running speed should be done by increasing one or both of these parameters, keeping in mind the good running technique (Aip Syarifuddin, 1992).

This study aims to determine whether there is a relationship seta prediction on the factors of anthopometri and physical ability to the achievement of long jump style squatting. Anthropometric factors are leg length and Body Mass Index (BMI), whereas in the ability of physical condition is the body flexibility and running speed.

METHODS

In this research the researcher use correlational research method by using approach approach survey method with test and measurement. Tests and measurements were performed to obtain an idea of the extent and relationship of leg length predictions (X1), Body Mass Index (X2), Body Flexibility (X3) and Running Speed (X4) to the squat style long jump achievement (Y).

Measurement instruments to be used in this study are as follows: Measurement of limb length using midline measuring instrument. Measurement of body mass index by measuring body weight and height by using measuring instruments stratu meter and scales. Measurement of back flexibility using the flexibility test test with sit and reach. Running speed measurements were measured using a 40 meter run track and measured with a stopwatch. Jogkok style long jump performance measurements using a squat style long jump test using a meter gauge.

Implementation of data analysis research, after data obtained from the results of further measurement analysis with regression techniques. But before performing the test of analysis first done a number of test requirements to determine the feasibility of data. The prerequisite test consists of a test of normality and a linearity test. After the prerequisite test, the next analysis is hypothesis test that is correlation coefficient analysis, multiple linear regression, F test and t test.

RESULTS AND DISCUSSION

Based on the data of test result and limb measurement, body mass index, body flexibility, running speed, and squat style long jump performance conducted in May-June 2017 with sample of 60 students trained SMA Negeri in Pekalongan Regency, group of research variables obtained analysis results for limb length variables obtained at least 70, maximum value 90, mean 78.6 with standard deviation 4,4501; for body mass index (BMI) variable, the value of at least 17, maximum value 29,4, mean 21,6 with standard deviation 2,8177; for variable body flexibility obtained a minimum value of 23, max value 47, mean 34.4 with standard deviation 5,5945; for running speed variables obtained a minimum value of 4.2, maximum value 6.6, mean 5.3 with standard deviation 0.6533; whereas for the variable achievement of long jump style squat obtained minimum value 3,2, max value 5,2, mean 4,4 with standard deviation 0,4330.

The results of normality test data performed on each group using SPSS 19.0 application through Kolmogorov-Smirnov test are as follows (**table 1**).

Table 1. Tests of Normality

	Kolmogorov-Smirnova		
	Statistic	Df	Sig.
Leg length	.104	60	.174
Body mass index	.079	60	.200*
Body Flexibility	.092	60	.200*
Running Speed	.111	60	.051
Long Jump Achievement	.100	60	.200*

From the normality test results in **table 1** found that the limb length variables obtained value of significance of 0.174 where the value is greater than 0.05 which means that the data on the limb length variables are normally distributed. In the body mass index (IMT) normality data, the value of 0.200 is obtained which is greater than 0.05, which means that the data on body mass index (IMT) variables are normally distributed. For variable flexibility togok obtained value of significance of 0.200 where the value is greater than 0.05 and has a normal data distribution. While the variable running speed obtained by the value of significance of 0.51 where the value is also greater than 0.05 which means the value of the data distribution is normal. And on the variable

Table 2. Regression Linearity Test

Independence Variable	Dependence Variable	F	Sig. (linearity)	Sig. (Deviation from Linearity)	Linearity
Leg Length (X1)	Long Jump Squat Style Achievement (Y)	0,543	0,119	0,907	Linier
Body Mass Index (X2)		2,230	0,005	0,157	Linier
Body Flexibility (X3)		1,035	0,000	0,447	Linier
Running Speed (X4)			0,000	0,130	Linier

of long jump achievement is got significance value 0,200 where the value is normal distribution.

From the result of **table 2** it can be seen that in the relation of long limb variable (X1) with the achievement of long jump style squat (Y) got the sig value. (linearity) 0.119 and sig. (deviation from linearity) 0.907, this proves that the variable has a significant linear relationship. On the relationship of body mass index variables (X2) with the achievement of long jump style squatting (Y) obtained sig value. (linearity) 0.005 and sig. (deviation from linearity) 0.157, this proves that the variable has a significant linear relationship. In the variable relation of body flexibility (X3) with long jump performance of squat style (Y) got sig value. (linearity) 0.000 and sig. (deviation from linearity) 0.447, this proves that the variable has a significant linear relationship. In the relation of variable running speed (X4) with the achievement of long jump style squatting (Y) got sig value. (linearity) 0.000 and sig. (deviation from linearity) 0.130, this proves that the variable has a significant linear relationship.

Table 3. Correlation Coefficient Analysis

Summary Model				
Model	R	R Square	Adjusted R Square	Std. Error of the Estimate
1	.715a	.511	.475	.3137

The result of correlation coefficient analysis can be seen in **table 3** obtained value R = 0,715 and value R2 = 0,511. Based on these results it can be stated that there is a significant relationship between the length of the legs, body mass index, body flexibility and running speed simultaneously with the achievement of long jump style squatting on students trained SMA Negeri in Kabupaten Pekalongan with the value of data analysis that is 0.715.

Table 4. Correlation Significance Test Results

ANOVA[b]					
Model	Sum of Squares	df	Mean Square	F	Sig.
Regression	5.649	4	1.412	14.352	.000a
Residual	5.412	55	.098		
Total	11.062	59			

Hypothesis test for variable limb length **table 4**, body mass index, body flexibility and running speed simultaneously using F test with 5% significance level obtained that significance value (0,000) <0.05 and Fcount = 14,352> Ftable = 2,540, then from test the hypothesis is accepted which means that there is a significant relationship between the length of the limb, body mass index, the flexibility of the body and the simultaneous running speed of the squat style long jump achievement.

While the hypothesis test for each predictor variable is obtained that **table 5**: limb length variable to the achievement of long jump squat style significance value (0.005) <0.05 and tcount = 2,915> ttable = 2,004, then from the test the hypothesis is accepted which means that there is a significant relationship between the length of the limbs against the long jump performance of the squat style; variable of body mass index to the achievement of long jump squat style value significance (0,002) <0,05 and tcount = -3,223> ttable = 2,004, hence from the test hypothesis accepted which mean that there is significant relation between body mass index to achievement

Table 5. Test Analysis of Multiple Regression coefficient

Coefficients[a]					
Model	Unstandardized Coefficients		Standardized Coefficients	t	Sig.
	B	Std. Error	Beta		
(Constant)	3.711	.859		4.319	.000
Leg Length	.027	.009	.278	2.915	.005
Body Mass Index	-.049	.015	-.318	-3.223	.002
Body Flexiibility	.026	.008	.330	3.274	.002
Running Speed	-.234	.069	-.352	-3.382	.001

of long jump squat style; the variable flexibility of body on the jumper long jump performance of significance value (0.002) <0.05 and tcount = 3.274> ttable = 2,004, then from the test the hypothesis is accepted which means that there is a significant correlation between the flexibility of body to the squat style long jump performance; while the running speed variables to the long jump performance of the squat style of significance value (0.001) <0.05 and tcount = -3.382> ttable = 2,004, then from the test the hypothesis is accepted which means that there is a significant relationship between the run speed against the long jump style achievement squat.

The result of regression coefficient correlation analysis from research can be written that simple linear regression formula is Y = 3,711 + 0,027 X1 - 0,049 X2 + 0,026 X3 - 0,234 X4. The interpretation of the above regression is as follows: Constanta (a), this means that if the limb length variable, body mass index, body flexibility and running speed have zero (0), then the value of the squat style long jump variable is 3.711.

Length coefficient value of 0.027. This implies that the limb length variable has a positive relationship with the long jump performance of the squat style which means that every increase of limb length of one unit then the jumper style long jump performance will rise by 0.027 meters with the assumption that the other independent variables of the regression model are fixed. The coefficient value of body mass index is -0.049. This implies that the body mass index variables have a negative relationship with the jumper style long jump performance which means any decrease in body mass index of one unit then the jumper style long jump performance will rise by 0.049 meters with the assumption that the other independent variables of the regression model is fixed . Together coefficient value of body equal to 0,026. This means that the variable flexibility of body has a positive correlation with the long jump performance of the squat style which means that each increase of flexibility of one unit body then the jumper style long jump performance will increase by 0,026 meters with the assumption that the other independent variable from the regression model is fixed. The value of the run speed coefficient is -0.234. This implies that the variable running speed has a negative relationship with the achievement of long jump style squat which means any decrease in the speed of one unit run then the jumper style long jump performance will rise by 0.234 meters with the assumption that the other independent variables of the regression model is fixed.

Discussion of the results of this study provides further interpretation of the results of data analysis has been done previously. Based on the hypothesis testing has yielded the conclusion of analysis that can be exposed.

In this study it was found that long jump athletes who had different leg lengths that were one long short in achieving a leap would be farther with long limbs. Each increase of limb length of one unit then the achievement of long jump style squatting will rise by 0.027 meters. Leg length is a strength advantage, because with a good long legs and explosive does not rule out the effect on muscle strength. The longer the muscle is stronger to move (Warsito, 2001). Viewed from biomechanics that long limbs have a longer or longer range. Thus, long legs have longer or longer swings, which can help achieve maximum jump spacing. The advantage of long legs is possible to increase the length of steps that can be done (Aip Syarifudin, 1996).

In the body mass index analysis also has a role in predicting the skip long jump style. Means any decrease in body mass index of one unit then the achievement of long jump style squats will rise by 0.049 meters Body weight and height is a part in biometrics that can affect the achievement of sports achievement. Adisasmita (1992) says that: The attractiveness of the earth caught at a point called "weight points". The weight is located at the waist, slightly below the navel.

At the time of a good landing on the long jump the squat style is a continuation of the squat style hovering pattern. Of course, should get the distance as far as possible, namely at the largest horizontal distance between the heel and center of gravity. So at the moment before touching the sand, both legs / limbs straightened / stretched forward and body bent forward (Jarver, 20015). The role of back spacing in the long jump is seen when the body whips forward as it flies. Good formation will provide a boost to mastery of techniques when performing long jump techniques especially when flying in the air. In this study the variable body flexibilit has a positive relationship with the achievement of long jump style squat which means any increase in flexibility togok one unit then the jumper style long jump performance will rise by 0.026 meters.

Running speed variables have a negative relationship with the achievement of long jump style squat, which means any decrease in the speed of one unit run then the achievement of long jump style squats will rise by 0.234 meters. According to Jess Jarver (1982) the leap away depends on running speed, strength and acceleration at take off (moving the horizontal speed to angular or vertical movement). The purpose of running before this jump is to increase maximum horizontal acceleration during take off.

Achievements that are optimal to achieve can be obtained by always paying attention to a fast technique, so that will produce a distance leap that far-away.

The results of this study can be seen that there is a relationship and prediction between the length of the leg, body mass index, flexibility togok and running speed together against the long jump style squatting. And it has a positive relationship on leg length variables and body flexibility, in other words if the value of limb length and body flexibility the greater, the greater the jump results in the long jump style squatting. While the variable body mass index and running speed have a positive relationship, which means if the body mass index and running speed is smaller then the greater the jump results in the long jump style squat Thus in this study if an athlete has a long leg, ideal body in this case has a low body mass index, large body flexibility and has a fast running ability it will get maximum jump results. So it can be concluded that between leg muscle strength, body weight and height influence and support in achievement of skip long jump jump results. And still there are other factors that affect the results of the long jump jump style squat not included in this study.

CONCLUSION

Based on the results of the research and the results of data analysis conducted, this study gives the conclusion that the variable length of the legs, body mass index, body flexibility and running speed have a partial or simultaneous relationship and become a predictor variable of squat style long jump performance on students trained SMA Negeri Regency of Pekalongan. The conclusions of this study are:

1. There is a significant correlation between the length of the limbs to the jumper style long jump performance with a prediction of 0.027
2. There is a significant relationship between the body mass index on the performance of long jump style squatting with a prediction of -0.049.
3. There is a significant correlation between the flexibility of body to the long jump performance of squatting style with prediction of 0,026.
4. There is a significant relationship between the running speed of the jumper style long jump performance with a prediction of -0.234.

REFERENCES

Ade Mardiana, Purwadi dan Wira Indra Satya. 2009. Pendidikan Jasmani dan Olahraga. Jakarta : Universitas Terbuka.

Adisasmita, Yusuf. 1992. Olahraga Pilihan Atletik. Jakarta: Depdikbuid.

Amirudin, P.S. 2016. Kontribusi Aspek Anthropometri dan Kapasitas Fisik Dominan Terhadap Prestasi Lompat Jauh Gaya Scheneppe. Kediri: Universitas Nusantara Pgri Kediri.

Hamlin, M.J and Sugiyama, Koji. 2013. Relationship Between Physical Fitness and Body Mass Index in 11 and 12 year Old School Children. New Zeland: Lincoln University. Japan: Shizouka University.

Ilham, Syaifudin, 2016. Hubungan Fleksibilitas Togok dan Panjang Tungkai Terhadap Kemampuan Lompat Jauh Gaya Schnepper. Kediri: Universitas Nusantara PGRI Kediri.

Jarver, Jess. 2005. Belajar dan Berlatih Atletik. Bandung: Poiner Jaya.

Kementerian Pendidikan dan Kebudayaan RI, 2014. Pendidikan Jasmani, Olahraga, dan Kesehatan - Edisi Revisi. Jakarta: Kementerian Pendidikan dan Kebudayaan RI.

Marwanto, Hadi. 2007. Sumbangan Daya Ledak Otot Tungkai dan Panjang Tungkai dengan Hasil Lompat Jauh Gaya Jongkok pada Siswa Putra Kelas XI SMA Negeri 13 Kota Semarang Tahun Pelajaran 2006/2007.

Sajoto, M. 1998. Peningkatan dan Pembinaan Kondisi Fisik dalam Olahraga. Semarang. Effhara Daharsa Prize.

Suharno, H.P.1993. Metodologi Pelatihan. Yogyakarta: IKIP Yogyakarta

Syarifudin, Aip. 1992. Atletik. Jakarta: Depdikbud

Warsito. 2001. Hubungan Panjang Tungkai dan Kekuatan Otot Tungkai Terhadap Hasil Lari 100 Meter pada Siswa Putera Sekolah Dasar Negeri Kelas VI di Kecamatan Pekalongan Timur Kota Pekalongan Tahun Pelajaran 200/2001. Semarang : UNNES

Wiarto, Giri. 2013. Atletik. Yogyakarta : Graha Ilmu.

The Utilization of the Environment as a Medium Instruction by Physical Education Teacher in the Coastal

Umar Nurzaman[1✉], Sulaiman[2], Agus Widodo Suripto[3]

Jurusan Pendidikan Jasmani, Kesehatan dan Rekreasi Fakultas Ilmu Keolahragaan, Universitas Negeri Semarang, Semarang, Indonesia[123]

Article History

Keywords:
The Coastal Environment; Media of learning; a Place of Learning.

Abstract

The purpose of this research is to know the types and ways to utilize the environment as a medium of learning from junior high school teachers in the coastal area of Kebumen Regency. This research method using qualitative research approach with data technique using interview technique, observation, and documentation. The research instrument uses interview guides and photo documentation. The results of environmental research are used as a place of learning in the coastal area Kebumen District, village buildings, beaches, and roads around the school. The environment used as learning media for Physical Education consists of paper assignment, modification of ball from coconut husk, perforated vessel made from used bucket, paint bucket cover and wood board for supporting learning. The conclusion of this research is the teacher of the coastal area surveyed Kebumen uses various ways to utilize the environment as a place of learning and learning media such as field to learn the big ball game and small ball game, while beach and school access road to learning athletics.

✉ **Correspondence address :**
Dusun Jerotengah Rt01/Rw08, Krakal, Alian, Kebumen 54532
E-mail: umarnurzaman88@gmail.com

INTRODUCTION

Physical education, health and sports is the main medium of education using physical activity or physical. Setiawan Aji (2012) is the Association of physical education pedagogy in the world of motion and physical appreciation. According to the Ega Trisna Rahayu in his book learning strategies of physical education, physical education is an educational process that utilizes the physical activity has been planned aims systematically to develop and improve individual organically, neoromuscular, perceptual, cognitive, and emotional, within the framework of national education (Ega, 2013). Physical Activity tailored to the selected objectives to be achieved and the capabilities of the students. The selected physical activity is emphasized in a variety of physical activities are reasonable, physical activity that requires little effort as a recreational activity and physical activity or in desperate need of hard effort such as for sporting activities coaching or achievements.

Physicaleducation, healthh and sports have the same goals with the goals of national education that is to equip students with skills or a useful life skill as a provision in the live the life at a later date. According to Aris Shoimin, "the education system in Indonesia should be in focus on the success of learners with the guarantee ability directed at life skill that can sustain the future well-being of the learners themselves to his family as well as the his future with a decent life in society "(Shoimin, 2014). One of the ketercapaian PJOK learning objectives is to equip students for skilled, responsive and capable of resolving the problems encountered in the environment of place of residence

The environment is where the activity of people's lives every day. Each region has different environmental characteristics. So the pattern of life of communities in each region will be different as well. The existence of the PJOK benefit from learning environment as a medium of instruction or as a place to learn it will be able to equip the student's skills in daily life in the neighborhood. The appropriate time to equip student skills is on the first level of secondary schools. A learning experience in the subjects of physical education of sports and health is directed to foster the growth of physical and psychic to be better development, at the same time shape the patterns of living lifelong healthy and fit. The Professional Physical Education teacher is very important role in order to achieve the Physical Education learning. As revealed by Herka Maya. J (2005) explains that a teacher who is a professional teacher who has high competence in teaching. They can design or designing a learning activity in any condition. Be it a minimal infrastructure, environment that is less conducive, even learners who have a background of affective abilities, cognitive, psychomotor, and different physical. In the use of media of instruction, teachers are required to always creatively exploit it or create the media. (Suherman, 2000) Physical Education learning with utilization of environment in every area. It is adapted to the geographical condition of an environment where learning takes place.

Kebumen Regency has 221 Junior High Schools (SMP) in every district, 24 of which are coastal area schools. The school is located in eight coastal subdistrict, subdistrict covering Ayah, Buayan, Puring, Petanahan, Klirong, Buluspesantren, Ambal, and Mirit.

Researchers have conducted the initial observation in some. There are SMP 1 Ayah, SMP 2 Ayah, SMP Negeri 1 Petanahan, SMP Negeri 1 Ambal and SMP PGRI 1 to find out the condition of the environment around the school. The results of these observations are presented in **Table 1.** below.

Table 1. The Results of the Environment Observation Around the School

School	the Environment Observation Around the School
SMP 1 Ayah	The village access road Rice fields The field village The beach
SMP 2 Ayah	The village access road The hills/karst The field village The beach
SMP PGRI 1 Ambal	The field village Rice fields The Streets of the village
SMP Negeri 1 Ambal	Ambal beach Coir handicrafts places The field village
SMP Negeri 1 Petanahan	Pertanahan beach The field village Sub gymnasium Argo tours

The observation result of early junior high school in the coastal area has no place for craft made extensive Physical Education learning. While the surrounding school environment there is a long beach, coir, handicraft industry and argue tours of plantations. The field village, and the access road to the school which can take advantage of as a medium or as a place of learning.

Based on the condition, researchers interested in conducting research on the utilization of instructional media or the environment as a place to learn Physical Education junior high school (SMP) in the coastal of Kebumen. Researchers want to find out more about the utilization of the environment in coastal areas as a medium of instruction or as a place to learn.

With respect to the background of the problems that have been expressed can be formulated some problems, the first is the environment anything that functions as a medium of instruction or places of learning by teachers of physical education and sports, health in high school the first coastal of Kebumen?, and the second is how teachers make use of the environment as a medium of instruction in the middle school PJOK district coastline area Kebumen.

The purpose of this research is to know the kind of environment that is utilized as a medium of instruction, or a place to learn from the teacher Physical Education in the coastal County of Kebumen, and to find out how teachers make use of the environment as a medium of instruction in the middle school PJOK district coastline area Kebumen.

METHODS

Research design is the blueprint that determines the execution further. Design research lays out the what, why, and how, the issue was examined by using the methodological principles. (Gulo, 2000) this research is research that is qualitative, because it intends to research and enter information as many of a certain incident. This research intends to find out and find as much information as the number of a particular incident and try to give you an idea of how big the level of creativity of Physical Education teachers in utilizing the environment as a medium Physical Education learning in junior high school, especially in coastal districts Kebumen. This research uses qualitative with data retrieval using interview techniques and observations.

The research subject is the retrieval technique with purposive sampling, namely choosing or selecting on the basis of criteria of terntentu created a number based on the purpose of research (Kriyanto, 2010). In the study of the subject is the teacher of the existing Physical Education in the coastal of Kebumen. The selection of the subject research was chosen based on the place of his junior high school (SMP). Starting from a school close to the beach, to a school far from the beach but still in the coastal County of Kebumen. The following is a list of schools that will be made the subject of research i.e. SMP Negeri 1 Mirit, SMP Negeri 1 Ambal, SMP Negeri 2 Ambal, SMP PGRI 1 Ambal, SMP Negeri 1 Petanahan, SMP Negeri 1 Ayah dan SMP Negeri 2 Ayah.

Qualitative data analysis starting from the analysis of various data that has been collected either researcher interviews, observation, and documentation. The data is then classified into particular categories-categories. Classification or pengkatagorian considers the validity (kevalidan), with attention to the competence of the subject, the degree of auntentisitasnya and do triangulation as a source of data (Kriyanto, 2006).

The data analysis process begins with a gather researchers throughout the whole data information obtained from interviews, observation and documentation. On analysis of data concerning the competence of the teacher Physical Education concerning the utilization environment of coastal areas as a medium of instruction. Researchers classify the data into categories of teacher competence, the competence, the competence of personality pedagogy, professional competence, and social competence. Researchers do a triangulation method, i.e. clarify data obtained with interviews, and documentation with the method of observation. Observations to test the validity of the data is done by observing the teachers learning activity.

This research uses qualitative-descriptive type. This research type is based on the basic question of ' how ' (Gulo, 2000). If the exploratory research conduct exploitation against the symptoms or an event, descriptive studies trying to dig deeper into why the symptoms or an event occurs. Thus the findings of researchers a broader descriptive and exploratory research was more detailed **Table 2.** of results Data retrieval based on standards of Competency learning Curriculum.

RESULTS AND DISCUSSION

Understand And Practice The Concept Of Motion Skill Fundramental The Small Ball Game

On the standard of competence this matter Physical Education teacher that utilizes the environment as a place of learning is the Physical Education teacher in SMP Negeri 1 Petanahan by making use of learning material for Badminton gymnasium. Other matters of Physical Education teacher SMP Negeri 2 Ambal utilizing the existing environment that is coir used to fill small plastic balls in a ball

Table 2. Table of results Data retrieval based on standards of Competency learning Curriculum

Standards Of Competence	Result
Understand and practice the concept of fundamental motion skills great ball game	The purpose of the school taken data research process selecting material dala ball big football games by utilizing the existing village field around the school
understand and practice the concept of fundamental motion skills small ball game	SMP Negeri 2 Ambal choose material ball kasti and softball by modifying the SMP Negeri 1 Petanahan SoftBall choose badminton material by utilizing Petanahan subdistrict Gymnasium as a place of learning
Understand and practice the specific motion path, run, jump, and throw in a variety of simple games and or traditional	The materials run by making use of the way around the school i.e. SMP Negeri 1 Ayah, SMP Negeri 1 Ayah, SMP Negeri 1 Mirit, SMP PGRI 1 Ambal. Then SMP Negeri 2 Ambal and SMP Negeri 1 Petanahan using shore athletics for material number run sprint
Understand and practice the concept of exercise increased degrees of physical fitness that relates to the health (durability, strength, body composition, and flexibility) and measurement of results	SMP Negeri 2 Ambal using MFT measurement techniques (Multi Fitness Test) by utilizing media audio loudspeakers and utilising wooden boards used as delimiters between students

or balls kasti softball. In addition, utilizing recycled paper for paper assignments. The paper describes the task instructions and directives to perform a movement.

Understand and practice the specific motion path, run, jump, and throw in a variety of simple games and or traditional

This competency standard material chosen by making use of the surrounding environment is utilizing the shore used a running track. Physical Education Teacher which makes use of the beach as a running track is SMP Negeri 1 Ambal dan SMP Negeri 1 Petanahan. A trip to the beach students and teachers bersepada with a distance of 2 kilometres. In addition to utilizing the shore as a place of learning, of physical education teachers SMP Negeri 1 Mirit, SMP PGRI 1 Ambal, SMP Negeri 1 Ayah dan SMP Negeri 2 Ayah utilize the access roads around the school environment to be a running track.

How to make use of the environment as a medium of instruction By Physical Education Teacher the ways of Physical Education teacher in the coastal region in utilizing the environment as a medium of instruction are as follows:

1. SMP Negeri 1 Ambal

1) Utilizes the field village in ways students are invited towards the field, then following up on the course the students collected and teachers provide a description of the material to be conveyed.
2) Ambal beach by way of the teacher walked into the classroom in advance to give you referrals Ambal heading to the beach, then students and teachers together to use the bike. After arriving at the beach students doing warm-up and teachers assisted by one of the students to make a running track using the cone. Next the teacher gives explanations and specific about the heating of material running 400 m sprint after that, students practice run and has is taken

2. SMP Negeri 2 Aal

1) Wastes sabapa used to fill small plastic balls are used for small ball game material namely softball and kasti.
2) Former paper wedding invitations and former foolscap paper used for tasks which contains instructions and commands to troubleshoot a movement. Close the bucket of paint that is already perforated made cone and ball container kasti in learning.
3) Laptop and speakers used to test the fitness of students by using measurements of the MFT.

3. SMP Negeri 1 Mirit

1) The school field used to run 400 meters. The length of the circumference of the page throughout the 80 meters. So the students surrounding the school grounds as much as five times a round.
2) The field of the village dimanfaatkannya to the big ball game that is football. The location of the field adjacent to the school, so the teacher directly invites students to direct toward spaciousness and directly describes the material.

4. SMP PGRI 1 Ambal

The field village used for ball games big and small ball game. Teacher invites students walking towards the field with distance from the school approximately 1 km. after arriving in the field of teacher ordered students to make the team and son bermainan. While students volleyball game melakukanm Princess along with the teacher.

5. SMP Negeri 1 Petanahan

1) Petanahan Gymnasium Subdistrict use to study Physical Education advance permission to Manager gor subdistrict. A study conducted at gor is a big ball game futsal ball smaller and the game of badminton. Futsal learning material presented is about basic techniques passing and control. While the material is shadow and badminton badminton game.
2) Petanahan Beach is used for athletic material as like to run sprints, Javelin throwing and discus throwing. The distance between the school and the beach approximately 2 km, so to get to there students and teachers use the bike.

6. SMP Negeri 1 Ayah

1) Village road used the teacher explains material run medium-haul or long distance. After the teacher explains material route and run mempraktikannya with the students begins warming up first. The length of the route to surrounding villages around the school is approximately 300 metres away.
2) Ball-tailed paper is used with each student got a job to bring and collect the paper and made into balls.

7. SMP Negeri 2 Ayah

1) Village road used to run surround the settlement residents around the school. The first study was conducted with students doing the warming up in the schoolgirl. After that, students do a run in accordance with the number to sort her absence.
2) BSC Gombong pool used for swimming material. Learning swimming is carried out twice in one semester. The distance from the school toward the pool about 5 km. So to go to the pool using a public transportation village. The entrance ticket to the swimming pool and transport rent paid each student. To alleviate such teachers create a policy so that each week the student contribution fee of Rp. 1000.00.

Learning Media Types

According to research in the journal Nurseto Tejo describes the kinds of learning media according to the form of the information used, can separate and classify media in five major groups, namely the visual media, visual motion media, media audio, audio visual, media and audio visual media motion. The process used to deliver the message, whether through direct vision, optical projection, projection electronic or telecommunications. By analyzing the media through the form of representation and the way it has, we get a format of classification which includes the seven media group publishers, namely: 1. printed materials, graphics, and still images 2. A silent projection media 3. Media audio, 4. Audio visual media silence, 5. Live Audio visual media/film, 6. Television media, and 7. Multi media (Nuurseto, 2011).

Learning media is any form of stimulus and provided teachers to push students learn fast, precise, easy, correct and not going verbalisme. The learning experience can be obtained through: a) the situation and condition, b) observe objects in the form of replacement props, c) Reading materials moulds such as magazines, newspapers, books and so on. Rowntree (1974) in his Rosdiani (2013) learning media grouped as follows:

a. Human Media interaction
b. Media Reality
c. Pictorial
d. a written Symbol
e. sound recording

Based on the data in field results obtained data about the media that is used by teachers of Physical Education in Kebumen Regency, the coastal region in accordance with the theory advanced by Rowntree as follows :

1. Human media interaction

Media type used by all informants in this study. This looks at the time informant 2, 3, 4, 5, 6, and 7 convey verbally introductory material on altetik run. The informant explains techniques run the gamut from start up to run motion, as well as explain the road route around the school or the beach as a running track. Meanwhile, informant 1 in addition to convey introductory material Multi Fitness tests on the physical fitness test material, the informant also inserts material biology of plant respiration is around.

2. Media Reality

Informant 1 and 6 using media reality in a way making multiple groups. Each group presented the game has didiskusikannya, while another group looked at it. While the informant 7 using the media reality is by example directly to the movement of students passing at football games.

In addition to using the media reality in the form of a human (students or the informant), in another reality media researcher observations used in the form of the path to run and field to play soccer. A running track in the form of the beach used by the informant 3 and 7. 3 using informants Coast Ambal, while informants 7 using Petanahan Beach. The second informant used the beach as a running track due to the close proximity and also the beach surface is flat and is suitable as a running track. Meanwhile the informant 2, 4, 5, and 6 using the roads around the school as a running track. This is because of the contour of the coast berbatuan so it is not suitable as a running track. There is also a school which is quite far from the beach.

3. Media Pictorial

Pictorial media by informant 1 by giving a task to students using the kelompokKartu task cards containing instructions or instructions to make a movement or a game done in a group. Pada kartu yang berwarna merah, masing-masing nomor memiliki petunjuk yang berbeda-beda dan akan digilir untuk semua kelompok (dalam bentuk sirkuit training). Sementara kartu berwarna hijau terdapat lebih dari satu petunjuk yang ada pada setiap kartu.

4. a Written Media

A written media used by all informants, namely in the form of a module that is given to each student.

5. Sound Recording Media

The media recorded voice used by informant 1, namely by giving material of physical fitness with Multi Fitness Test.

Based on expert opinion and the results of the findings, the situation can be conclude that those types of media of instruction consisting of Human media interaction, media reality media, pictorial, and written media, and sound recording media used by Physical Education of Junior High School in the coastal region as a medium of instruction.

The Role, Function And Benefits The Media Learning Physical Education

The role and function of the tools and learning of physical education media are: 1) improve the quality of human resources capable of competing and cooperation in the era of globalization. 2) improve the skills and physical quality to support daily activities. 3) increase self-reliance in following intrakulikuler or extra lessons and learn at home (Rosdiani, 2013). Media teaching can heighten the learning process of the students in the teaching which in turn heightens the learning outcomes expected to be achieved. The benefits of learning media in the learning process of students include: a) the teaching would be more attracted the attention of students so as to cultivate the motivation to learn. b) teaching materials will more clearly its meaning so that it can be better understood by the students, and allows students to master learning objectives better. c) learning methods will be more varied, not merely verbal communication through the utterance words by teachers, so students don't get bored and not run out of steam, when teachers teach to every hour lesson. d) students will be doing more learning activities, for not only listening to descriptions of teachers but also perform other activities such as observing, perform, demonstrate and others (Nana. S and Ahmad Rifai, 2015).

From the results of the interview, the situation can be drawn the conclusion that the functions and role of the media learning is to assist students in understanding the intent of the material presented by the teacher so that the media can help learning success. In addition the role and function of the media learning is learning and evaluation of materials for the determination of the subject matter of the next learning and media will make students happy, joyful and healthy.

The Utilization Of The Environment As A Medium Of Instruction Or As A Place To Learn

The concept of learning facility modifications as well as the media of instruction sets forth the conditions and environment of the school which can be utilized as a means of teaching and media prasaran, physical education sport and health. Beside that, it also described how to create a simple means of procurement or which may be developed/ manufactured from materials that exist around the environment students (Rosdiani, 2013).

Other opinions according to Regine. A in his journal, entitled "*the influence of Model environmental education Learning-based Pools Towards mastery of the concept of environmental education for prospective primary school teachers*," explains one of the learning models are expected to increase mastery of the concept of environmental education for prospective teachers are learning outside the classroom (outdoor). Environmental education learning outside the classroom with engaging students to blend with nature and doing various activities of learning that leads to the realization of student behavior to care for the environment through the stage of understanding, awareness, caring, responsibility, and behavior (MOE, 2005). Model-based environmental education learning pool has karekteristik as follows: a) the Learning Activity examines the problems of the environment of the school. b)

Learning using learning facilities that exist outside of the classroom and in the classroom. c) emphasis on the aspect of the attitude of care with cognitive aspects, besides the school environment and performance (Risda Amini and Munandar. A, 2010).

This is in accordance with the findings of researchers in the field of learning that utilizes the environment as a place to learn and as a medium of instruction. Like learning that is delivered by Physical Education Teachers 3 informant SMP Negeri 1 Ambal utilizes Ambal Beach as the place of a running track a distance of 400 m. In addition to utilizing the beach as a place of learning, the teacher invites students to care about the environment of the beach by way of picking up/take the trash around the coastal environments. A similar case is also used by teachers of Physical Education of SMP Negeri 1 Petanahan i.e. informant 7 in an interview explaining that in learning that utilizes the environment as a place to learn he is utilizing Sports districts and Buildings Petanahan Beach. GOR sub utilized for learning ball games big and small ball game i.e. futsal and badminton. While on the beach petanahan utilized for athletic learning i.e. run sprint, long jump throwing discs while the informant 2 informants, 5, and 6 utilize access roads around the school environment as a place of learning within a running track athletics.

Other Learning results in the pass by informant 1 Physical Educationteachers in SMP Negeri 1 Ambal almost makes all the learning material Physical Education utilizing the environment as a medium of instruction. diantanya modification of ball kasti using small plastic ball filled with ground coconut fibers from the rest of the results making a doormat. Next media modification is utilizing a paint bucket lid perforated core for use as a cone, or a container of ball kasti. The next medium that is utilized is the former dimanfaat bucket as a hollow vessel in learning athletic number run.

The real findings and theory from some experts on the utilization of the environment as a medium that is by learning how to modify the ball softball with coir, then use a bucket of used to be a hollow vessel, utilizing unused paper to make a paper assignment, and take advantage of close buckets of paint into a cone. In addition, to equip students will be aware of, understand and attention as well as the responsibility for Physical Education teachers of surroundings in the coastal region engage their students learning to perform around the school environment such as the beach, and access the roads around the school.

CONCLUSION

Based on the results of research on "the utilization of the environment as a medium of learning By teachers of Physical Education of Junior High School in the Coastal County of Kebumen" some conclusions can be drawn as follows:

The type of environment that functions as a medium of instruction or as a place of learning by teachers of Physical Education of Junior High School in the coastal of Kebumen is as follows, first place learning environments that are utilized in the form of the field village, beaches and streets around the school environment. Then the environment that functions as a medium of learning include paper assignment that made of paper invitations that are unused anymore and the ball tailed made from paper, then plastic ball filled with coir, bucket the former made a hollow vessel, cover the bucket of paint and wood Board be used as a means of learning.

How is done by Physical Education teachers in Junior High School in the coastal District in Kebumen utilizes the environment as a learning medium or place of study. The field village in kebumen Regency's coastal area is used for learning the game a large ball and a small ball game. While the beaches and roads around the school environment utilized to study athletics. Learning that utilizes media environment in coastal areas include the assignment, paper made from the rest of the paper used and unused paper invitations, paper task contains instructions or instructions to perform a movement or make a movement or a game. Then there is a small plastic ball filled with grain of coir. This small plastic balls used in games a small ball that is the earliest known softball game kasti and modifications. While the former bucket of paint that made a hollow vessel. Bucket or a hollow vessel is used on athletic material i.e. number run short distances (sprint). So this water filled vessels then students ran while carrying a bucket of water until the finish line.In addition, the lid of the paint bucket and wood boards are used as a means of supporting the learning process.

REFERENCES

Aji, S,. Hermawan P.R, dan Harry Promono. 2012. Pengembangan Model Pembelajaran Kids Athletic Melalui Pendekatan Lingkungan Pantai. Journal Active. Vol. 1. No. 4. ISSN 225-6773.

Amini, R dan Mundandar, A. "Pengaruh Model Pembelajaran Pendidikan Lingkungan Berbasis Outdoor Terhadap Penguasaan Konsep Pendidikan Lingkungan Bagi Calon Guru Sekolah Dasar". Jurnal Penelitian Pendidikan Vol. 11, No. 1, April 2010: 412-565.

Aris, S. 2014. 68 Model Pembelajaran Inovatif dalam Kurikulum 2013. Yogyakarta: Ar Ruzz Media.

Ega, T, R,. 2013. Stratengi Pembelajaran Pendidikan Jasmani "Implementasi pada Pembelajaran Pendidikan Jasmani, Olahraga, dan Kesehatan". Bandung: Alfabeta.

Gulo, W. 2000. Metodologi Penelitian. Jakarta: Grasindo.

Herka Maya. J. 2005."Pemilihan Media Visual dalam Menunjang Pembelajaran Pendidikan Jasmani di Sekolah Dasar. Jurnal Pendidikan Jasmani Indonesia. Vol. 3. No. 1

Kriyanto, R. 2009. Teknik Praktis Riset Komunikasi. Jakarta: Prenada Media

Kusumawati, M. 2015. Penelitian Pendidikan Jasmani Olahraga dan Kesehatan. Bandung: Alfabeta

Nurseto, T. 2011. Membuat Media Pembelajaran yang Menarik. Jurnal Ekonomi dan Pendidikan. Vol. 8. Nomor 1

Rosdiani, D. 2013. Perencanaan Pembelajaran dalam Pendidikan Jasmani dan Kesehatan. Bandung: Alfabeta

Sudjana, N dan Ahmad Rifai. 2015. Media Pembelajaran.Bandung: Sinar Baru Algensindo.

Suherman, A. 2000. Dasar-Dasar Penjaskes. Jakarta: Depatemen Pendidikan Nasional Direktorat Jendral Pendidikan Dasar dan Menengah Bagian Proyek Penataan Guru SLTP dan Setara D- III.

31

Modification of Hitball Games in Physical Education, Sports, and Health Learning in School

Roas Irsyada[1]✉, Uen Hartiwan[2]

Jurusan Pendidikan Jasmani, Kesehatan dan Rekreasi Fakultas Ilmu Keolahragaan, Universitas Negeri Semarang, Semarang, Indonesia[12]

Article History

Keywords:
Modification;
Small Ball Game.

Abstract

A small ball game is one of the materials contained within the scope of elementary school learning. The kind of small ball game such as Kasti, Rounders, Softball and Baseball. How the result applied of small ball game modification on Physical Education learning process 4th grade on elementary school. This research is a development research that aims to produce products in the form of Hitball game using procedural development model. The type of data used is qualitative and quantitative. The game of Hitball, has contributed to an increase in the student's pulse rate by 50.97%. In addition, the results of the pulse rate of learners after learning can increase by 73.80% of the maximum pulse rate. From the result of the research, it is concluded that the game of Hitball is in accordance with Core Competencies and basic competencies of Physical Education on Elementary Class IV and can increase the intensity of student movement which is indicated by the increase of the average pulse as much as 50,97%..

✉ **Correspondence address :**
Gd f1 lantai 2 Jalan Sekaran, Sekaran, Gunung Pati, Sekaran, Gn. Pati, Kota Semarang, Jawa Tengah 50229
E-mail: roaspjkr@mail.unnes.ac.id

INTRODUCTION

Physical education is the foundation for continuous sports coaching, which is an indispensable learning process for cognitive and social development (Rusli Lutan, 2004). Physical education also plays a role in stimulating involvement in sports and physical activity, laying the foundation for healthy living along the life and involvement in the social life of society (Rusli Lutan, 2004). Education is incomplete without physical education, and there is no physical education without media of motion. Motion as a physical activity is a natural foundation for man to learn to know the world and himself. According to Rusli Lutan (2001) that Physical Education is a series of subject matter that gives a real contribution in everyday life in an effort to increase the growth and development of physical and spiritual learners. Therefore the implementation of Physical Education should be more developed to a more optimal direction so that learners will be more innovative, skilled, creative, and have the freshness of physical and healthy life habits and have knowledge and understanding of human motion. Therefore, as one component of education which must be taught in schools, physical education has a very strategic role in the formation of the whole person (Toho Cholik Muthohir, 2007).

Pangrazi (2004: 4) states that penjakjasorkes are the stages of a public education program that contributes to the overall growth and development of the child, especially through movement experience. This is a learning program that gives attention to all the domain of learning, namely: (1) psychomotor, (2) cognitive and (3) affective.

Objectives Physical education in schools one of them is to provide motion skills for learners, in the hope that existing movement skills to be developed and enhanced into the development of specialist motion of certain branches according to the talents, interests and potentials of learners. The objective is contained in Article 25 paragraph 3 of Law no. 3 of 2005 on National Sport System. The contents of article 25, paragraph 3 are as follows: "Development and development of educational sports at all levels of education provides the freedom to learners to perform sports activities in accordance with the talent and interest".

The implementation of Physical Education in the Curriculum 2013 focuses on student interests. The Penjasorkes material in the 2013 curriculum for SD can be seen from the Core Competencies (CC) and Basic Competencies (BC) at different grade levels. The following will be shown Core Competence (CC) and Basic Competence (BC) for fourth graders (four) Primary School contains about small ball game material.

Table 1. Core Competence (CC), Basic Competence (BC), and Learning Material Physical Education Elementary School Class IV

KI	KD
4. Present factual knowledge in clear and logical and systematic language, in aesthetic work in movements that reflect healthy children, and in actions that reflect the child's faithful behavior and noble character	4.2 Practicing variation and combination of locomotor, non-locomotor, and manipulative base motion patterns in small ball games based on the concept of motion in various games and or traditional small ball sports

Small ball game is one of the material in physical education subject in elementary school level. The form of small ball game that is often used is kasti. The game uses some basic techniques of throwing, capturing, and hitting the ball. These three basic techniques require accurate targeting and good coordination between eyes and hands that are not owned by primary school-aged children. In capturing techniques, they tend to still have fear in doing these basic techniques. The purpose of small ball games is to develop all the domains of both cognitive, affective, and psychomotor through a team game activity that is applied through the activity of practicing variations and combinations of basic techniques of small ball games both throwing, hitting and catching. One type of small team ball game is a game of kasti, where there are techniques of throwing, catching and hitting.

The precision is needed when going to throw and catch the ball. But this is still rarely done because students tend to perfunctory when throwing and catching the ball. In addition to the technique of spanking the ball, in the game often the students are not about the ball. The small size of the ball and focusing the eyes on the moving ball can not be combined with the swing arm to hit the ball using a ball beater with a small cross section as well. So the impact of the ball with the baton has not happened and the stage of hitting the ball is often missed.

Based on the above background, in learning penjasorkes less optimal student movement intensity because the learning process is not done through complex motion activities and not optimal in developing the three domains in learning (cognitive, affective, and psikomotor). Researchers want to facilitate students in performing basic techniques of throwing, capturing, and hitting in a small ball game. How is the role of the Hitball learning model in small ball game material subjects of physical education elementary school students? This study aims to produce Hitball game products that can be used as a media teacher physical education in delivering the material in small ball game learning. The development of Hitball game products is an effort in improving the complex motion skills of learners in small game ball games subjects physical education elementary school students.

The results of this study are expected to contribute as follows a) As stock experience in the field of research in developing a sport. b) Increase scientific development especially related to sports game development products. c) As a basis for the development of research results in the future. d) As a medium in learning Physical education in general and small ball games in particular. e) As an encouragement and motivation to the pemas teacher to modify a game that aims to create a new form of game so as to attract learners to follow subjects Physical education.

METHODS

This research is a development research that aims to produce products in the form of Hitball Game which is in accordance with the growth and development level of elementary school students. According to Borg and Gall in Sugiyono (2009), Research and development is a method or method used to develop or validate the products used in education and learning.

This development research uses a procedural development model, because this model is descriptive, that is a procedure that describes the steps that must be followed in producing the product. According to Wasis (2004) in each development can choose and find the most appropriate step for his research based on the conditions and constraints faced. Research and development seeks to produce a component in the education system through development and validation steps. It further mentioned that the research and development procedure basically has two main objectives: 1) developing the product, and 2) testing the effectiveness of the product in achieving the goal.

Developmnet Procedures

Procedures or research and development steps should not use standard steps to be followed, but each development can choose and determine the most appropriate step for its research based on the conditions and constraints it faces. Based on these opinions then the procedure used in the development of this Hitball game includes five steps, namely: 1) Conduct analysis of product to be developed 2) Developing Hitball Game start product 3) Expert Validation 4) Field Trial 5) Product Revision 6) Data Type

The data used in this research are qualitative and quantitative data. Qualitative data is obtained from interviews in the form of criticism, advice from expert physical education and oral and written learning experts as a constructive input for product revision materials. While quantitative data obtained from pulse taking before and after learning, influence the use of products and games learners.

1)Data Collection Instrument

Instruments used in product development in the form of interviews, observation, questionnaires, documentation, pulse, and game learners in playing the game Hitball. Questionnaires used by experts in the form of a number of aspects that should be assessed feasibility. The items used in the questionnaire include the quality of a Hitball game, as well as general comments and suggestions if any.

2)Data Analaysis Technique

Data analysis technique used is percentage to analyze and assess the subject of developer in assessing level of eligibility, quality, and acceptance of product in the form of data of psychomotor, cognitive, and affective aspect.

Hitball game products are said to overcome obstacles in the teaching of small ball games marked with the results of the average calculation of quality assessment questionnaires filled by experts Physical education (lecturers) and learning experts (physical education teachers). The analysis technique used is descriptive analysis technique in the form of percentage.

Increasing the physical intensity with the game product indicator can make the learner move marked by the increasing of pulse after following small game of ball game. Analysis of data used to determine the increase in physical intensity is to know the results of pulse measurement of learners before and after follow the learning (using the product).

RESULTS AND DISCUSSION

The data obtained from the questionnaires

by skilled experts and learning experts is a guideline for declaring whether a small ball hitball modification product can be used for small-scale trials and large-scale tests. The following is the result of filling out a questionnaire from the experts of Penjas and the learning expert.

Table 2. Average Score Results Expert Score

Experts	Results Average Score Assessment
PE Experts I	3,35
Learning Experts I	3,26
Learning Experts II	3,32

Looking at the results **table 2** the average score of the questionnaire scores conducted by each expert Physical education and learning experts obtained an average score of 3.31 (three point thirty-one) or in the "good / proper / clear" rating category. Therefore, it can be concluded that the game of Hitball for learning small ball game of Elementary School can be used for small-scale trials.

Implementation of small-scale testing of Hitball game products can be done well, but there are some obstacles that make this game can not be played to the fullest. The following are the obstacles that come after Hitball game products are tested on a small scale:

Table 3. Constraints and Constraints on Small Scale Trials

Revised Reasons	Repairing Suggestions
Too easy to turn off the opponent	The batter is turned off by means of the ball rolled over the safe line and captured by the defensive player.
Distance base 10 meters too far	The base distance is brought closer from the safe line to 8 meters
Unclear Field Boundaries	The field boundaries are clarified using cones and lines

(Source: 2017 Research)

The analysis technique used is the percentage for analyzing and assessing teachers Physical education in assessing the level of product quality against Hitball game products.

The results of research on teachers of physical education related to the acceptance of Hitball game products for learning Elementary Physical Education, obtained a description of aspects (1) the suitability of products with Competence Standards, basic competencies, and characteristics of learners, (2) the effect of the product on the improvement of cognitive domain, (3) the effect of the product on the improvement of the affective domain, (4) the effect of the product on the improvement of the psychomotor domain, (5) the effect of the product on the enhancement of the learner's activity, and (6) the feasibility of Hitball game product. From these six points the results obtained that the game Hitbal very good and appropriate for students so it can be used as a medium of motion in the physical education of small ball games.

The results of the pulse count of 40 learners are as follows:

Pulse Rate	Before Learning	After Learning
AVERAGE	79,35 times/ minute	155,66 times/minute

(Source: 2017 Research)

From the data shows an increase in pulse rate of 50.97%. In addition, the results of the students' pulse rate after learning has increased by 73.80% of the maximum pulse rate. These results also indicate compliance with the recommended exercise intensity that is 60-90% of the maximal pulse rate.

Based on data analysis, a hitball permeation can be used as a medium for small ball games. The result is because Hitball includes all the motion indicators of small ball game and softball ball. The basic motion of throwing the ball, catching the ball, and hitting the ball is very easy for students in this game so the game can run effectively.

The game of Hitball, has contributed to an increase in the student's pulse rate by 50.97%. In addition, the results of the pulse rate of learners after learning can increase by 73.80% of the maximum pulse rate. These results also indicate compliance with the recommended exercise intensity that is 60 - 80% of the maximum pulse rate.

Increased pulse rate can be used as an indicator of increased physical intensity of learners. Physical intensity may increase due to pulse response due to physical activity of learners when playing a game of Hitball. The pulse of this response can be a measure of the increase in the pulse of learners in achieving the intensity of the exercise suggested. An increase in the average pulse response of 73.80% of the activities performed, is one indicator that the game Hitball can increase the physical intensity of learners in the learning process small ball game.

CONCLUSION

From this research can be drawn conclusion, among others: 1) Has the creation of game products Hitball game that can be used as a medium of motion small game material in learning pemas in school. 2) a hitball game can overcome the problems that arise from the learning of small ball material related to the mastery of basic techniques of throwing, capturing, and hitting the ball. This can be seen from the observation of the implementation of research where students can perform such basic techniques well so the game goes well. 3) Hitball games can increase the intensity of student movement in small ball learning. This is indicated by the increase in the students' pulse rate.

REFERENCES

Moh. Fahmi. 2017. Permainan "Happy Bouncing Ball" Untuk Pembelajaran Tenis Meja Bagi Siswa Kelas V Sekolah Dasar. Active : Journal Of Physical Education, Sport, Health, and Recreation. https://journal.unnes.ac.id/sju/index.php/peshr/article/view/14536. Diakses 6 Juli 2017. 14.46.

Mutohir, T. C., & Maksum, A. (2007). Sport development index, alternatif baru mengukur kemajuan pembangunan bidang keolahragaan. Jakarta: PT Indeks.

Pangrazi ,2004. Program pendidikan umum : Depdik¬bud

Lutan, R., & Suherman, A. (2004). Kebugaran Jasmani. Direktorat Jendral. Jakarta.

Rusli Luthan dan Adang Suherman. 2001. Perencanaan Pembelajaran Penjaskes. Jakarta : Depdikbud.

Sugiyono. 2009. Penelitian Pendidikan. Bandung : Alfabeta.

32

Interplay Among Physical Characteristics Play Position and Shooting Accuracy of Elite-Female Basketballers

Olufunmilola Leah Dominic[1]✉, Chioma Esther Whoba[2], Adetayo Ebun Talabi[3], Surajudeen Tosho Bakinde[4], Sikiru Adewale Adeoye[5], Tajudeen Olarewaju Ibraheem[6], Iliasu Yakubu Seidina[7]

Department of Human Kinetics Education, University of Ilorin, Nigeria[1234567]

Article History

Keywords:
Physical Fitness; Performance; Speciality; Training

Abstract

This study was conducted to examine effect of specialty and training frequency on physical fitness profile of Federal Capital Territory Abuja Karate Team. Descriptive correlational research design with stratified and purposive sampling was adopted to study 16 out of 30 karatekas (male, n = 9; female, n = 7); age, 28.4 ± 7.0 years. Data were collected using stopwatch, punch pad, kicking pad, karate belt, training bag and measuring tape after informed consent. SPSS 20.0 was used for data analysis with frequency, percentage, mean, t-test and multiple regression with 0.05 alpha level. No significant difference between the fitness profiles of kumite and kata and kata only group; t = .803, MD = 1.467, df = 14, p = .435 and 2 = 4% (0.04), and 95% CI = -5.38 to 2.44. Those who trained 3 days/wk. had higher fitness profile than those who trained daily, t = 2.32, MD = 3.37, df = 14, p = .039, 2 = 30% (0.30) and 95% CI = -6.54 to -0.19. Training frequency had greater influence on their fitness profile = .65, p =.01. Training frequency of 3-4 days/wk. and regular assessment of physical fitness using SKFT batteries was recommended.

✉ **Correspondence address :**
E-mail: lolafunmidom@gmail.com

INTRODUCTION

Studies have documented that no any two individuals will shoot in exactly the same way because of each individual having unique structural body and way of displaying skills. The unique movement and stylistic interpretations of individual player, accounts for multiple patterns of movement and paths of projection that determine whether shooting is successful or not (Çetina, & Murat, 2014; Joseph , 2015). However, a good player is one who is both accurate and precise by shooting the same way each time and making it in the basket (Arcidiacono, P., Kinsler, J., & Price, J , 2017 ; Lab-Write, 2005).

Physical (height and weight), anthropometric (body lengths) and physiological differences, age and level of experience are identified factors predisposing to variability in performance whether of success or failure of athletes during competition (Er ulj, F., & Štrumbelj, E., 2015 ; Apostolidis & Zacharakis, 2015). Tsarouchas et.al 'study in 1990, found some differences within good shooters in which some had 'low' elbow technique while others used a 'high' elbow technique in their shooting form and these have been found to depend on individual's unique structure and function, assets and liabilities. Studies by Padulo.,et all (2015), burns (1990) and Malone (1999) explained that skilled shooters are not born, but instead can develop with proper training using scientific approach as a necessity (Brancazio, 1984; Sekulic .et.all, 2017). The general observations of researchers are that one of the reasons for low performance in shooting is that most players do not learn the proper technique differentiating between strong and weak team (Shaoliang, Alberto, Miguel-Angel, Hongyou, Bruno, & Jaime, 2017). However, if the correct technique is consistently learnt and practiced overtime, accuracy and precision of shots become very high in performance.

The invention and development followed by the evolution of the rules and tactics of the basketball game resulted in the three basic playing positions designated as centre, forward, and guard (Miller & Bartlett, 1996, te Wierike, 2017) with the expected contribution to the team's scoring. Centres are mostly the tallest players (Dominic, 2005; Shaoliang, 2017) and normally playing close to the basket in order to utilize their heights to the greatest benefits of the team, whereas the major assignment Guards who are mostly the shortest players is to originate attacking patterns, a role which requires them to dribble the ball up the court (Krause, 1991; Miller & Bartlett, 1996; Abdelkrim . et .all , 2010) causing them to stay further away from the basket. The Forwards mostly are of medium stature, and their role incorporates aspects of those of both centres and guards. They are also expected to help guards in setting up attacking patterns and centres in defending opponents close to the basket. They also contest rebounds from missed shots, playing both the left and right hand side of the court between the zone and the side lines (Coleman, 1975; Miller & Bartlett, 1996, ; Abdelkrim . et .all , 2010). Players in all the three positions are expected to contribute to their team's scoring.

Height or stature and its reach play crucial role in sports, especially in basketball playing ability and scoring where height is also used as one of the indices for talent hunting. Oranugo's study, (1995) revealed that age, height, weight and body composition have significant relationship with winning in elite competitions. This has implication for training, tactical and strategic development for optimal performance. However, we investigated if these relationships or contributions could be significant in shooting performance.

Pojski ,. et all, (2011) reported findings which have shown that free throw percentage, field goals and three-point shots distinguish winning and losing of basketball teams (Trnini , et al, 2002; Pojski,. et al, 2009) while players who could score in all stages of the game under different conditions are essential for shooting accuracy and winning (Pojski, et al, 2011). The study was therefore undertaken to determine the interplay among physical characteristics, position played and shooting accuracy of Nigerian elite female basketball players.

METHODS

The research design was descriptive correlation using three by one by three factorial design (3x1x3) which permitted the categorization of players according to playing role/position (guards, forward, and centre) of three categories based on position played only and successful shots at three shooting distances which are the common shooting zones. Shooting at 2.74m, 4.67m and 6.40m distances represented at least the zone of each of the player during play (Miller & Bartlett, 1996).

The sample of the study comprised 14 of the 15 National champions for the Zenith Female Basketball league who completed the measurement and were in Camp preparing for an international club championship. The participants had played at national and international competitions and had varying basketball experience and proficiency. All the players are right-handed, and their age ranged from 19 to 25 years which is comparative to previous studies (Eddings, 1996, Rojas. et.al, 2000). Informed consent and permission from team handlers were obtained before taking part in the study. The coaches objectively rated the players from 1-15 according to their shooting ability (CRSPA).

Bio-data included age, competition played and levels of play, years of experience, categories of exposure, training exposure. The height, weight were measured and BMI was calculated. For accuracy test, the method of Landin .,et all ,1993 ; Button, et al (2006) for accuracy test were adopted for the study. Before the measurement were collected, The measurement procedure included general and specific warm up, followed by shooting trials and a pre-test of 10 trials for each type of shot were conducted in order to classify the relative ability of each of the participant in comparison with the coach's rating. For the data collection, each participant was then video recorded taking 30 experimental trials, in three blocks of ten (14 participants x three blocks x ten shots per block) for each of the shooting perimeters, for the 3 shooting distances. The outcome of the scores of experimental shots was not video recorded, but were kept by the experimenter according to an objective rating system (Landin,. et all , 1993; Button, et al, 2006).

The researchers used the accuracy tests to measure and to compare players 'performances in shooting accuracy and also in relation to physical characteristics of height, weight and BMI. 5- Point scale was used as adapted from Landin,. et all (1993) and Button,. et al (2006) basketball free throw scoring system..

The weight was measured using bathroom scale calibrated in kilogramme. The height was obtained using two-calibrated metre-rulers stationed on the wall and both used for BMI determination. The descriptive statistics of percentage, ranking and mean were used to describe the data, Pearson's Product Moment correlation ('r') was used to test for significant relationships between the shooting accuracy at the different shooting distances and physical characteristics. For inter-individual data analysis, one way ANOVA was used to find significant variability between the group trials in shooting accuracy. The level of significance was set at 0.05.

RESULTS AND DISCUSSION

The range age of the players by play position were guards- 20-22years; forwards-21-24 year' and centre- 18-25years of age. The physical characteristics of the female elite basketballers showed weight range of the guards-60-68kg; for-

Table 1: Participants' Scores and Percentages of Shooting Accuracy at Three Shooting Distances

Position of Play	Participant	2.74m shot		4.67m shot		6.40m shots		CRPSA	OPPSA	ORPSA	YE
		Score	%	Score	%	Score	%		%		
G1	Guard 1	124	82.67	135	90.0	115	76.67	4th	83.11	6th	5
G2	Guard 2	133	88.67	128	85.33	114	76.0	2nd	83.33	5th	8
G3	Guard 3	136	90.67	143	95.33	116	77.33	3rd	87.78	1st	8
G4	Guard 4	122	81.33	127	84.67	116	77.33	5th	81.11	9th	5
G5	Guard 5	122	81.33	131	87.33	109	72.67	10th	80.44	10th	9
F6	Forward 1	124	82.67	137	91.33	115	76.67	7th	83.56	4th	8
F7	Forward 2	110	73.67	120	80.0	109	72.67	12th	75.33	14th	9
F8	Forward 3	130	86.67	128	85.33	112	74.67	11th	82.22	7th	11
F9	Forward 4	132	88.0	121	80.67	113	75.33	9th	81.33	8th	8
F10	Forward 5	127	84.67	127	84.67	101	67.33	14th	78.89	12th	8
C11	Centre 1	128	85.33	139	92.67	120	80.0	1st	86.00	2nd	9
C12	Centre 2	126	84.0	136	90.67	117	78.0	6th	84.22	3rd	5
C13	Centre 3	118	84.0	133	88.67	110	73.67	8th	80.22	11th	5
C14	Centre 4	118	78.67	120	80.0	106	70.67	13th	76.44	13th	4

CRPSA: Coach's Ranking of Players shooting ability; **OPPS**- Overall Percentage of players shooting accuracy; **ORPSA**- Overall ranking of players shooting accuracy; **YE**=Years of experience

wards 67-85kg and centres 75-80kg. For height, guards were between 1.65-1.68m; forwards 1.75-1.88m and centre 1.88-1.93m. The BMI revealed range of 19.87-22.04kg/m2 for guards; 21.22-24.05kg/m2 for forwards; and 20.78-22.21 kg/m2 for centre players.

Research Question (RQ) 1: How accurate are the shots of female elite Nigerian basketball players?

Table 1 shows the score and percentage of accuracy shots of the participants at three distances with the subjective ranking by the coaches and objective ranking as determined by the accuracy testing. In 2.74m shooting performance, except forward 2(73.67%) who had 9 years' experience and centre 4 (78.67%) with only 4 years, all the participants scored above 80% and only C1 in 4.67m shot forward 5 who had 8years of experience scored the lowest (67.33%). Other participants' range fell between 70.67-78.0%. The result showed non- group domination in the shooting perimeters, as the ranking was shared between the guards, forwards and centre players (see table 1). Summarily, all the players have very 'good' score percentages in comparison with elite and international players.

Research Question (RQ) 2: Are there any relationships between physical characteristics and shooting accuracy of Nigerian female basketball players?

We further hypothesised that there is no significant relationship between physical characteristics (height, weight and BMI) and shooting accuracy of the female basketball players.

Table 2: Correlation Matrix of Physical Characteristics and Shooting Accuracy at Three Shooting Distances

	Wt	Ht	BMI	2.74m	4.67m	6.40m
Wt	1	0.857*	0.370	0.030	-0.181	-0.041
Ht	0.857*	1	-0.002	0.156	-0.026	.154
BMI	0.370	-0.002	1	-0.069	-0.188	-0.196
2.74m Shot	0.030	0.156	-0069	1	0.425	0.373
4.67m Shot	-0.181	-0.026	-0.188	0.425	1	0.595*
6.40m Shot	-0.041	0.154	-0.196	0.373	0.595*	1

*Correlation is significant at the 0.05 level (2-tailed) = p value >0.497

Table 2 indicates significant relationship between weight and height only, and independently both are insignificant with BMI establishing that neither height nor weight can predict BMI independently. No significant correlation was found between any physical characteristic and distance shooting but indicated between 4.67m and 6.40m shooting accuracy (p.val.> 0.497) demonstrated by both being distant shots from the basket. The insignificant correlation establishes height generally as factor of athletic ability, jump height, height release ratio but not paramount for accuracy of the shot.

RQ3: Does positional play (such as guard, forward, and centre) of the female basketball players differentiate their shooting accuracy at 2.74m, 4.67m and 6.40m distances?

We further hypothesized that: Position of play (guard, forward, centre) will not significantly d+ifferentiate shooting accuracy at the three shooting distances (2.74m, 4.67m and 6.40m).

Table 3: One-way ANOVA for position of play and shooting accuracy at the three shooting Distances

Shooting Accuracy	Sum of Squares		df	Mean Square	F-ratio	Prob
2.74m	Between Groups	111.214	2	55.607	1.085	.372
	Within Groups	564.000	11	51.273		
	Total	675.214	13			
4.67m	Between Groups	54.600	2	27.300	.535	.600
	Within Groups	561.400	11	51.036		
	Total	616.000	13			
6.40m	Between Groups	44.464	2	22.232	.884	.441
	Within Groups	276.750	11	25.159		
	Total	**321.214**	**13**			

F(2,11) = 3.98>0.05 *Significant.

The result of the ANOVA (**table 2**) shows that position of play does not significantly differentiate between shooting performance of the categorised players at the three shooting distance perimeters.

DISCUSSION

Generally, all the participants' scores at 2.74m (73.67- 90.67%), 4.67m (80.0-95.33%), and 6.40m (67.33-80.0%) demonstrate elite and international level. The score levels of the players favourably compared with elite international free throw shooters (78 ± 8) who were studied by Hudson (1982) and also when compared with the three national players studied by Button et al. (2006) of which only the senior players scored 90% while the two remaining shooters scored 70% and 66% respectively. Similarly Button et al's participants on

5 points scale experiment score for 30 free throws scored 114, 116 and 112 in order of performance; while the lowest score was 120 and the highest 143 for this study for the middle distance experimental shot. The above showed that the participants are highly skilled players in shooting. Apart from Hudson (1982) who studied female shooters in free throw in Elliot (1991), Eddings included only two females among his 22 participants,. the female compared favourably with other studies. Similarly, this study proved no gender differential when it comes to shooting accuracy and performance, implying that tactical and technicalities of skill difference might be only due to learning and integration processes involved in adaptation and training. Furthermore, other physiological factors could be determinant factor of differences found and not the technical aspect of shooting.

Tsarouchas,et al., (1990) used accuracy as a strategy to classify the elite players in their study. They espoused that the 'good' shooters were those who shot above 80% while 'poor' shooters were those whose ratings are below 65%. Comparing our participants' shooting accuracy to previous studies, they could be rated as highly skilled players. However, this study group performed well in the middle distance than the short distance and long distance shots. This might have occurred because most of the basketball players shoot consistently within this range for the uncontested shot (free throw) and mostly practiced it as penalty shot. Basketballers perform well in this shot than the jump shot because it is a closed skill that requires specific consistent segmental angular configuration, velocity and ball projection (All Africa Games [AAG], 2003). Furthermore, majority of the players could score 10 out of 10 in the middle distance shot. However, the performance of Guard 3 (1st) and 2 (2nd) was not expected in 2.75m shot because they tend to play more at the top of the key rather than at the perimeter zone which is a common area in which the forward and centre players predominantly operate and not the guards (see table 1). This enlightens more on the role and effect of practice and training rather than position of play zones on performance especially as it relates to shooting. This further has implication for strategies and conditioning of beginners and promising players by teachers and coaches when laying foundation for skill acquisition especially in relation to attacking the rim for making points and optimal performance. Though tactical and strategic patterns of training are essential for positional adaptation, but this should not be made rigid when it comes to offensive playing techniques especially with high level of shooting accuracy and performance being the goal of basketball as a sport. Coaching in this direction will prevent shooting potentials of players' being incapacitated.

The findings on the relationship between physical characteristics and shooting accuracy revealed that shooting accuracy does not depend solely on height and weight of the shooter though they are significant for general athletic prowess and playing ability especially when it comes to reach plays and take offs in basketball shooting. Furthermore, height and weight of the basketball players are of significant advantage for higher release height and release height ratio (Hudson, 1982; Eddings, 1996; Miller & Bartlett, 1993 and 1996) and essential for training, tactical and strategic development but not specific for prediction of shooting accuracy (Okuneye & Osman, 1996; Ackland, et.all., 1997; Dominic, 2006; Shahdadi, & Alisoufi, 2016) as established by this study. Hudson (1974) founded that velocity of wrist flexion just prior to release was one of the best predictors of shooting accuracy. By implication, physical characteristics might be of advantage in reducing the distance of projection of the ball to the basket but does not significantly contribute to the accuracy of the shot. It is deduced therefore, that there are general factors of performance of basketball as a sport and specific factors for specific skill and specific technique in each of the skill. This calls for specificity of training to optimise player's performance in specific shot and not by play position as observed in training programmes.

Differentiation was sought among the participants based on the position played on the court in order to discover if it might determine performance level at the three shooting distances using ANOVA (see table 3). The findings demonstrated that role differentiation is imperative to determine perimeter of play especially in defensive and strategic positioning for offensive plays and short skill, but not for accuracsy at different distance. The guards were expected to perform poorly in the 2.74m shots and better in 6.40m shots but this was not found to be so confirming shooting accuracy not determined by their play position, rather by other factors relating to training and practice. Centre came 1st in the long distance shot (6.40) as against the general expectation from guards as based on play position while G3, G2 and F1 came first, 5th and fourth respectively in the short distance shot (4.67m) (see table 1). This therefore calls for understanding by teachers, coaches and sports scientists that shooting is a specialized skill which requires special consideration and technicalities for athletes, coaches and athletic trainers when it comes to conditioning for optimal performance.

CONCLUSION

We concluded that the female players are highly skilled in shooting accuracy performance and compared favourably with other elite and international players confirming good technique. Height, weight and BMI are insignificantly related to shooting accuracy at three predominant shooting distances in basketball. Play position does not determine shooting accuracy in relation to shooting distances. Since height and weight especially are not directly related to shooting accuracy, shooting accuracy performance at three distance zones should also be added to variables for talent hunting and team selection since optimal product in any basketball contest is the ability to outscore the opponents at the final whistle.

REFERENCES

Ackland, T. R., Schreiner, A.B and Kerr, D.A 1997. Absolute size and proportionality characteristics of World championship Female basketball players. Journal of Sports Science, 15 (5); 485-90. https://doi.org/10.1080/026404197367128

All African Games Basketball Game Statistics (AAG,) 2003. Basketball Games Statistics of Nigeria team.

Abdelkrim, N. B., Chaouachi, A., Chamari, K., Chtara, M., & Castagna, C. (2010). Positional role and competitive-level differences in elite-level men's basketball players. The Journal of Strength & Conditioning Research, 24(5), 1346-1355.

Arcidiacono, P., Kinsler, J., & Price, J. (2017). Productivity spillovers in team production: Evidence from professional basketball. Journal of Labor Economics, 35(1), 191-225.

Apostolidis, N. & Zacharakis, E. 2015.The influence of the anthropometric characteristics and handgrip strength on the technical skills of young basketball players. Journal of Physical Education and Sport, 1-10. DOI: 10.7752/jpes.2015.02050

Brancazio, P. 1984. Sport Science. New York, Simon and Schuster.

Burns, F. T. 1990. Teaching components for shooting improvement in National Wheelchair Basketball. Symposium for Coaches. Athletes and Officials (pp. 79-83). University of Alberta: Rick Hansen Centre.

Button, C., Macleod, M., Sanders, R., and Coleman S. 2006. Examining Movement Variability in the Basketball free-Thrown Action at Different Skill Levels Department of Physical Education, Sport and Leisure Studies. pp.1-29.

Çetina, E and Murat, S. 2014. Analysis of jump shot performance among 14-15 year old male basketball player. Procedia - Social and Behavioral Sciences 116, 2985 – 2988. doi:10.1016/j.sbspro.2014.01.693

Coleman, B. 1975. Basketball: Techniques, Teaching, and Training. London: Kaye and Ward.

Dominic, O. L. 2005. Evaluation of the body proportions of Kwara State basketball players. Journal of Physical and Research, 11(2), 1580-1587.

Dominic, O. L. 2006. The relationship between physical characteristics and shooting ability of Kwara state basketball players. Journal of Education Research and Development, 3: 167-172.

Eddings, M. R. 1996. Effect of manipulating angle of projection on height of releaser and accuracy in basketball free throw: A biomechanical study. Unpublished Masters Thesis, California State University, Chico.

Elliot, B. 1991. The jump shot: a comparison of male and female shooting techniques. Sports Coach; (Oct-Dec.) p. 39-45.

Er ulj, F., & Štrumbelj, E. (2015). Basketball shot types and shot success in different levels of competitive basketball. PloS one, 10(6), e0128885.

Hudson, J. L. 1974. A computerized cinematographical analysis pf college women in basketball one-handed free throw. Master's Thesis, University of Purdue.

Hudson, J. L. 1982. A biomechanical analysis by skill level of free throw shooting in basketball. International Symposium of Biomechanics in Sport, J. Terauds, Delmar, CA, Research Center for sports, Academics Publishers, 95-102.

Joseph, J. G., Geiser, T. D., & Abnett, A. C. (2015). U.S. Patent No. 9,017,188. Washington, DC: U.S. Patent and Trademark Office.

Krause, J. V. 1991. Basketball Skills and Drills. Champaign, IL; Human Kinetics.

Lab-write-improving Lab reports 2005. Descriptive lab selfGuide. Retrieved on 20/08/2014. www.ncsu.edu/labwreite/Experimental/accuracy-precision.htm

Landin, D. K., Herbert, E. P. & Fairweather, M. (1993). The effect of variable practice on the performance of a basketball skill. Research Quarterly for Exercise and Sport, 6, 232-237.

Malone, L. A. 1999. Relationship between performance characteristics and player classification in wheelchair basketball. Unpublished Ph. D Thesis. University of Alberta. Retrieved from Online National library of Canada pdf – NQ39563.

Miller, S., & Bartlett, R. M. 1993. The effects of shooting distance in the basketball jump shot. Journal of Sport Science, 11, 285-293.

Miller, S. & Bartlett. R. M. 1996. The relationship between basketball shooting kinematics, distance and playing position. Journal of Sports Science, 11, 243--253.

Oranugo, J. B. C. 1995. Morphological Considerations as means of selecting Basketball players for the 1996 Olympics Games in Atlanta, USA NASSM 6, p.135-140.

Padulo, J., Attene, G., Migliaccio, G. M., Cuzzolin, F., Vando, S., & Ardigò, L. P. (2015). Metabolic optimisation of the basketball free throw. Journal of sports sciences, 33(14), 1454-1458.

Pojski , H., Šeparovi V., U i anin, E. 2009. Differences between successful and unsuccessful basketball teams on the final Olympic tournament. Acta Kinesiologica, 3 (2): 110 114.

Pojski , H., Šeparovi , V., & U i anin, E. 2011. Reliability and Factorial Validity of Basketball Shooting Accuracy Tests. Sport Scientific and Practical Aspects, 8, 1: 25-32.Internationaic

Rojas, F. J., Caper, M., One, A & Gutierrez 2000. Kinematic adjustments in the basketball jump shot against an opponent. Ergonomics, 43(10)1651-1660.

Sekulic, D., Pehar, M., Krolo, A., Spasic, M., Uljevic, O., Calleja-González, J., & Sattler, T. (2017). Evaluation of Basketball-Specific Agility: Applicability of Preplanned and Nonplanned Agility Performances for Differentiating Playing Positions and Playing Levels. The Journal of Strength & Conditioning Research, 31(8), 2278-2288.

Shahdadi, A & Alisouf, N. 2016. relationship between anthropometric characteristics and jump shot skill in female basketball players. European Journal of Physical Education and Sport Science, 2(6) 112-122. http://dx.doi.org/10.5281/zenodo.232591

Shaoliang, Z Alberto, L, Miguel-Angel, G, Hongyou, L, Bruno, G. & Jaime, S. 2017. Players' technical and physical performance profiles and game-to-game variation in NBA, International Journal of Performance Analysis in Sport, 17:4, 466-483, DOI: 10.1080/24748668.2017.1352432.

te Wierike, S. C. M., Elferink-Gemser, M. T., Tromp, E. J. Y., Vaeyens, R., & Visscher, C. (2015). Role of maturity timing in selection procedures and in the specialisation of playing positions in youth basketball. Journal of sports sciences, 33(4), 337-345.

Trnini , S., Dizdar, D., Lukši , E. 2002. Differences between winning and defeated top quality basketball teams in final tournaments of European club championship. Collegium Antropolgicum, 26 (2): 521–531.

Tsarouchas, L, Kalamaras, K., Giavroglou, A. and Prassas, S. 1990. Biomechanical analysis of free throw shooting in basketball. In E. Kreighbaum & A. McNeill (Eds), Biomechanics in Sport VI. pp. 551-560. Bozeman, MT: Montana State University.

33

Health Implications of Physical Activity Participation of Second Cycle School Students

Moses Monday Omoniyi[1]✉, Asamoah Richmond[2], Doku Abigail Oforiwaa[3], Afrifa Daniel[4], Asamoah-Mensah Anthony[5], Deku Prince De-Gualle[6], Tiguridaane Isaac Azo[7]

Department of Sports and Exercise Science, Faculty of Allied Health Sciences, College of Health sciences, Kwame Nkrumah University of Science and Technology, Kumasi, Ghana[1234567]

Article History

Keywords:
Physical activity; Sedentary lifestyle; Students

Abstract

The general objective of the study is to investigate health implications of physical activity participation of second cycle school students in Kumasi, Ashanti region of Ghana. This exploratory research recruited 660 SHS students (mean aged=16.51 ± 18.41 years). Age, height, weight, waist to hip ratio, BMI, systolic and diastolic blood pressure and resting energy expenditure were measured. Physical activity involvements were identified using modified SQUASH questionnaire. The prevalence of sedentary lifestyle due to the introduction of modern technological implements in learning, recreation and occupation play significant roles among the causes of cardiovascular risk factors globally. In Ghana, senior high school (SHS) students partake in physical activity (PA) as part of their physical education programme but there is scarce information on the health implications of such participation. This study examined the health implications of PA participation of senior high school students in Kumasi with emphasis on gender, weight, BMI, heart rate, waist to hip ratio and blood pressure. This study concluded that second cycle school students are physically active with incidences of overweight, obesity and morbidity. The PA program and time spent by those overweight, obese and morbid should be re-designed to prevent cardiovascular risk factors.

✉ **Correspondence address :**
E-mail: mmomoniyi.chs@knust.edu.gh

INTRODUCTION

Physical activity (PA) plays an important role in prevention of non-communicable diseases (NCDs) such as cardiovascular diseases, overweight and musculoskeletal disorder (Baldew et al, 2015). It is an established fact that regular (≥3 times per week) moderate intensity PA such as brisk walking, dancing and gardening decrease the risk of NCD (Gulati & Anoop, 2014) . PA is commonly recommended as an important lifestyle in prevention of hypertension but worldwide prevalence of hypertension is projected to increase to 60% by 2025(Diaz & Shimbo, 2013). PA lowers blood pressure and assists in weight management and a reduction in visceral fat (Tchernof & Jean-Pierre, 2013). People of all ages can improve the quality of their lives and reduce the risks of developing coronary heart disease, hypertension, some cancers like; colon cancer and breast cancer, and type 2 diabetes with participation in moderate PA and exercise (Roper et al, 2016). Daily exercise will also enhance one's mental well-being and promote healthy musculoskeletal function throughout life (Gillen & Jenna, 2012). Although habitual PA is an attainable goal to a healthier life and significant health benefits can be obtain by a correct and graded PA throughout the week (Gillen & Jenna, 2012). Fitness programs involving progressive increase intensity of exercise will elicit greater cardio-protective benefits. There is a growing understanding of how levels of PA positively affect cardiovascular, musculoskeletal, respiratory, endocrine function, and mental health (Pontzer & Herman, 2016). Physical inactivity increases the risk of many chronic conditions, such as cardiovascular diseases, type 2 diabetes, obesity, colon cancer, breast cancer, dementia and depression (Egan, Brendan, Juleen & Zierath, 2013). The World Health Organization (WHO, 2000) recommends PA of at least 150 min per week at moderate intensity, or high-intensity physical activity of at least 75 min per week, in order to gain health benefits. Moderate and high-intensity PA can be combined to achieve the recommended amount of PA (El, Walid, Sakari, & Steve, 2017).Overweight and obesity are the major risk factors for increased morbidity, disability, and premature mortality from cardiovascular disease (mainly hypertension, heart disease and stroke), type 2 diabetes, musculoskeletal disorders (osteoarthritis and chronic back pain) and some cancers (breast, and colon) (Msyamboza, Kapaki, Damson & Titha, 2013). It is estimated that the burden of hypertension is attributable to obesity and is approximately 80% for men and 60% for women with respect to their physical activities but has a ratio of 32:14mmHg per pound respectively (Lam et al, 2015). Using body mass index (BMI) as an anthropometric measure, overweight category (BMI ≥ 25 kg/m2) is associated with approximately 30% higher for overall mortality and 40% higher for cardiovascular mortality of which is considered as a health problem for second cycle schools (Patel & Sen, 2016). Despite well-documented evidence that physical activity is beneficial to children, average fitness levels of children in the advanced world have declined. Lack of physical activity has been associated with childhood obesity: obesity raises the risk for type 2 diabetes mellitus, insulin resistance, heart disease, high blood pressure, metabolic syndrome, and other health related disorders. Type 2 diabetes, once uncommon in childhood, now represents 8% to 45% of all diabetes reported in children and adolescents,(Katz et al., 2010)

It is recommended by Health and Human Service that children and adolescents should engage in 60 minutes of physical activity per day, meeting this recommendation can improve cardiorespiratory fitness, muscular strength, blood pressure, and can decrease depressive symptoms in children in a short amount of time (Health and Human Service, 2010). Despite the known benefits, research shows a significant. Epidemiological findings have reported a decrease in physical activity as autonomy increases throughout middle and high school, this decrease in physical activities is associated to many factors including the gain of greater gain autonomy relative to their daily lives, psychosocial and residency (location, i.e. on or off campus housing) and greater time demands (e.g. work, class time) as well as different access to places to be active, (Calestine, Bopp, & Bopp, 2017).

The general objective of the study is to investigate effect of health implications of physical activity as a correlate of demographic profiles in second cycle students in Kumasi, Ashanti region of Ghana.

The study specifically sought to:

1. Determine demographic profiles status of second cycle school students.
2. Examine the level of blood pressure, heart rate and resting energy expenditure of the students.
3. Investigate the relationship between demographic profile and health implications of physical activity involvement in second cycle school students.
4. Investigate the relationship between blood pressure, heart rate, resting energy expen-

diture and physical activity involvement of the students.

5. Investigate the relationship between demographic profile and physical activity involvement of the students based on gender and class level.

METHODS

This exploratory research design recruited 660 Senior High School students in Ghana (mean aged=16.51 ± 18.41 years. Following a verbal discussion with the various head of the schools, letter of introduction was handed over to them and consent of parent in case of minor was sought. The data collected was divided into Demographic information; age, height, weight, waist to hip ratio and BMI and resting energy expenditure, systolic and diastolic blood pressures. The types of physical activity the students involve themselves were measured using modified SQUASH questionnaire. Convenient sampling technique was used in recruiting students because of the busy academic schedules of some students.

RESULTS AND DISCUSSION

Questionnaire guide with questions on health enhancing physical activity as correlate of body composition and anthropometric profile was developed. The questionnaire consisted of three parts; the first part included questions on demographic information, the second part included anthropometric and physiological measures such as height, body mass index, weight, and Waist-hip ratio and the third part included questions on health enhancing physical activity pattern of senior high school (SHS) students on frequency of physical activity participation (items) such walking or cycling, and duration for each activity within a week.

Weight and height was measured to the nearest 0.1 kg and 0.5cm respectively using a Health-O-Meter, floor type, model RGZ-16O. In measuring weight, the scale was placed on an even firm floor. Participants stood on the scale with shoes removed, both feet at the center of the scale with weight evenly distributed, looked straight ahead so that the line of sight was parallel to the floor and the weight of the participant was recorded. In measurement of height, the participants removed their shoes, bulky clothing, hair ornament, and unbraid hair that could interferes with measurement. Participants stood on the base of the health-o-meter with feet flat and together, legs straight, arms at side and shoulders level. Participants looked straight ahead so that the line of sight was parallel to the floor and height was recorded. BMI was calculated as weight (kg)/height2 (m2) and used to categorize BMI-measured weight status: underweight (BMI ≤ 18.5), normal weight (BMI 18.5–24.9), overweight (BMI 25.0–29.9) and obese (BMI ≥ 30) (WHO, 1995). Waist circumference (WC) was measured midway between the inferior angle of the ribs and the supra-iliac crest (WHO, 2011) to the nearest 0.5 cm using a non-stretchable but flexible measuring tape (ISAK, 2001). During the measurement, participants stood in an upright position, with arms relaxed at their side, feet evenly spread apart and body weight evenly distributed in accordance with the WHO expert consultation report on waist circumference and waist-to-hip ratio (WHR) (Mogre, Nyab & Aleyira, 2015). Abdominal obesity will be determining as a waist circumference >102 cm in male and >88 cm in female according to the World Health Organization cut-off points and risk of metabolic complications for Waist circumference (WHO, 2011).

Resting Energy Expenditure (REE) Equation: Males: 50.9xBW(kg) + 25.3xHt(cm) – 50.3xA(y) + 26.9); Females: (51.2xBW(kg) + 24.5xHt(cm) – 207.5xA(y) + 1629.8); Where BW is body weight, Ht is body height and A is age. Each REE value was converted from kilojoules and expressed as kilocalories by dividing each value by 4.186.

RESULTS

Majority of the participants in this study were between the ages of 16 and 18, followed by the 13-15. Out of the 660 participants 276, 237 and 147 were SHS 1, 2 and 3 students respectively. Majority of the participants recorded 75% as normal weight, followed by 20% as overweight, 4% as obese and 1% as morbid.

Table 1. Descriptive statistics of demographic profiles

Demographic Profile	Mean	Standard Deviation	Rating
Age(years)	16.5	1.84	NA
Height(m)	1.63	3.23	NA
Weight(cm)	60.11	1.35	NA
BMI	22.62	2.14	Normal
Waist to hip ratio	0.81	0.03	Normal
Heart rate / min	73.22	0.93	Normal
Systolic Blood ressure(mmHg)	121.2	1.93	Normal

Diastolic Blood ressure(mmHg)	76.88	1.25	Normal
Resting Energy Expenditure(C)	.77	3.25	Normal

The results of the participants showed that, they have normal heart rate, waist to hip ratio, systolic and diastolic and resting energy expenditure.

Table 2. Chi-Square Distribution of Physical Activities Participation

Physical Activity Involvements	Response	N (%)	P-value
`Do you engage in physical activities?	No	46 (7.0)	.000
	Yes	614 (93.0)	
Which of these activities do you regularly participate?	Soccer	145 (23.6)	.000
	Basketball	44 (7.2)	
	Running	153 (24.9)	
	Volleyball	71 (11.6)	
	Jogging	96 (15.6)	
	Others	105 (17.1)	
How many times per week do you engage in physical activities?	1-2	153(24.9)	.000
	3-4	240 (39.1)	
	5-6	90 (14.7)	
	7 above	131 (21.3)	
How long do you spend in performing these activities or sports?	30-45mins	192(31.3)	.000
	1 hr	120(19.5)	
	2 hours	234(38.1)	
	3 and above hours	68(11.1)	
Where do you long spend in performing these physical activities?	Home	227 (37.0)	.000
	School sports field	234 (38.1)	
	Sports recreational Centre	155 (24.9)	
With whom do you normally do your physical activities	Alone	139 (22.6)	.000
	School peers	266 (43.3)	
	Parents and relatives	104(16.9)	
	Other People	111 (17.1)	
When do you usually do your physical activities?	Morning	199(31.8)	.000
	Afternoon	135(22.0)	
	After evening meals	100(16.3)	
	Any convenient time	184(30.0)	
When are your reasons in participating of sports or physical activities?	Good Health	328(54.4)	.000
	Competition	133(21.7)	
	To lose weight	141(23.0)	
	To gain weight	12(2.0)	

About 93% of the respondents engage in some physical activity with the most being running (23.2%), soccer (22%) and jogging (14.5%). Majority (36.1%) engage in these activities 3-4 times per week with a modal duration of 30-45 minutes per session. The school sports field was the most cited place for which these physical activities take place but slightly fewer also said they do it at home, school peers (40.3%), activities (30.2%) but 27.9% cited any convenient time. 100(15.2%) engage in this activities after evening meals.

Table 3. Passive Activities

Activities	Response	N (%)	P-value
On average, how long do you watch TV/DVD/Video per day	30-45mins	85(12.9)	.000
	1 hour	193(29.2)	
	2 hours	191(28.9)	
		161(24.4)	
Do you use a computer?	No	96(14.5)	.000
	Yes	553(83.3)	
If you do, how long do you spend using this computer?	30-45mins	50(7.6)	.000
	1 hour	172(26.1)	
	2 hours	188(28.5)	
	3 and above	145(22.0)	
On average, how many hours do you sleep in a day?	2-3 hours	105(15.9)	.000
	4-5 hours	18127.4)	
	6-7 hours	284(43.0)	
	8 hours and above	61(9.2)	
What are your reasons for not participating in active sports or physical activities?	I have no time	192(29.1)	.000
	No suitable facility	168(25.5)	
	Not important	97(14.7)	
		108(16.4)	

Majority of the respondents watch television, DVD or videos for an average of 1 hour per day. About 84% own a computer with 28% of those spending 2 hours per day on their computers whilst 15.9% spend between2 and 3 hours. Modal sleep time for the participants of this study was between 6 and 7 hours with only 9% sleeping for above 8 hours per day. The most mentioned reasons for participation in physical activities were good health, followed by to lose weight, competitions and to gain weight in that order. Reasons for not participating in included lack of time (29.1%), No suitable facilities (25.5%), not important (14.7%) and others (16.4%).

Table 4. Association between Body Mass Index and Physical activities

BMI Classification	Physical Activities	
	No (n=46)	Yes (n=614)
Normal	23 (50.0%)	480 (78.2%)
Overweight	9 (19.6%)	109 (17.8%)
Obese	14(30.4%)	25(4.1%)
Morbid	0	5(0.8%)

DISCUSSION

Most students do PA 614(93%), majority in soccer 145(23.6%) at least 3 - 4 times in a week 240(39.1%) for two hours 234(38.1) in school 234(38.1%) with their peers 266(43.3%) in the morning 199(31.8%) and at convenient time 184(30.0%) which affirms Allender and co's study that, for young children and teenagers, pressure to conform to social stereotypes is a key motivator as well as children see enjoyment and social interaction with peers as reasons to be physically active (Allender, Cowburn, & Foster, 2006). The study recorded that the reasons of participation in physical activity been good health for majority 328(54.4%) as similarly observed by Boozer that physical activity and health related quality of life were significantly related (Boozer, 2017), followed by losing weight 141(23.0%) which is in agreement with the benefits of participating actively in physical activities (Calestine et al., 2017), competition 133(21.7%) and gain weight 12(2.0%). It is also observed in this study that majority of the students 480(78.2%) and 23(50.0%) both who actively participate in PA however most of the students who do not actively participate in PA found themselves in the overweight and obese range and those who do not actively participate in PA respectively fall within the normal BMI range compared to their counterparts who actively participate in PA, similarly studies have shown that physical activity and health related quality of life were significantly related (Boozer, 2017; Calestine et al., 2017).

CONCLUSION

This study concluded that second cycle school students are physically active. However, some of them are overweight, obese and morbid. The PA program and time spent by those overweight obese and morbid should be re-designed to prevent cardiovascular (CV) risk factors.

REFERENCES

Allender, S., Cowburn, G., & Foster, C. 2006. Understanding participation in sport and physical activity among children and adults : a review of qualitative studies, 21(6), 826–835. https://doi.org/10.1093/her/cyl063.

Baldew S. M., Ingrid K. S. K., Christel S. C. F., Jerry R. T., Luc V., & Veronique C. 2015, Self-reported physical activity behavior of a multi-ethnic adult population within the urban and rural setting in Suriname, BMC Public Health Vol. 15, No. 1, p. 485.

Boozer, S. 2017. Effect of Physical Activity on Quality of Life for College Students : A Comparative Gender Study by. Honors Theses, 526. Retrieved from http://aquila.usm.edu/honors_theses/526

Calestine, J., Bopp, M., & Bopp, C. M. 2017. College Student Work Habits are related to Physical Activity and Fitness. International Journal of Exercise Science, Vol. 7, 10, 1009 –1017

Diaz K. M. & Daichi S., Physical activity and the prevention of hypertension, Current hypertension reports, Vol. 15, No. 6, p. 659-668.

Egan B. & Juleen R. Z., 2013, Exercise metabolism and the molecular regulation of skeletal muscle adaptation, Cell metabolism Vol. 17, No. 2, p. 162-184.

El A., Walid S. S., & Steve D., 2017, Correlates of achieving the guidelines of four forms of physical activity, and the relationship between guidelines achievement and academic performance: Undergraduate students in Finland, Central European journal of public health Vol. 25, No. 2 p. 87.

Gillen J., 2012, Low-volume, high-intensity interval training: A practical fitness strategy, Wellspring, Vol. 23, No. 4, p. 1-4.

Gulati S., & Anoop M., 2014, Sugar intake, obesity, and diabetes in India. Nutrients Vol 6, No.12, p. 5955-5974.

Health and Human Services, 2010. The Association Between School-Based Physical Activity, Including Physical Education , and Academic Performance, 2010(April).

ISAK (2001). International Standards for Anthropometric Assessment. Underdale, S.A.; International Society for the Advancement of Kinanthropometry.

Katz, D. L., Cushman, D., Reynolds, J., Njike, V., Treu, J. A., Walker, J., … Walker, J. (2010). Putting Physical Activity Where It Fits in the School Day : Preliminary Results of the ABC (Activity Bursts in the Classroom) for Fitness Program, 7(4).

Lam B. C. C., et al. 2015, Comparison of body mass index (BMI), body adiposity index (BAI), waist circumference (WC), waist-to-hip ratio (WHR) and waist-to-height ratio (WHtR) as predictors of cardiovascular disease risk factors in an adult population in Singapore, PLoS One, Vol. 10, No. 4 p. e0122985.

Mogre V., Nyaba R., Aleyira S., & Sam N. B. 2015, Demographic, dietary and physical activity predictors of general and abdominal obesity among university students: a cross-sectional study. Springerplus, Vol. 4, No. 1, p. 226.

Msyamboza K. P., Kathyola D., & Dzowela T. 2013, Anthropometric measurements and prevalence of underweight, overweight and obesity in adult Malawians: nationwide population based NCD STEPS survey, Pan African Medical Journal, Vol. 15, No. 1.

Patel, S & Sen, D J., 2016, Get slim to fulfill the dream. World Journal of Pharmacy and Pharmaceutical Sciences. Vol 5, No. 8, p. 14-24

Pontzer H., Brown M. H., Raichlen D. A., Dunsworth H., Hare B., Walker K., & Plange-Rhule J. 2016, Metabolic acceleration and the evolution of human brain size and life history, Nature, Vol. 533, No. 7603, p. 390.

Roper JL, Harding EM, Doerfler D, Dexter JG, Kravitz L, Dufek JS, Mermier CM. 2016, The effects of gait retraining in runners with patellofemoral pain: A randomized trial, Clinical Biomechanics, Vol. 35 p. 14-22.

Tchernof A., & Jean-Pierre D., 2013, Pathophysiology of human visceral obesity: an update. Physiological reviews, Vol. 93, No. 1, P. 359-404.

World Health Organisation. 2011. Waist Circumference and Waist-Hip Ratio: Report of a WHO Expert Consultation, Geneva, 8–11 December 2008. Technical report, World Health Organization.

World Health Organization. 1995, Physical status: the use and interpretation of anthropometry. Report of a WHO Expert Committee. World Health Organ Tech Rep Ser, 854, p. 1–452.

The Effect of Touch of The Ball in Small Side Games on The Improvement Vo2max Amateur Football Players

Ketut Chandra Adinata Kusuma[1], I Kadek Happy Kardiawan[2]

Jurusan Pendidikan Kepelatihan Olahraga, Fakultas Olahraga dan Kesehatan, Universitas Pendidikan Ganesha,Indonesia[12]

Article History

Keywords:
Small Side Games; Two Touch; Free Touch; VO2max

Abstract

The aims of this study was: (1) the effect of training the small side games 4v4 two-touch game against VO2max, (2) the effect of training small side games 4v4 free touch against VO2max, and (3) the different effect between small side games 4v4 two touches and small side games 4v4 free touch against VO2max. This research is an experimental research with a modified pre-test – post-test group design. The subjects of this research were 32 amateur football players. MFT was used to measure VO2max in data collecting technique. The data were analyzed by using t-statistical calculation assisted with SPSS 16.0 at 0.05 significance level. The result shows the exercise of small side games 4v4 two touches affected to VO2max (sig value = 0.000), training of small side games 4v4 free touch affected to VO2max (sig value = 0,016) and there are some differences between two touches and free touch training. Coaches are suggested to use small side method in order to improve the VO2max of their players.

Correspondence address :
E-mail: chandra_ketut@yahoo.com / happy.kardiawan@yahoo.com

INTRODUCTION

Based on the competition analysis when competing shows that football is a sport that is classifield as high intensity sports (Alexandre, et.al, 2012). During the game, each player will be find a jump situation, dribbling the ball, shooting the ball, running at different speeds, running with the ball, run in a direction, sliding tackle, controlling the ball under pressure opponent. That situation shows that many factors influence each player (physical, technique, tactics) and the importance of developing these conditions to achieve performance during the match. In this context, the preparation of football players before participating in the competition requires training that matches the demands of the actual match (Reilly in Rodenaz, 2015). Physical conditions are very important as a foundation in supporting other performance for each players. Bad physical conditions will certainly have a bad impact on the appearance techniques and tactics.

According Sajoto (1995:8) there are ten types of physical coditions, which need to be developed among other strength, endurance, muscular power, speed, flexibility, agility, coordination, balance, accuracy, and reaction. Good endurance is one of the physical conditions that must be owned by each player, without reducing the role of the other nine physical conditions. Based on the research stated that non-goalkeeper players usually run as far as 10-12 km in one match. The midfielder position becomes the player with the longest running distance of 12 km in every match. The logical consequence is that each player has a minimum VO2max level in the good category.

However, based on the observations result at Undiksha FC, one of the amateur clubs that competed in League 3 PSSI, showed the average VO2max results of the players who were not good enough when referring to Prima Pratama standard. Excluding the goalkeeper, the average VO2max of the Undiksha FCC players is 42,5 ml/kg/min. The implication of the above is that it is difficult for Undiksha FC players to be able to play with high pressing during defence, or control the ball primed for 90 minutes during offence.

VO2max is the ability of human respiratory organs to breath as much oxygen as possible during training (Sukadiyanto, 2011: 83). VO2max or also called maximum oxygen use is the fastest tempo in which a person can use oxygen during exercise. VO2max is very important to support the work of a muscle by taking oxygen and channeling it to all muscle tissue that is active, so that it can be used for metabolic processes.

According to Irianto (2004: 23) endurance of the heart or also called cardio respiratory is the functional ability of the lungs and heart im supplying oxygen for muscle work for a long time. A person who has good lung and heart endurance will not be quickly exhausted after work. Quality of lung and heart endurance is exspressed as VO2max, which is the maximum amount oxygen that can be consumed in ml/kgbb/minutes. In football games the ability of good aerobic endurance or high VO2max is highly prioritized.

Small Side Games (SSGs) becomes a popular training method by many amateur and professional teams as an effective method for aerobic exercise by combining technical, tactical and physiological exercises (Rampini et,al. 2007). SSGs method require each player to actively move with high intensity, because players play in a space that is not large and each player touches the ball more frequently. Hill-Haas, et.al (2011) defines small sided games as a game played in field with a size that more than football generally uses modified rules and involves a players that are smaller that actual number of players. Advantages in the Small Side Games methods: (1) many technical elements are contained, tactics and physicality in one exercise, (2) in this exercise there are opponents playing so that it is like a real game and there is an element of mental training.

There are several studies that the influence of the game model of the goal model, and the number of players on the intensity of play on SSGs (Rodenas, et.al. 2015). The game model is the amount of touch to the ball that is allowed for each player. Whereas the number of players arranged is 4 versus 4, 5 versus 5, 6 versus 6. It turns out that the fewer the number of players involved, the higher the internsity of play shown from the height of the player's Hrmax.

Katis (2009) also revealed the effect of SSGs on the formation od physical conditions and the performance of young football players. Dellal A, et.al (2011) also briefly researched the effect of the number of contact with the ball with SSGs 4 versus 4 models which showed that with a smaller number of ball contacts it would increase the Maximum Heart Rate (HRmax) of each player. So, the less the number of the ball touches by the player and the less number of players involved there will be an increase in Hrmax each player.

Based on this, the researcher is interested in revealing "The Effect of The Number of Touches of Balls in Small Side Games on Increasing VO-2max of Amateur Football Players". Although this was once researched by Dellal A, et.al but the research subject at that time was an international elite players. Whereas for amateur players there have been no results related to this report and no one has measured the effect of VO2max on the perpetrators.

METHODS

This type of research is experimental. The design of this study uses the modified pre test-post test group design (Kanca, 2010: 87).

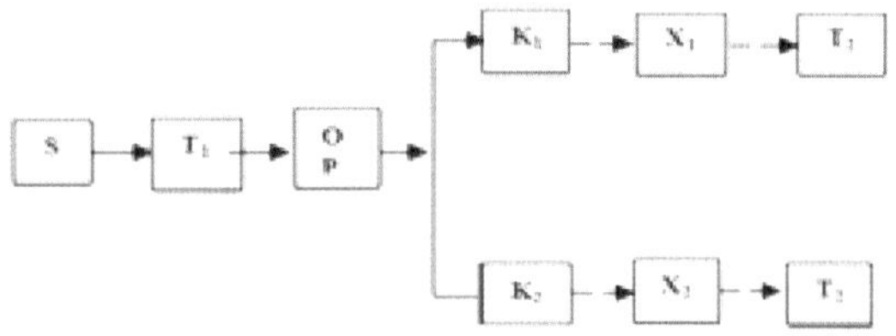

Picture 1. The modified pre test-post test group design

The population of this study were all Undiksha FC players who competed in the League 3 PSSI Association of Bali Province in 2018 totaling 32 people, not including the goalkeeper. The population was involved in the study, the research subjects were 32 goalkeepers. Because all of these members include population reseach. So that the 32 reseach subjects were given a pre test namely the Multistage Fitness Test (MFT) first, then divided into two groups using ordinal pairing techniques. Group 1 which will be given training on small side 4v4 games with two touches and group 2 will be given small side 4v4 games with free touches. After the two group were given training 23 times the meeting continued with a post test using the MFT. Data analysis using the t test, but before testing the hypothesis the normality test was first performed using Kolmogorov-Smirnov and Levene's Test Of Equality Error Variance test to test homogeneity at 5% significance level.

RESULTS AND DISCUSSION

Testing the normality of data distribution is done to ensure that the research subject is normally distributed. To find out the normality of data distribution, the Kolmogorov-Smirnov formula is used at a significance af 0,05. If sig> 0,05 the data is said to be normally distributed. Conversely, if sig< 0,05 the data is not normally distributed. Based on the analysis that has been done using SPSS 16.00 for Windows the results are obtained as shown in the following **Tabel 1**.

Tabel 1. Test the normality of data distribution

	Kolmogorov-Smirnova		
	Statistic	**Df**	**Sig.**
Pre test two touch	.200	16	.087
Post test two touch	.154	16	200*
Pre test free touch	.158	16	200*
Post test free touch	.158	16	200*

Based on **Tabel 1** above, it can be seen that for all the significance variables in the Kolmogorov-Smirnov test is greater that 0,05. Thus, all data distribution is normally distributed.

The variance homogeneity test is carried out by grouping based on the given test model. The homogeneity test of variance between groups was carried out with the help of SPSS 16.00 for Windows using Levene's Test Of Equality Error Variance, statistical hypothesis tested in homogeneity testing is as follows.

Ho : the variance in each group is the same (homogeneous)

Ha : the variance in each group is not the same (not homogeneous)

With the testing criteria used is if Ho p>0.05 where the data has the same variance if the significant number generated is more that 0.05. summary results of data homogeneity calculation using SPSS 16.00 for windows can be seen in the following **Tabel 2**.

Tabel 2. Summary of The Results Homogeneity Test of Variance Test of Homogeneity of Variances

Data group	Levene Statistic	Df1	Df2	Sig.
VO-2max	0,060	1	30	0.808

Based on **Tabel 2** above, the Levene's test results show that the p>0,05, then accept Ho. So that it can be concluded that the variance in each group is the same (homogeneous).

The research hypothesis that has been stated states that there is an effect of the results of small side games on VO2max. Hypothesis testing using t test with the help of SPSS 16.00 for Windows. The results of the analysis with t test are presented in **Tabel 3** below.

Based on **Tabel 3** above, a significant value of 0,000 is obtained p<0,05. This result is used as a basic in the decision. The decision taken is to reject Ho and accept Ha. This result states that the-

Tabel 3. Paired Samples Test

	Paired Differences					t	df	Sig. (2-tailed)
	Mean	Std. Deviation	Std. Error Mean	95% Confidence Interval of the Difference				
				Lower	Upper			
Pair 1 wotouch – twotouch	-3.96250	1.71109	.42777	-4.87428	-3.05072	-9.263	15	.000
Pair 2 freetouch – freetouch	-1.90625	2.82382	.70595	-3.41096	-.40154	-2.700	15	.016

re is a training effect for small side games against VO2max. So it can be concluded that there is a significant influence between small side games and VO2max training.

Based on the testing of the first hypothesis it turns out that there is a significant effect of the training of 4v4 two touch small side games on VO2max ($p < 0.05$). The small side 4v4 two touch training exercise is a 4 versus 4 game simulation training with the rules that every player is allowed to touch the ball for a maximum of 2 times in a row. so that in this training can increase speed, agility in the game and of course increase endurance. Based on Arcos's research, Asier Los et.al. (2015) also states that SSGs have a significant effect on improving aerobic fitness and are better than interval training methods. Rodenas, et.al. (2015) also suggested that the modification of the game model, the goal model, and the number of players in SSGs affected the intensity of playing for elite young players. Modification of the number of players means that the smaller the number of players involved the higher the heart rate (HRmax) the players involved. The training of small side games 4v4 two touch has the advantage that all players are more active in moving to carry out cooperation in attack and the passing must be precise and accurate. Dellal, et. al. (2011) also revealed that there was a faster increase in Heart Rate (HR) players who performed SSGs one touch (1T), two touch (2T) than players who performed SSGs free play or free touch.

Based on the second hypothesis testing, there was a significant influence from the training of small side games 4v4 free touch on VO2max ($p < 0.05$). Small side games 4v4 free touch training is a 4 versus 4 game simulation training with the rules of play for each player is not limited to the maximum number of touches with the ball, so that in this exercise there will be more dueling, HR response also increased (Dellal, et. Al. 2011). This small side 4v4 free touch training training is very beneficial because it can create space and also disrupt the opponent's guard.

Based on the testing of the third hypothesis, there was a significant difference in the effect of training in small side 4v4 two touch games with small side games 4v4 free touch on VO2max. Whereas the small side games 4v4 two touch training is greater than the small side 4v4 free touch games. Two touch SSGs characters require each player to move more or in other words, each player cannot linger over the ball. So that every player has very little active rest time. HR automatically increases each player very fast compared to free touch. Free touch SSGs can linger on the ball for a long time, so that other players who don't control the ball can take a longer active break which directly reduces the HR of each player.

CONCLUSION

Based on the results of data analysis and discussion above, it can be concluded that the number of ball touches in small side games affects the increase in VO2max of amateur soccer players. So that it is expected that football coaches and football extracurricular coaches can implement the exercise to increase the VO2max of their players / students.

REFERENCES

Alexandre, D., da Silva, C. D., Hill-Haas, S., Wong, D. P., Natali, A. J., de Lima, J. R. P., & Karim, C. 2012. "Heart rate monitoring in soccer: Interest and limits during competitive match play and training, practical application". Journal of Strength and Conditioning Research. 26. 2890–2906.

Arcos, Asier Los., Vazquez, J. S., Martin, J., Lerga, J., Sanchez, F., Villagra, F., Zulueta, J. J. 2015. "Effects of Small-Sided Games vs. Interval Training in Aerobic Fitness and Physical Enjoyment in Young Elite Soccer Players". PLoS ONE 10(9): e0137224. doi:10.1371/ journal. pone.0137224.

Dellal, A., Lago, C., Wong, D.P., Chamari, K. 2011.

"Effects of the number of ball contacts within bouts of 4 vs 4 small-sided games". Int J Sports Physiol Perf. 6(3). 322-333.

Hill-Haas, S. V., Dawson, B., Impellizzeri, F. M., & Coutts, A. J. 2011. "Physiology of small-sided games training in football: A systematic review". Sports Medicine. 41. 199–220.

Irianto, Djoko Pekik. 2004. Bugar dan Sehat Dengan Olahraga. Yogyakarta : Andi Offset.

Kanca, I Nyoman. 2010. Metode Penelitian Pengajaran Pendidikan Jasmani dan Olahraga. Singaraja: Universitas Pendidikan Ganesha.

Katis, A., Kellis, E. 2009. "Effects of small-sided games on physical conditioning and performance in young soccer players". Journal Sports Science and Medicine. 8(3). 374-380.

Muzakir, Doddy Rachman. 2013. "Para Pekerja Keras Di Liga Champion". Tersedia pada http://lab-bola.com/para-pekerja-keras-di-liga-champions/. Diakses pada tanggal 27 November 2017.

Rampinini E, Impellizzeri, F. M., Castagna, C., Abt, G., Chamari, K., Sassi, A., Marcora, S. M. 2007. "Factors influencing physiological responses to small-sided soccer games". Journal Sport Science. 25(6). 659-666.

Rodenas, J. G., Calabuig, F., Aranda, R. 2015. "Effect of the Game Design, the Goal Type, and the Number of Players on Intensity of Play in Small-Sided Games in Youth Elite Players". Journal of Human Kinetics. 49. 229-235

Sajoto, Mochamad. 1995. Peningkatan dan Pembinaan Kekuatan Kondisi Fisik. Semarang : Dahara Prize.

Sukadiyanto dan Muluk, D. 2011. Pengantar Teori dan Metodologi Melatih Fisik. Bandung: Lubuk Agung.

35

Benefits of Roller Derby: The Roller Girl Perspective

Barbara A. Masberg[1], **Andrea Eklund**[2]

Department of Family and Consumer Sciences Central Washington University[12]

Article History

Keywords:
Roller Derby; Flat Track; Benefits; Empowerment; Bout

Abstract

Roller derby consists of two teams vying for points played on a flat oval track wearing quad skates. The specific research questions asked were: What are the characteristics of roller derby league members? What are the motivations of women who join roller derby leagues? What are reasons for continuing to participate? Do roller derby participants identify specific characteristics of the sport that distinguish it from other sports? Are there specific benefits from roller derby women seek and receive? An on-line survey was used and qualitative data were analyzed (n=1597). Based upon the data, a typical respondent is Caucasian, 20 to 40 years of age, heterosexual, in a married/domestic partnership, and has a post-secondary degree. Reasons for joining included looking for a new way to get exercise, add something new and different to my life, and roller derby might fit my personality. For continuing, the following reasons were ranked as important; roller derby adds richness to my life, I like the idea of overcoming obstacles as a team, and I like the social interaction. Because of participation, they benefited several ways including a positive opinion of self, health improvement, increased relationships, and an added outlook.

Correspondence address :
E-mail: Barbara.Masberg@cwu.edu

INTRODUCTION

Roller derby originated in the1930's as roller skating marathons. By 1937, roller derby had evolved into a physical competition between two teams with associated media and spectators. Roller derby has had many boom-and-bust cycles with its popularity peaking in 1949 with 55,000 fans watching a competition in Madison Square Garden (Coppage, 1999). There were several short-lived attempts to revitalize the sport since that time through theatrical television programs, which were short-lived. In 2003, the Texas Rollergirls league gained media attention and launched league formation in other towns (Coppage, 1999; Kearney, 2011; Mabee, 2007). In 2006, Roller Derby Worldwide (2012) had 160 leagues registered on its database. Today, Roller Derby Listing reports 1,917 registered leagues (Derbylisting.com, 2018).

The main purpose of this research was to increase understanding of why roller derby members are attracted to this sport and continue to participate. The specific research questions asked:

(1) What are the characteristics of roller derby league members?
(2) What are the motivations of women who join roller derby leagues?
(3) What are reasons for continuing to participate?
(4) Do roller derby participants identify specific characteristics of the sport?
(5) Are there specific benefits from roller derby women seek and receive?

Most of the current research findings about roller derby are found in feminist literature, which contextualizes the meaning of the sport for women. Storms (2008) suggests that roller derby is another window through which to understand the evolution of feminism in America as women seek alternative ways to experience their bodies and gender. Peluso (2010) concluded that roller derby threatens the gender order status quo due to the formation of a league identity of shared values creating solidarity to the point of having the members "guard the boundaries of the community from outsiders" (p. 132). Roller derby is empowering and has a diffusion effect wherein empowered women empower others, improve self-confidence, sexuality, and empowerment. (Peluso, 2010 p. 76). Carlson (2010) revealed that roller derby provides a venue for women to emphasize femininity whilst also being aggressive. Authors (Eklund & Masberg; 2014; Strubel & Petrie, 2016) found that body image and self-esteem improved with involvement. Nevertheless, others point out that size does matter as the attitude toward size or bigger is better changes based upon the level of competition of the roller derby team (Draft, 2017). Injuries and the "willingness to play through" mentality is prevalent in roller derby for a variety of reasons, to not let down their teammates, playing time, and so they do not appear weak (Madrigal & Robbins, 2017, p. 185).

Pavlidis (2012) states that roller derby is ". . . an enabling space where female subjectivities and collective belonging can be played with" (p. 173). In Cotterill's ethnographic study, seven themes emerged regarding the reasons for participating in roller derby: "outlet for aggression, escape from daily constraints, camaraderie, exercise, empowering women, self-fulfillment and love of the sport" (p. 33). Rowlette (2015) supported these themes with her results that identified areas that were important when participating in roller derby: "(1) intimidation during the initial skating experience, (2) challenges of learning new skills, (3) developing and maintaining relationships, (4) feelings of strength, and (5) relieving built-up stress (p. 42)".

Finley (2010) offered the idea that intragender relationships developed through roller derby may provide an impetus for "gender maneuvering" in other settings. The interactions between women seem to transform women to "athletes and supporters of other women activities as teammates" (p. 381). Finley (2010) viewed the roller derby subculture as something that "challenges the gender relations of sport (p. 380). Using the do-it-yourself (DIY) organization and being "by the skater for the skater" causes struggles with the amount of time required for bouts and management as well as the financial expense (Beaver, 2012). However skaters choose to continue to be self-managed in order to have control over their league. Other research addresses roller derby and media exposure that points out that through the broadcasting of roller derby there are other models of empowered women. (Kearney, 2011, p. 297).

Involvement and relationships are shown to be integral motivators for joining and continuing in the sport. The culture experienced by current participants may be different from future participants as the sport settles on operation and management norms (Filip, 2016)

Roller Derby Basics

Roller derby is a high contact sport played on a flat or banked oval track wearing four wheeled roller skates. Each team is composed of Blockers, a Pivot, and a Jammer. Each game or bout is comprised of two 30-minute periods of play and each jam is 2 minutes long. Points are earned when the Jammer passes each opposing player. A Pivot keeps the pack together and directs play. Blockers either block opposing Jammers or assist their own Jammer through the pack. There are four main types of blocks: (a) the booty block uses the derriere; (b) the shoulder check, a hit to the side of the body using the shoulder and ribs; (c) the hip check; and the (d) sternum check, using the back of the shoulder to hit the sternum. Hitting or using the lower leg, forearm, elbow, or head to block is illegal. (Coppage, 1999; Deford, 1971; Finley, 2010; Mabe, 2007; Peluso, 2010).

The Women's Flat Track Derby Association (WFTDA, 2018) has established minimum skill requirements and other standards for the sport. Every skater is required to wear a helmet, wrist guards, elbow pads, knee pads, a mouth guard, and quad roller skates (Delano, 2010; Mabe, 2007; Peluso, 2010; WFTDA, 2018;)

Starting out interested women recruit others and seek volunteers to be a leader or manager, and others to serve on committees. A league may have 10 to 130 members. Each league has bylaws and policies, which may include practice and bout-attendance requirements, codes of conduct, new skater policies, skating and bout rules, dismissal policies, and insurance requirements. (Beaver, 2012; Mabe, 2007; Peluso, 2010).

New members are called fresh meat and train for 60 to 90 days to learn the rules and how to move on skates. Fresh meat are tested on their skating ability and knowledge of the rules. They then join league practices and are placed on a team (personal communication, May 28, 2012).

Roller derby requires considerable time commitment. A typical weekly schedule could be made up of two to four practices, one scrimmage, a league committee meeting, and a bout. Most leagues have an attendance requirement, attendance at 75% of practices, or 12 out of 16 practices in one month (Barbee & Cohen, 2010).

METHODS

The investigators developed an on-line survey. The survey instrument contained closed-ended and open-ended questions. Roller derby members both reviewed and pilot tested the survey instrument. A final draft was created, and was published to Qualtrics for data collection.

This research used cluster sampling. A mailing list of roller derby leagues was obtained through Roller Derby Worldwide (2012). At the time of this study, 615 leagues were listed in the United States. This list contained links to either a league Facebook page, or a league website. Phone numbers were used to obtain e-mails. Leagues not included were junior or coed leagues or had invalid contact information.

The implementation process involved sending 583 e-mails with a request to pass along the request to their league members. Respondents self-selected and 1,597 league members from 481 leagues responded to the survey. Demographic data and closed-responses were analyzed using SPSS software. The responses to the open-ended questions were coded to identify patterns (categories and themes) in the data (Saldana, 2016).

RESULTS AND DISCUSSION

Table 1 outlines the demographic characteristics of the respondents. A Roller Girl is Caucasian/White, Heterosexual, between the ages of 20 and 40 years, has earned a degree from a college or university, is married or in a domestic partnership and has one to two children living with her. Respondents were members of a league located in every state in the United States and the District of Columbia:

The length of time as a member and the number of bouts revealed the participants' involvement (see **Table 2**). The highest portion of respondents (35.7%, n= 570) were members for one year or less. The number of bouts in which they had participated reflected fresh meat, zero bouts, (21.9% n=349) and a very well-seasoned member who had more than 15 bouts (24.3% n=388). Respondents rated their skating ability before starting roller derby and then rated their current skating ability on a 10-point scale from 1-low ability to 10-high ability. Skating ability before starting roller derby and their current skating ability, mean score of 3.75 (SD=2.30) and 7.18 (SD=1.57) respectively.

Respondents were asked to rank a list of reasons for initially deciding to join roller derby (1= most important), **Table 3**, as well as a list of reasons for continuing to participate (**Table 4**).

The aggregated mean was used to indicate the more important items. Other comments made were "always wanted to do roller derby", or it looked like "fun" (n=52, 37.1%). Stress reduction and wanting to hit people (n=23, 16.4%) was mentioned along with respondents having some type of connection or need for connection (n=21, 15.0%) such as a friend was trying out, involvement in the community, looking for social interaction after moving to the area, or just "attention".

Table 1: Characteristics of the Respondents

Age of the Respondents	#	%
18 to 19 years	11	0.77%
20 to 29 years	554	38.96%
30 to 39 years	653	45.92%
40 to 49 years	192	13.50%
50 to 59 years	12	0.84%
Total	1422	100.00%

Race or Ethnicity	#	%
White/Caucasian	1384	86.9
Hispanic/Latina/	95	6
Other	49	3.1
Asian / Pacific Islander / Asian American	24	1.5
Black / African American	21	1.3
Native American	19	1.2
Total	1592	100

Current Relationship status	#	%
Married / Domestic Partnership	782	49.2
Single	374	23.5
Cohabitating (not married or domestic partnership)	340	21.4
Separated / Divorced	90	5.7
Widowed	5	0.3
Total	1591	100

Sexual Orientation	#	%
Heterosexual	1240	77.6
Bisexual	199	12.5
Homosexual	96	6
Other	55	3.4
Total	1590	99.6

Highest Education Level	#	%
Some high school	4	0.3
Completed high school or GED	72	4.5
Junior College/Community College/Trade School (Associate's Degree)	160	10.1
Some college/university	334	21
Two year degree	119	7.5
Four year degree	565	35.5
A graduate degree (e.g. Masters, Ph.D. or an M.D.)	336	21.1

Current Profession or Type of Employment	#	%
Professional/technical	478	30.30%
Manager/official/proprietor	183	11.60%
Student	152	9.60%
Clerical	139	8.80%
Teacher	113	7.20%
Service worker	113	7.20%
Homemaker	84	5.30%
Sales	71	4.50%
Health Care	64	4.10%
Crafts/trades	40	2.50%
Unemployed	36	2.30%
Owner	31	2.00%
Laborer	24	1.50%
Artist	24	1.50%
Military	11	0.70%
Operator	7	0.40%
Retired	6	0.40%
Total	1576	100.00%

Approximate Annual Household Income	#	%
Less than $25,000	291	18.6
$25,000 to $49,999	470	30.1
$50,000 to $74,999	348	22.3
$75,000 to $99,999	216	13.8
$100,000 to $124,999	103	6.6
$125,000 to $149,999	58	3.7
$150,000 to $174,999	32	2
$175,000 to $199,999	16	1
$200,000 to 224,999	11	0.7
$225,000 to $249,999	6	0.4
More than $250,000	12	0.8
Total	1563	100

Table 2. Roller Derby Profile Information

Length of Time Participating	#	%
1-6 months	262	16.4%
6 months to 1 year	308	19.3%
1 to 2 years	497	31.2%
2 to 3 years	218	13.7%
3 to 4 years	122	7.7%
4 to 5 years	82	5.1%
More than 5 years	105	6.6%
Total	1594	100.0%

Participation in Number of Bouts	#	%
Zero	349	21.9
1 bout	140	8.8
2-5 bouts	308	19.3
6-10 bouts	284	17.8
11-15 bouts	128	8.0
more than 15 bouts	388	24.3
Total	1597	100.0

Table 3. Reasons for initially joining roller derby

List of reasons	Mean	SD
Looking for a new way to get exercise	3.81	2.379
Add something new and different to my life	4.22	2.669
Roller Derby might fit my personality	4.61	2.896
Meet new friends	4.93	2.450
Improve my overall health	5.08	2.285
The competition	6.09	2.594
Work on becoming more athletic	7.15	2.287
Needed a challenge	7.22	3.037
Feel like I belonged to something	7.33	2.849
Want to skate	7.77	3.921
Idea of accomplishing something as part of a group or team	8.63	2.826

The more important reasons to continue to participate were a bit different as the social aspect game out (see Table 4). Other comments contained more insight, "I love it" (n=21, 21.7%), roller derby was an outlet for stress (n=12, 12.4%), the "big crazy family" and other relationships (n=11, 11.3%) and they were accomplishing something "I keep getting better at it, why stop"(n=11, 11.3%).

Table 4. Reasons for continuing in roller derby

Reasons for continuing	Mean	SD
Roller Derby has added richness to my life	3.56	2.323
I like the idea of overcoming obstacles as a team	4.56	1.927
I like the social interaction	4.67	2.109
I find I like the competition	5.40	2.383
I get an opportunity to express myself in a new way	5.56	2.941
I enjoy the support of team members	5.65	2.238
I like working on improving my skating	5.82	2.571
I like the exercise	6.55	3.600
Roller Derby has changed my outlook on my life	6.55	3.605
I like the effort and perseverance involved	7.18	2.774
I love it, It's fun,	21	21.65%
Outlet for stress or "hitting people legally"	12	12.37%
Relationships; "a big crazy family", "community/sisterhood", "parties",	11	11.34%
Accomplishment	11	11.3%

The pragmatic reason for beginning the sport, exercise, was subsumed by such reasons as social interaction, richness and overcoming obstacles. Henderson et al., (2002) have pointed out creating positive environments for women's leisure is important. The sport is attractive to the respondents as it is for adult women and roller derby allows all women no matter their size, skating skill, age, or profession to participate.

A key to roller derby's popularity could be the inclusivity of the sport. The respondents liked that roller derby did not include minimum skill level requirement. A skater may become a member with no skating ability but must make the effort to meet a skating proficiency. The reason for continuing in the sport is as one woman said, "I love the mental challenge of pushing myself to new limits". The physical and mental effort seems to be a benefit of the sport, the satisfaction with a sweaty workout, and the chance to "hit someone". Roller derby offers a "career track" or progression of development from Fresh Meat, through a training period, then to probation, and finally choosing a derby name and number when joining a team. The DIY aspect offers members the opportunity to improve skills. Respondents noted the impact of gaining skills to apply to their professional lives.

To explain the attraction of roller derby the question was asked; "What makes roller derby different from other sports?" **Table 5** contains the major categories that emerged from the data; (1) General Characteristics (2) The Self, (3) Relationships, (4) Inclusivity; and (5) Perceptions of the sport; and (6) No opinion (Did not do sports, do not do other sports, do not like sports). The number of phrases analyzed was 2,891 (n=1,531; 95.9%; mean responses= 1.89).

Table 5. How is roller derby different from other sports?

Response	#	%
The Play	786	27.2%
Self	742	25.7%
Relationships	481	16.6%
Inclusivity	440	15.2%
Perception of the Sport	350	12.1%
Did not do sports, do not do sports, do not like sports	92	3.2%
Total	2,891	100.0%

The actual play is different. Roller derby strategy and playing offense and defense at the same time and the fact that roller derby is a full contact sport for women was paramount. Skating, the commitment needed, and mentoring occurring were seen as different. The individual outcomes of participating in the sport (The Self) were seen as different from other sports (n=742, 25.7%). Many felt roller derby empowered them and they gained "fun" and enjoyment. Roller derby adds enriching experiences and becomes a "lifestyle". Learning new skills is something different as well as having the opportunity to further develop those skills and become "good at it."

Relationships were a keystone. The depth and scope of these relationships ranged from a friendship, a social circle, sisterhood, "family", and team accomplishment. The feeling of belonging extended beyond the individual's team and the league to the larger roller derby community. This belonging included the Inclusivity of the sport. Women of all ages, fitness levels, skill levels, body types, and professions may join and contribute. Women join with no skating ability and are able to become competent and join a team in the league. Roller derby is a sport for adult women, "women over 22".

Perception of the Sport is "intense exercise", and roller derby necessitates perseverance and pushing yourself beyond your limits, endurance, and "fierceness"

The effect on the respondent (empowerment, fitness, skill development, self-esteem) differed from other sports. These conclusions mirror Cotterill's (2000) findings whereby roller derby provided an outlet for aggression, escape from daily constraints, camaraderie, exercise, empowering women, self-fulfillment, and love of the sport". It is logical to conclude that other sports for these women were not empowering, did not allow for skill development and did not improve self-esteem. These aspects should be fostered and developed in sports participant; a sport should be empowering! The overwhelmingly positive affect of roller derby on the respondents necessitate more research. Could this be why roller derby is popular?

An open-ended question, "how has roller derby affected your life" resulted in 4,073 coded phrases (n=1567; 98.1% response rate), a mean of 2.6 phrases per respondent. Nine categories emerged from the data (see **Table 6**).

Table 6. How has roller derby affected your life

Response	#	%
Positive opinion of self	1,157	28.4%
Health	1,019	25.0%
Relationships	777	19.1%
New Outlook	404	9.9%
Skills	265	6.5%
Takes a lot of time	191	4.7%
Affecting other parts of their life	160	3.9%
Negative comments	44	1.1%
Negative effects on body	37	0.9%
Travel	19	0.5%
Total	4,073	100.0%

The most numerous comments addressed how they feel about themselves; opinion of self. These were positive comments as they had increased confidence or felt more empowered; "gets me out of my shell, pushes my comfort level". Some found the new confidence and empowerment translated to their work and personal lives. There was an increase in self-esteem, "I feel better about myself" especially acceptance of the body. Others enjoy the challenge and sense of accomplishment from meeting goals, getting results, and achievements both personally and as a team. Many comments reflected an increased self-efficacy; "I never thought I would succeed in derby, but I have, and I've found that I'm more willing to take big life risks, such as switching career paths."

The physical being, and personal health were benefits including all aspects of the individual; "physicality", mental, emotional, overall health, and weight loss; "I was in shape before, but now I'm more muscular", "I've lost 30 lbs.", and No more asthma." Roller derby also positively affected the ability of respondents to overcome negative life events such as a death, divorce, addiction, and addressed illness such as diabetes and depression.

The connection and support of league members had a major impact on the lives of the respondents. The relationships gained included; a network, a community, friends, a social life, and "a family". These relationships and the support gained granted them the ability to accomplish things, gain confidence and overcome challenges. "The friendships you build during the process of blood, sweat and tears are there for a long time."

Effusive remarks were made such as "I love everything about it" or "it has changed my life" indicating they had gained a new outlook. Respondents also felt roller derby added something new and different to their lives as roller derby "was something to look forward to in their lives" or roller derby was "something out of the ordinary". The respondents have gained new skills including skating, leadership skills, and working as a team. Additionally, coaching, mentoring, training, and business operation skills transferred, to their work lives.

The obligations of roller derby affected their non-roller derby family. Several mothers indicated the "me time" offered by roller derby provides an outlet that results in better interactions at home. Roller derby could become a focus of family activity as daughters have joined junior leagues, husbands have become referees, and other friends and family have become fans. Self-confidence increased, which benefited their careers, however, problems, developed within the family; ". . . has strained non-derby relationships". Some mentioned problems with the marriage after joining "my husband resents me for "getting out", but others say roller derby has improved their marriage.

Besides the strain on relationships, the respondents disclosed other negative effects on their lives including their work, time, financial resources, and bodies through injuries. Roller derby "takes over" their time and time demands are further exacerbated by league management duties. Problems were noted but not enough to want to give up roller derby. Some respondents have "cut back" on their time given to the sport. Injuries and physical pain affected the lives of very few, 37 respondents (0.9%), but most did not let it slow down participation for too long

The impact on the respondents' lives revealed praise for the sport and the effect their participation had on their physical and mental well-being, family relationships, and plans. There are costs and the respondents commented on the tradeoffs they made with family and friends, the injuries, and time commitment; "about 90% of what I do on any given day has something to do with roller derby." At what point do the costs outweigh the benefits? What negotiation occurs so roller derby can remain part of one's life? These are questions for a deeper investigation. Individual benefits must offset the "costs" as many saw improvement in health, fitness, family interaction, empowerment, self-esteem, and professional life.

The Physical Activity Council's annual participation study (2018) indicated participation in many areas of active participation is either flat or declining and the inactivity rate is increasing. In fact they report that the top 2 reasons for non-participation are "Having someone to take part with" and "having a friend take me along" As Putnam (2000) states in Bowling Alone, "Americans have had a growing sense at some visceral level of disintegrating social bonds" (p. 287). Why is the sport of roller derby gaining membership while other sports have been flat or losing participants? Is roller derby the antithesis to Bowling Alone?

The grass roots design of roller derby results in members being invested and passionate about the sport, their league, and teammates. The survey asked participants to use five words to describe roller derby and their chosen words typify this investment and passion. Firstly, the building of a "Community", with "family", "friends", and "sisterhood" creates a new social environment. In roller derby, the social aspect seems to be more important. The term collective has cropped up in the literature as something that emerges from women participating in activities such as roller derby (Pavlidis, 2012). The collective could provide room for "gender maneuvering" in other settings typified by skills and confidence gained from roller derby being used to make changes in their lives and to improve career opportunities. Mentorship and support practiced as part of roller derby could extend into other arenas whereby mentorship becomes a norm rather than something trained. It would become non-threatening to the mentor.

Success in roller derby could mean climbing the roller derby career track, playing on elite teams, or being able to "beat" someone. It is competitive. This view is shared by many respondents; they like the competitive aspect of the sport and accomplishing something as a team. Perhaps for many success is being part of the roller derby community with such intrinsic rewards as fun and an outlet for emotion and "I keep getting better at it, why stop." The reasons for continuing in the sport transformed from the reason for initially joining the league.

Roller derby creates an environment of teamwork, relationships, teaches skills, provides an outlet for stress, and consists of many components including the physical, strategies, and creativity. Participants gain prolific tangible (i.e. the physical changes to their bodies) and intangible (i.e. the mental aspect and relationships formed) benefits. Roller derby participation is increasing while the trend in other sports is flat or decreased participation. Is this a new model for activities? Should a culture be formed to provide an outlet for individuals to create space for themselves? A persona allows an individual to try other behavior and gain insight into the effect of that behavior. It has resulted in the empowerment of women. It is important to note the "adult" aspect whereby a sport is learned in a supportive environment as an adult. It has a career so there is somewhere to use the skill once learned. Many times adults take introductory courses and when the class ends the opportunity for continued practice and participation ends as well. An individual who does not progress well still participates and belongs in the league. Roller derby is a sport for "adult women" is attractive as there are no other options.

Our work environments are changing as more individuals work from home. Regular telecommuting increased 115% since 2005 (Lister & Gardner, 2017). Telecommuting is approximately 2% of the United States workforce. It is estimated that 45% of the U.S. workforce has a job that is compatible with telecommuting (Global Workplace Analytics, 2012). Additionally, there are home-based businesses and mobile employees. Thus, a staff that works face to face will be unique. As our workplace becomes more mobile, our offices disperse, and individuals work alone, personal interaction will be explored in other venues. In roller derby personal interaction has been shown in this research as paramount to members. How will sport and leisure activities provide "face time" with others?.

CONCLUSION

The main purpose of this research was to increase understanding of why roller derby members are attracted to this sport and continue to participate. This research provides a look at who a roller derby member is through their demographic characteristics and their roller derby longevity and skill level. The reasons for joining were exercise oriented but grew to social and relationship reasons. The benefits indicated were geared toward the social and improvement in self esteem and professional skills. The sport is different from other sport in that it allows for an unskilled participant to excel and be encouraged. Thus, why are derby members attracted to the sport and continue is because of the structure of the sport itself but also the organization and comradery gained. Through the structure and organization, the participants are addressing their needs for a "family"!.

REFERENCES

Barbee, J & Cohen, A (2010). Down and derby, the insider's guide to roller derby. Berkley: Publishers Group West.

Beaver, T. D. (2012). "By the Skaters, for the Skaters" The DIY ethos of the roller derby revival. Journal of Sport and Social Issues, 36(1), 25-49. doi: 10.1177/0193723511433862

Carlson, J. (2010). The female significant in all-women's amateur roller derby. Sociology of Sport Journal, 27(48), p. 428-440.

Coppage, K. (1999). Roller derby to roller jam: The authorized story of an unauthorized sport. Oxford, MS: Squarebooks.

Cotterill, M.S. (2010). Skating the metaphorical edge; An ethnographic examination of female roller derby athletes. (Master's Thesis) Retrieved from the University of Delaware library http://dspace.udel.edu:8080/dspace/handle/19716/9789?show=full

Deford, F. (1971). Five strides on the banked track: The life and times of the roller derby. Boston: Little Brown & Company.

Delano, B. (2010). Roller derby more than fishnets and flair. American Fitness, 28 (5), 45.

Derbylisting.com (2018) Roller derby list. Retrieved from http://derbylisting.com/dl/grid/

Draft, A. (2017). Sizing up skaters: An interrogation of body discourses in elite women's flat track roller derby. Women in Sport and Physical Activity. 25(1), 20-29. https://doi.org/10.1123/wspaj.2015-0031

Eklund, A., & Masberg, B. (2014). Participation in roller derby, the influence on body image. Clothing and Textiles Research Journal, 32(1), 49–64. doi: 10.1177/0887302X13511295

Filip, M. (2016) Motivation in high-level roller derby; Athletes' experienced peer motivation climate and basic psychological needs. Master's Thesis Retrieved from: http://umu.diva-portal.org/smash/record.jsf?pid=diva2%3A1114417&dswid=-1068

Finley, N. J. (2010). Skating femininity: Gender maneuvering in women's roller derby. Journal of Contemporary Ethnography, 39(359). doi: 1177/0891241610364230.

Global Workplace Analytics (2012). The latest telecommuting statistic. Retrieved from http://www.teleworkresearchnetwork.com/telecommuting-statistics

Henderson, K.A., Hodges, S., & Kivel, H. (2002). Context and dialogue in research on women and leisure. Journal of Leisure Research, 34(3), 253-271.

Kearney, M. C. (2011). Tough girls in a rough game. Feminist Media Studies,11(3), 283-301. http://dx.doi.org/10.1080/14680777.2010.535309.

Lister, K. & Gardner, K. (2017). The 2017 state of telecommuting in the United States employee workforce. Retrieved from http://globalworkplaceanalytics.com/telecommuting-statistics

Mabee, C. (2007). Roller derby: The history and all-girl revival of the greatest sport on wheels. Speck Press: Denver, Colorado

Madrigal, L. & Robbins, J. (2017) Roller derby: Experiences with injury and pain in players' behavioral repertoires. Journal of Sport Behavior, 40 (2), 171-190.

Pavlidis, A. (2012). From Riot Girls to roller derby? Exploring the relations between gender, music and sport. Leisure Studies, 31(2), 165-176. https://doi.org/10.1080/02614367.2011.623304

Peluso, N. M. (2010). High heels and fast wheels: Alternative femininities in neo-burlesque and flat-track roller derby. (3464369 Ph.D.), University of Connecticut, Ann Arbor. ProQuest Dissertations & Theses Global database.

Physical Activity Council (2018) 2018 Physical Activity Council participation report. Retrieved from http://www.physicalactivitycouncil.com/

Putnam, R.D. (2000) Bowling alone: The collapse and revival of American community. New York: Simon & Schuster

Roller Derby Worldwide. (2012). Derby roster. Retrieved from http://www.derbyroster.com/index.php

Rowlett, J. T. (2015). Skating for strength: The experiences of skating in women's flat track roller derby. (1591127 M.A.), Clemson University, Ann Arbor. ProQuest Dissertations & Theses Global database.

Saldana, J. (2016). The coding manual for qualitative researchers. Los Angeles: Sage Publications.

Storms, C. E. (2008) "There's no sorry in roller derby": A feminists' examination of identity of women in the full contact sport of roller derby. The New York Sociologist, 3, 66-86. doi=10.1.1.603.9559

Strubel, J. & Petrie, T.A. (2016). "Bout Time! Renegotiating the body in roller derby. Sex Roles 74(7-8), 347-360. https://doi.org/10.1007/s11199-015-0490-0

Unlisted (1936). Roller derby. Time, 27(5), 26.

Women's Flat Track Derby Association (WFTDA). (2018). http://wftda.com/

Profile of Physical Fitness Level of Students - High School Students in Trenggalek Regency Based on TKJI

Henri Gunawan Pratama[1] **, Khamim Hariyadi**[2]**, Rohmat Febrianto**[3]

STKIP PGRI TRENGGALEK, Indonesia[123]

Article History

Keywords:
TKJI; Kabupaten Trenggalek; Fitness; Health; physical activity

Abstract

The era of globalization was currently existing cultural shifts, in terms of communication, transportation and technology which have an impact on the lack of physical activity and sports activities of youth participants.. This study aims to determine the level of physical fitness of X (ten) grade high school students in the district of Trenggalek. Research uses a qualitative approach through a series of tests and measurements based on TKJI. The population of this study were all students of class X (ten) who had just entered the high school level. The study was conducted in 9 schools that had received recommendations and permits from the school with a total sample of 1,264 research students from public and private high schools. The results of research that have been done that the physical fitness level of students in the District of Trenggalek at the high school level of class X, 61% are in the category of Less inversely proportional to the level of fitness of students who are in the Medium category of 13% and good 1% based on TKJI. Whereas for the body mass index results 54% in the Normal level and 12-16% included in the category of Light and light skinny. The conclusion of this study is that there is a need for physical education learning that can maximize physical activity activities and sports activities of students in daily life.

Correspondence address :
E-mail: henrigunawan92@gmail.com

INTRODUCTION

Sports in the life of the Indonesian nation is part of the nation's achievements that grow and develop in line with the times. Therefore sports have a large share and is one of the media for the development of Indonesian people as a whole (Ma'arif, 2015).

While the main problem facing physical education today is the change in cultural values, from the culture of motion to a culture of silence. The cultural shift was triggered by the impact of economic globalization, communication and transportation technology so that children tend to eliminate physical activity in various activities. (Kurniawan, 2016) Good physical fitness, can be achieved by doing regular exercise, is one of the factors needed to achieve high work productivity, because it is able to overcome the workload given to it. Physical fitness, or briefly called fitness, is a major factor for humans to be able to carry out their daily activities well. Measuring the level of fitness needs to be done for students, because efforts to improve and maintain physical fitness systematically will be easier to do through school. Improvement and maintenance especially for students must be strived so that they are always ready to carry out their activities without feeling tired. For students, physical fitness can improve learning achievement because with good fitness, they will be better prepared to receive lessons and will be healthy, fit and smart generations.

Previous research was conducted on STKIP PGRI Trenggalek students according to the results of research conducted it can be seen that 55% of female students are in the Medium category, while male students are 80% in the Lesser category. This may be because before the tests and measurements are carried out, they are not maximal or there is a sick person, thus affecting the power to carry out the test again. At the graduation rate given using the PAP method, all students of Health and Recreation Physical Education <60 with a percentage of 9% are declared not graduated with an average score of 55, while> 60 with a percentage of 86.6% are stated Pass with an average score of 77. Secara umum pendidikan jasmani sangat mempengaruhi kebugaran jasmani di tingkat anak-anak, akan tetapi saat menjelang dewasa persepsi mereka akan pendidikan jasmani mulai menurun (Frans C Trudeau and Roy J. Shephard ,2005:89-105). For this reason, we conducted a study to find out the level of health and fitness of students from an education level. We hold tests at the high school (SMA) level that have just entered the X (ten) class with the reason that this period is a period of growth, so that it affects the level of their health quite a lot. It is undeniable that the growth of hormonal levels at that time was very unstable, so that it could affect their weight and height. This condition is also related to nutritional status that can be known by the Body Mass Index (BMI).

METHODS

The use of methods that are in accordance with the objectives to be achieved is an absolute requirement required in a research process. In this study researchers used non-experimental research that is Evaluative. This research is a research that uses the procedure of collecting and analyzing data, aims to design, refine the results of the TKJI recommendations for physical and sports education teachers.

In accordance with this type of research, the main instruments are the TKJI data and the IMT data of the tenth grade (Ten) high school students in Trenggalek Regency. Equipped with assistive devices in the form of photo cameras, Field Survey Form Instruments, TKJI Test Assessment Forms, stopwatches, vertical jumps, pull-ups, body scales, height measuring instruments.

Collecting data in this study uses TKJI (Indonesian Physical Fitness Test) to determine the fitness level of students and also use BMI (Body Period Index) to determine the development of health and growth of students.

In this study there are two assessment methods, namely PAN and PAP. PAP is usually called criterion evaluation is a measurement that uses different references. In this measurement students are compressed with criteria that have been determined in advance in instructional goals, not with the appearance of other students. Researchers are more suitable to use PAP (Assessment Reference Reference) because researchers want students to get grades with their own abilities. To determine the value of each sample the researcher uses the formula:

$$\mathbf{X = (Sa/St) \times 100}$$

information:

Sa: Score Raw

St: Highest Score at

X : Skor

To Determine Graduation used

To Determine Graduation used Formula:

60% x 100 = 60

So the value of 60 and above is passed and the score below 60 is declared as not passing. The Research Procedure consists of 3 stages;

1.Location / Survey Mapping

- Search for information about the schools that will be used as research sites in Trenggalek Regency.
- Submit a letter of application to conduct test

and measurement research to the school
- Reconciliation with High School Physical Education teachers in Trenggalek Regency regarding tests and facilities and equipment needed during the study.
- Provide information to students regarding the schedule and activities of conducting test and measurement research

2. Test Preparation

Preparing equipment to be used during tests, height measuring instruments, scales, mattresses, Stop Watch, Vertical Jump, Test Assessment Instruments.

3. TKJI Test Implementation

-Sit Up Test
- Pull Up Test
-Vertical Jump Test
-Running 1200 and 1000 m run tests
-Implementation of a 50 m Sprint test).

RESULTS AND DISCUSSION

Results and discussion of this research (1) time of research utilizing physical education classes that have received permission from the school, (2) The duration of data collection is quite long from the field survey until data collection in schools is an average of 8 hours per day which is carried out for 3 months up to data processing (3) from the survey results that there are schools that meet the standard implementation of tests and there are which is not, for and the number of test participants consists of 1,264 students from 9 schools who have obtained permission, and (4) the following data that has been taken in this study will be explained from the **Table 1-6**.

Table 1. Physical Fitness Level Students of SMAN 1 Tugu

Category	Fitness	
	Total	%
Very less	8	13
Less	42	67
Average	0	0
Good	0	0
Very good	0	0
Absent	13	21

Table 2. The index of the body of students SMAN 1 Tugu

Category	IMT	
	Total	%
Skinny	8	13
Thin	7	11
Normal	30	48
Chubby	5	8
Very fat	0	0
Not active	13	21

What can be understood from the results of the data above is that for the physical fitness level of students can be said to be very less about 67% with a total of 42 students from a total of 63 students in class X. For IMT can be said to be good with an average of 48% Normal.

Table 3. Physical Fitness Level of Students of SMA 2 Karangan

Category	Fitness	
	Total	%
Very less	1	1
Less	57	63
Average	20	22
Good	4	4
Very good	0	0
Absent	9	10

Tabel 4. The index of the body of students SMAN 2 Karangan

Category	IMT	
	Total	%
Skinny	4	4
Thin	14	15
Normal	56	62
Chubby	6	7
Very fat	2	2
Not active	9	10

SMAN 2 Karangan shows that there are differences in data from several existing schools, it is known that the level of fitness is 22% and is good at 4%, although there are few but shows that there is a good change in the level of fitness at this school and is directly proportional to the BMI of 62% Normal.

Compared to these two schools, only between SMAN 1 Tugu and SMAN 2 Were far different in terms of their physical fitness and body index, when viewed in terms of geography, these two schools are in the same highlands or urban areas.

This study was not focused on the two schools alone, of the seven other schools the geographical location was not the same from the highlands, lowlands to coastal areas. If viewed from the geographical point of view, the level of physical fitness and body mass index are different and not the same. This happens because the physical activity done is not the same in each school, some schools in fact are more non-academic than their academic activities. This is shown in **Table 5&6** below.

Table 5. Physical Fitness Level of all students

Category	Fitness	
	Total	%
Very less	166	166
Less	778	778
Average	166	166
Good	16	16
Very good	0	0
Absent	148	148

Tabel 6. The index of the body of all students

Category	IMT	
	Total	%
Skinny	149	12
Thin	204	16
Normal	686	54
Chubby	49	4
Very fat	25	2
Not active	152	12

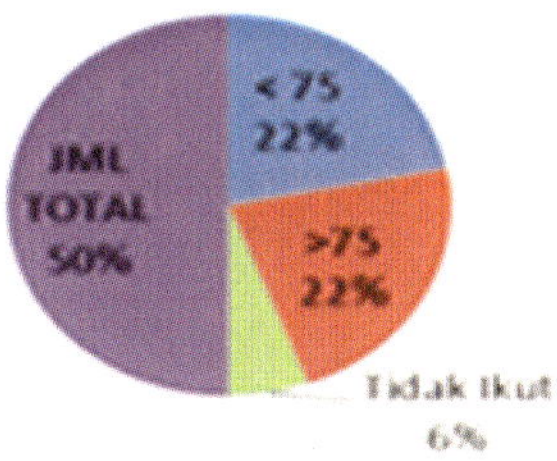

Picture 1. KKM values of students as a whole.

All of the data presented above that the physical fitness level of students in the District of Trenggalek at the high school level of class X, 61% are in the category of inversely proportional to the level of fitness of students who are in the medium category of 13% and good 1% and can be known from the Test Results Indonesia's Physical Fitness Level.

These results can be supported from several studies related to physical fitness Physical fitness has a function to support the ability and ability of each human being, which is useful in enhancing work productivity (Anon, 1971 a Anon 1991).

This means that the higher the status of one's physical fitness, the higher the work power of that person. This is in accordance with the results of research conducted on industries in America, which concluded that employees who were given physical fitness training programs turned out to be fresh workers who had high pesformance, productive in work, have a positive attitude towards fellow workers, less absent and more creative.

All of the percentages of the results of the Indonesian physical fitness test, when viewed from the criteria of completeness that has been determined, then for the minimal criteria students are balanced. KKM 75 of physical body minimum 22% and KKM> 75 by 2.

CONCLUSION

Based on the results of the Physical Fitness Test and Body Mass Index data, this advice needs to be understood by Physical Education teachers in schools to improve fitness, nutrition and KKM Assessment is well achieved for students.

Ideal category: Maintained, Perform daily activities as usual, Keep your body fitness by doing sports activities according to their respective hobbies, Set your diet according to 4 healthy 5 perfect, Avoid consuming alcoholic beverages, illegal drugs, free sex and cigarettes.

Skinny category : Increase the consumption of foods and drinks that contain fat in accordance with a healthy 4 diet 5 perfect, Do sports activities according to each hobby as a balance and fitness, adequate rest and reduce excessive activity, Avoid sleeping late at night (staying up late) , fruits containing sugar, Keep exercising lightly at least 3 times a week, Avoid consuming alcoholic beverages, illegal drugs, free sex, and cigarettes.

Healthy mild / thin categories : Consume more foods and drinks that contain carbohydrates and proteins, for example: rice, potatoes, eggs, shrimp. Do sports activities according to your hobbies as balance and fitness, adequate rest and reduce excessive activity, consumption of fruits that contain sugar, keep light exercise at least 3 times a week.

REFERENCES

Trudeau F and Shephard R.J. 2005. Contribution of School Programmes to Physical Activity Levels and Attitudes in Children and Adults: Sports Med 2005; 35 (2): 89-105

Kemenpora. 2009 : Parameter Tes PPLP edisi Yogya. Jakarta: Deputi Peningkatan Prestasi dan Iptek Olahraga.

Pratama,H.G 2015 : Evaluasi Tingkat Kebugaran Jasmani Mahasiswa Pendidikan Jasmani Kesehatan dan Rekreasi STKIP PGRI Trenggalek : Bravo s Vol 3 Nomor 4 hal 204-208

Kurniawan. A 2016 : Peningkatan Kebugaran Jasmani Melalui Modifikasi Permainan pada Siswa SMP Islam Gandusari : Bravo s Vol 4 Nomor 1 Hal 1-7

Ma'arif. I 2015 : Survei Perbedaan Tingkat Kebugaran Jasmani pada Peserta didik kelas VIII SMPN 4 Lamongan dan SMPN 1 Solokuro Lamongan : Bravo's Vol 3 Nomor 4 Hal 181-187

The Development Model of Learning Shot Put Oriented by Playing for Elementary School Students

Irwansyah[1]✉, Guntur Firmansyah[2]

Pendidikan Jasmani Kesehatan dan Rekreasi, Fakultas Pendidikan Ilmu Eksakta dan Keolahragaan
IKIP Budi Utomo, Indonesia[12]

Article History

Keywords:
Development; Learning Model; Shot Put; Play.

Abstract

Research development of aim products in the form of a model of learning-oriented bullets starting play in an effort to create a situation of active learning. The research method used is the method of research development (research and development), of the Brog and Gall which is divided into two stages, namely the early research (needs analysis) and development. Research conducted at SDN Klojen in Malang city. The instruments used were the questionnaire and interviews. Data were analyzed with a qualitative analysis techniques and quantitative descriptive. Based on the results of the expert analysis of the game, Physical Education in Elementary School, Learning experts and experts of athletics (Shot Put) assessing learning models Shot Put play orientation was at 88.75% category with good qualifications and a small group of trial results and large group shows that the model of learning was play orientation cartridges starting at 84.72% category with the qualification of "good" so that the shot put learning playing approach have can be used as a model for improve the quality of learning making learning active and fun.

✉ **Correspondence address :**
E-mail: gunturpepeng@gmail.com

INTRODUCTION

Study on the problems of physical education is a reasonable thing. However, any problem must be solved and look for a solution considering the physical education at school plays an important role in developing the potential and experience of motion students and students. The teacher is one of learning resources and spearhead in improving the quality of an education. Teachers as educators have the main task of educating, teaching, guiding, directing, train, assess and evaluate learners constantly need to improve the quality of professionalism constantly. In an era of ever-changing curriculum, organization of education requires teachers who are able to perform the task and create new learning strategies that can help solve the problems of the students in the class. Physical education is one of the teaching material that did not escape from problems in its implementation in accordance with the goal of reaching a basic curriculum on komptensi.

Implementation of the learning of physical education to achieve the desired goal, the teacher should devise learning process effectively. The more effective the teacher in teaching, then processed condition would be more supportive of the achievement of the learning objectives. However, it's all not be separated from the role of teachers as educators to increase the motivation and interest of students with a more interesting learning, so that students are able to regenerate the passion of learning actively.

External learning is learning that demands the role of teacher as one learning resource called teaching or teaching. Hakkatnya learning is a combination of the two activities, namely, the activity of the teaching and learning activities (Winarno, 2011:12). The activity of the teaching concerning the role of a teacher in the context of seeking creation of harmonious communication between the teacher of interwoven itself with learners. Learning is purposeful and intentional effort aimed by a person or group of people (including teachers and textbook authors) so that other people (including students), may obtain a meaningful experience. This effort is an activity based on the interests of the learners. (Walker, 2015; McCombs, 2000). In learning requires a good Groove so that what was on the study session is reached. The flow of the learning success will be an example on the situation and conditions of learning at the time it is called a model of learning. Own learning models are usually compiled based on various principles or theory of knowledge experts draw up a learning model based on the principles of learning theory, sociological, psychological, analysis time and other theories. Rusman (2011:113) mention that the learning model is a plan or pattern that can be used to shape curricula, designing learning materials, learning guide and processed or the other. According to the thinking Trianto (2007:1) "learning model is a planning or a pattern that is used as a guide in planning the learning in the classroom or learning in the tutorial".

Implementation of the learning of physical education taught in schools there are some sports games, among others, development activities, athletics, gymnastics, and rhythmic activities. Athletics is one of the sports that teach range from elementary to High School levels, as there are in the curriculum unit level education (KTSP) primary school (elementary school) class VI contained BSNP Athletics lesson is one that must be taught, in the process of lesson athletics has lots of numbers one number Shot Put. Shot Put number throwing from the sport of athletics is one of the kinds of skills menolakkan objects in the form of bullets as far as possible. The purpose of starting the bullet is to achieve the distance as repulsion, (Ambarwati et al, 2017; Ferry Fitriyanto, 2016:28;Yusuf, 2016:294). .

From an explanation of the notion of starting the bullet above can be obtained from the conclusion that the decline of cartridges is one of the sport of Athletics in the throwing athlete, defends iron ball throwing bullet weight as far as possible.

In rejecting the cartridges include 3 stages, namely 1) preparation; Straddle stand, relax the shoulders, wide position sideways from the direction of repulsion. The right hand holds the bullet and put on the neck under the jaw and stuck in the shoulder. Elbow left skewed to the front of the chest, a view towards repulsion, 2) Refused; Use the leg closest to the swinging leg throws as a sector to decline. At the time of swinging leg in front, swivel waist toward your hips and roll sector helped to push towards the front of the top, and the body leaning forward, fixed gaze towards repulsion, 3) end Attitude; The right foot is driven forward replacing the left foot as the object. The left leg straight back with your right leg, knees relaxed somewhat bent and fixed gaze towards repulsion, (Endang, 2010:22; Darmawan, 2018).

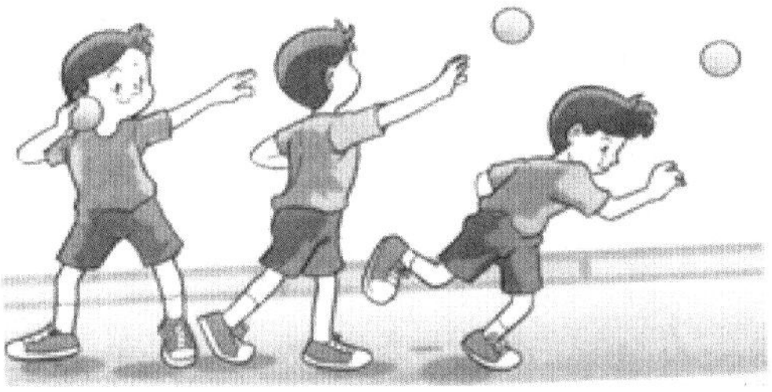

Picture 1. Shot Put Method (Endang, 2010:22)

The development patterns of motion base bullet can deny using the tools and materials of any kind, an important tool that we will use preferably spherical (Bahagia, 2010:66). This means that a teacher can utilize a variety of equipment, such as a ball. For students of elementary school teacher may use equipment that is not too heavy, for example tennis balls or Softball. One of the modifications of the equipment the bullet based on the size, shape and weight is an alternative learning Shot Put. (Priyo et al, 2013). Activity play in learning basic motion bullet starting can be done with a variety of formations, could use a formation one direction or face to face (Bahagia, 2010:67, Bakhrul,2013). If using the formation dealing penjas a teacher must provide sufficient distance and setting a turn throwing should be supervised to prevent an accident.

According to Maryani (2015:2018) based on studies of motion rejecting the bullet will have far less results in motion straight still kedepaan or repulsion of less than 42 degrees from the starting corner. Some research supports learning media learning activity decline in the Shot Put Rosita (2015) that mention that starting learning the bullet through the media in the form of a ball of plastic impact posisif that is able increase the interest and motivation of learning so that the learning outcome increases. Purwanto (2015) shot put through the learning approach of playing goal ball defends the sand can improve learning outcomes Shot Put

The starting teaching material is the bullet on physical education learning activities scope of athletics are less sought after by students. This is apparent from initial needs analysis results through dissemination of the question form and interview conducted in school SDN Klojen in Malang city in get data between other 80.10% students are not motivated when learning Shot Put, 85.70% of students feel it is hard When using the original cartridges that weighed 4-5 kg, 85.00%, students feel on learning that convey by the less fun, 75% of students wanting a lighter bullet, 97.00% of students agreed if the original bullet made of iron was renamed the bullet an imitation lighter with more secure construction (rubber ball, and a shower of balls), whereas 95.80% of students agreed starting learning model if developed bullet done with playing an activity fun.

Based on the above things, then researchers trying to formulate a problem as the following " How was the development of learning model of play-oriented Shot Put for fourth grade students of SD Negeri Klojen Malang ".

Through the research of the development of this model aims to tackle one of the problems of studying decline Shot Put the development of learning models Shot Put play oriented for grade IV SDN Klojen in Malang city.

METHODS

This research use the development model that follows the model of development research and development (Winarno 2007:48) in detail stages of research consists of ten phases which was later adopted by researchers into eight stages of implementation are: 1) do research which is the needs analysis through observation and interviews, 2) planning modelling bullets starting learning-oriented play, 3) product development as well as evaluating against the experts. The initial product of the already formed dijustifikasi by 1 person 1 person game expert expert health physical education and recreation, and 1 person learning experts, 4) next steps, products that have been tested by experts dijustifikasi cobakan on elementary school students by involving the 8 subjects 5 trials) first revision of the trial results and improve or perfect the trial results in accordance with the results of trials of small group, 6) field trials conducted on elementary school students by involving test subjects 40, 7) revised the trial results and improve or perfect the trial results in accordance with the results of field trials, 8) dissemination and implementation.

This research was carried out on SDN Klojen in Malang city. The subject in this study are students and students of class IV SDN Klojen in Malang city, who becomes the object of the research is in the study Shot Put-oriented learning through play for grade IV SDN Klojen in Malang city. This research began on 17 October 2017.

Data collection instruments used in the collection of data on research development this is the observation, documentation and dissemination of the now. After the data is retrieved and then conducted data analysis of any subject that includes test and evaluation experts with guidelines the following scoring (Creswell, 2010:278): "the answer to a have a value or score 4, Answer b has a value or a score of 3, Answer c has the value or score 2, Answer d to have value or score 1 "

a. To process data of the data analysis techniques used are descriptive and qualitative analysis techniques in the form of percentages:

b. a. qualitative Analysis was used to analyze the results of the review data collection experts using a qualitative approach. Qualitative data were analyzed using models, Miles and Huberman (Sugiyono, 2008:247-253) which consists of three steps, namely: "(1) Data reduction (2) Data display (3) Conclusion drawing"

c. b. descriptive Analysis in the form of a percentage used to analyze the results of data collection trial a small group and large group testing. Formula to manipulate data in the form of a descriptive percentage, (Sudijono, 2008:43) are as follows:

P = F/ N X 100%

Description :

f: frequency that is being sought —

N: Number of case (amount of frequency by the number of individuals)

P: Number percentage

According to the opinions delivered by Arikunto, (2006:344). "If the data is in the form of percentage, proportion or ratio, then a conclusion can be drawn, adjusted to the problem". The following categorization percentage categories that will be used are:

76%-100%	Good Category	used
56%-75%	simply Category	used
40%-55%	less good Category	not used
< 40%	not good Category	not used

RESULTS AND DISCUSSION

From this research obtained the results that can be seen in the table presenting data for the analysis of 40 students of SDN Klojen in Malang city (**Tabel 1**). Based on the recapitulation of the initial needs analysis results tally can be illustrated in the form of a bar chart as shown in Figure 2 below:

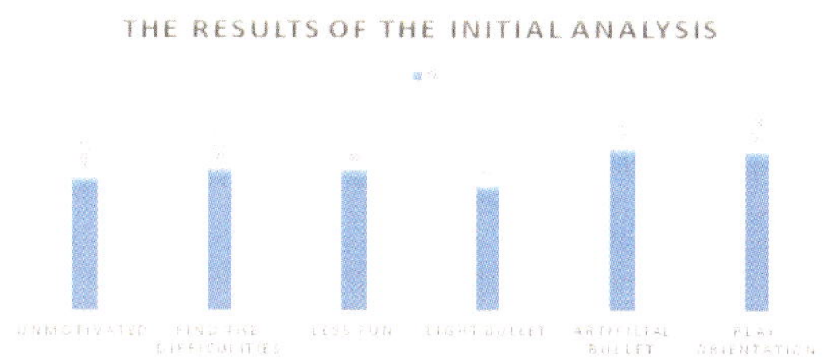

Figure 2. The Results Of The Initial Needs Analysis

Tabel 2. Presentation of Data evaluation (Expert) 1 Person game Experts

Expert	Score Minimum	Score Maximum	Result	Percentage
Game Expert	12	48	40	83,34 %

Based on **table 2** can be noted that the percentage of evaluation results from the expert game was 83.34%.

Tabel 3. Presentation of Data evaluation (Expert) 1 Person penjas SD Learning Experts

Expert	Minimum score	Maximum Score	Result	Percentage
Physical Education Learning in Elementary School	12	48	38	79,17

Tabel 1. Presentation of the results of the Data Analysis needs of 40 Students

Component	Discovery
Needs analysis of teacher through charging the now	1. obtained data that 80.10% of students learning Shot Put. 2. obtained data that 85.70% of students feel difficult when using original cartridges that weighed 4-5 kg 3. retrieved data that 85.00%, students feel on learning that convey by the less fun 4. retrieved data that 75% of students wanting a lighter bullet 5. retrieved data that 97.00% of students agreed if the original bullet made of iron was changed to a lighter clone cartridges with safer constructs (ball Curry, and the bath ball) 6. retrieved data that 95.80% of students agreed starting learning model if developed bullet done with an enjoyable play activity
Product Development	1.On the basis of needs analysis done product development started on 04 September 2017 2.Product development measures undertaken are: •Study the curriculum, learning implementation plan (RPP) and the syllabus on SD class VI Materials resist bullets •the collection materials/material in the form of book • Drawing up model starting game cartridges 3.The results of the 4 models starting game cartridges (1. rubber ball throwing game, 2. War game balls, Throwing game ban, 4. The game encourages the ball hanging)

Based on **table 3** can be noted that the percentage of the results of the evaluation of the expert learning penjas SD was 79.17%

Tabel 4. Presentation of Data evaluation (Expert) 1 Person Athletic Experts Shot Put

Expert	Minimum Score	Maximum Score	Result	Percentage
Shot Put Athletic	12	48	43	89,58%

Based on **table 4** can note that the average percentage of evaluation results from Athletics experts Shot Put was 89.58%.

Based on the evaluation results recap experts in obtaining results that can be illustrated in the form of a bar chart as shown in Figure 3 below:

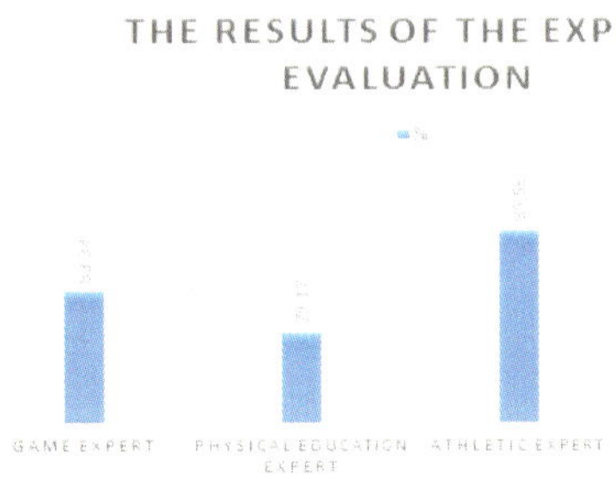

Picture 3. The Results Of Evaluation Experts

Tabel 5. Presentation of Data the results of the tests of the small groups of 8 students

Component	Minimum score	Maximum score	Result	Percentage
Small Group Trial	96	384	345	80,20

Based on **table 5** can be noted that the number of overall average percentage of a small group of trial results was 80.20%.

Tabel 6. Presentation of Data the results of the tests of the large group of 40 Students

Component	Minimum score	Maximum score	Result	Percentage
Large Group Trial	360	1440	1220	84,72

Based on **table 6** can be noted that the number of overall average percentage of trial results is a large group of 84.72%.

Based on the recapitulation of trial results in obtaining results that can be illustrated in the form of a bar chart as shown in Figure 4 below:

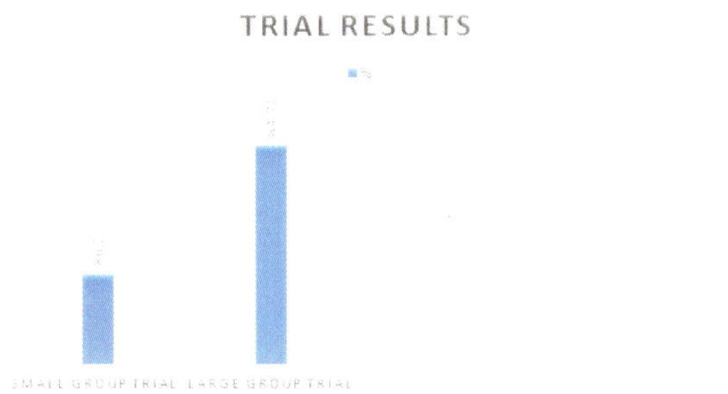

Figure 4. Product User Trial Results

DISCUSSION

One of the effective learning approach to learning is the approach play. Play and the game is the two terms are often used interchangeably, whereas someone who play it are doing a game and the game is played. Child's play child means doing a game. Motion in play is a vehicle for stimulating and motivating to encourage and stimulate critical thinking on the subject of learning. Motion spur children to think and find out why and how the against, so the play is an important part in the development and knowledge as well as the development of motion. A child can do with energetic physical activity but naturally and can enjoy the game with happy, (Bakhrul, 2013:5). Physical education as a vehicle to develop the potential of motion students noticed milestone learning so it will be tiered skills and knowledge. Learning materials resist bullets is one of learning material which contains basic motion development declined as the topic. The order of the stages of the learning will be very uninspiring and less attractive if not approached with the game it is in accordance with findings Ulum (2013). The results of the findings of the researchers that the model approach to some of the games that is throwing a rubber ball, a ball game, a war game throwing tires, push the ball Game. Will make learning Shot Put be passionate and interesting so that will improve student learning outcomes. This is because the model learned by the game approaches tailored to the characteristics of elementary school students of class VI. In accordance with the opinion of the Sanjaya (2015) stating that a learning approach to adjust to the conditions and characteristics of learners.

CONCLUSION

The conclusions obtained in the research of the development of the results of the analysis of the percentage specified that if the percentage of achievement on the interval 100-76.0% berklasifikasi both meaning model of learning-oriented bullets starting play decent used, thus the trial results on large group test overall aspects that are judged to have reached 84.72% the Product model of learning-oriented bullets starting play have been compiled berklasifikasi well and can/ feasibility as learning materials at grade VI SDN Klojen in Malang city.

REFERENCES

Arikunto. S. 2006. Prosedur Penelitian Suatu Pendekatan Praktek Edisi Revisi VI. Jakarta: Rineka Cipta.

Bahagia, Y. 2010. Pembelajaran Atletik. Jakarta : Direkorat Jenderal Pendidikan Dasar dan Menengah.

Bakhrul, U. 2013. Penggunaan Pendekatan Bermain Dan Berlomba Untuk Meningkatkan Efektifitas Pembelajaran Tolak Peluru Gaya Membelakangi Pada Siswa Kelas Iv Di Sd Negeri Petung Ii Kecamatan Pasrepan Kabupaten Pasuruan. PEDAGOGIA Vol. 2, No. 1 (diakses 16 Mei 2018)

Creswell, J. W. 2010. Research Desaign Pendekatan Kualitatif, Kuantitatif, dan Mixed. Pustaka Pelajar: Yogyakarta

Darmawan, A. D. (2018). Peningkatkan Pembelajaran Tolak Peluru Dengan Media Bola Tenis Pada Siswa Kelas Vi Madrasah Ibtida'iyah Psm Gambyok. Jurnal Koulutus, 1(1), 49-56.

Ambarwati, D. R et al, 2017. Pengaruh Daya Ledak Otot Lengan, Kelentukan Panggul, dan Koordinasiterhadap Keterampilan Tolak Peluru Gaya O'Brien. Available Online at http://journal.uny.ac.id/index.php/jolahraga Jurnal Keolahragaan, 5 (2), 2017, 207-215

Endang, 2010. Pendidikan Jasmani, Olahraga dan Kesehatan untuk SD/MI Kelas IV BSE. Jakarta: Pusat Perbukuan Kementerian Pendidikan Nasional.

Feri Fitriyanto. 2016. Peningkatan Kemampuan Tolak Peluru Dengan Pembelajaran Modifikasi Peluru Dari Bola Kasti Pada Siswa SDN Karang Pelem 1 Sragen Tahun 2016. Jurnal Ilmiah SPIRIT, ISSN; 1411-8319 Vol. 16 No. 2 Tahun 2016.

Maryani, E. 2015. Meningkatkan hasil Belajar Tolak PeluruMelalui Permainan Tolak Sasaran Pada Dinding. Journal Of Physical Eduction, Sport, Health and Recreations. Active 4 (8) (2015) hal 2017-2021 ISSN 2252-6773

Yusuf, M. 2016. Kontribusi Kekuatan Otot Tungkai Dan Daya Ledak Otot Lengan Terhadap Kemampuan Tolak Peluru Mahasiswa Fpok Ikip Mataram Tahun Akademik 2015/2016. JUPE, Volume 1 ISSN 2548 – 5555.

McCombs, B. L. (2000). Assessing the Role of Educational Technology in the Teaching and Learning Process: A Learner-Centered Perspective. In The Secretary's Conference on Educational Technology (pp. 2–17). Retrieved from http://eric.ed.gov.silk.library.umass.edu/?id=ED452830

Priyo, H., Ranu, B., & Rumini. (2013). Pengembangan Pembelajaran PENJASORKES Tolak Peluru Dengan Modifikasi Ukuran Berat Peluru, 4(4).

Walker, T. D. (2015). Differentiating Learning Outcomes: A Student- Centered Approach with Value Added Benefits. The Journal of the World Universities Forum Www.ontheuniversity.com, 8(4), 1835–2030.

Purwanto. 2015. Upaya Meningkatkan Pembelajaran Tolak Peluru Dengan Menggunakan Media Bola Pasir Pada Siswa Kelas V MI NU 01 Kemantran Kecamatan Kramatan Kabupaten TegalTahun Pembelajaran 2013/2014. Journal Of Physical Eduction, Sport, Health and Recreations. Active 4 (8) (2015) hal 1988-1991 ISSN 2252-6773

Rosita, I. Upaya Meningkatkan Hasil Belajar Tolak Peluru Melalui Media Bola Plastik Bekas. Journal Of Physical Eduction, Sport, Health and Recreations. Active 4 (8) (2015) hal 1978-1982 ISSN 2252-6773

Rusman. 2011. Model-model Pembelajaran Mengembangkan Profesionalisme Guru. Jakarta: RajaGrafindo Persada

Sanjaya, W. (2015). Perencanaan dan desain sistem pembelajaran. Kencana.

Sudijono. A. 2008. Pengantar Statistik Pendidikan. Jakarta: Grafindo Persada

Sugiyono.2008. Metode Penelitian Kuantitatif, Kualtitatif dan R & D. Bandung: Alfabeta.

Trianto. 2007. Model Pembelajaran Terpadu. Jakarta: Prestasi Pustaka

Ulum, B. (2013). Penggunaan Pendekatan Bermain dan Berlomba Untuk Meningkatkan Efektivitas Pembelajaran Tolak Peluru Gaya Membelakangi Pada Siswa Kelas IV di SD Negeri Petung II Kecamatan Pasrepan Kabupaten Pasuruan. PEDAGOGIA: Jurnal Pendidikan, 2(1), 14-35.

Winarno, M.E. 2007. Metodologi Penelitian dalam Pendidikan Jasmani. Malang: Fakultas Ilmu Pendidikan Universitas Negeri Malang.

Winarno, M.E. 2011. Metodologi Penelitian Dalam Pendidikan Jasmani. Malang: Media Cakrawala Utama Press.

Walker, T. D. (2015). Differentiating Learning Outcomes: A Student- Centered Approach with Value Added Benefits. The Journal of the World Universities Forum Www.ontheuniversity.com, 8(4), 1835–2030.

Throwing Game of Rubber Ball

Terms and how to play

1. number of participants: not limited to sharing in 2 groups
2. Tools and materials: 4 rubber balls, bucket, lime, marker, raffia rope
3. Time allocation: free
4. How To play:
   - Students enter within the throwing area
   - Each group appoints representatives to make a throw
   - Before the tosses, the ball is marked with lime first
   - Student throws forward as far as possible
5. Each student gets 2 chance of throwing
6. Unauthorized throw :
   - At the time of the Student performing the toss, pass through the boundary of the throwing area
   - Rubbers fall off the field
   - The ball falls in the middle of the line between 10 and 20 or 20 and 30 and so on
7. Determination of the winner: the highest score to be a winner

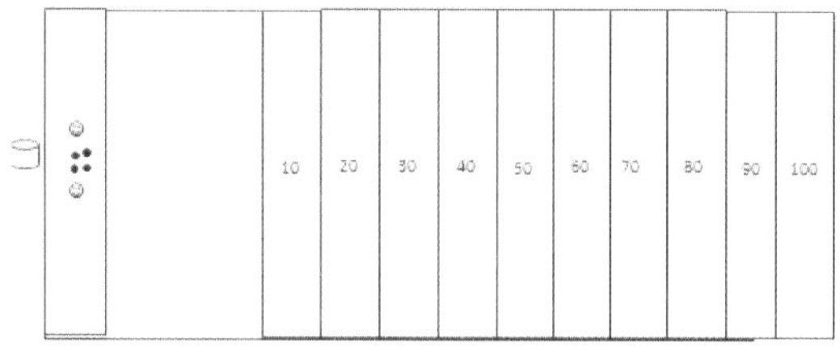

Game of Ball War

1. number of participants: not limited to sharing in 2 groups
2. Tools and materials: 2 baskets, 200 small plastic balls, lime
3. Time allocation: free
4. How To play:
   - Students enter within the throwing area
   - Each group appoints representatives to make a throw
   - Before the tosses, the ball is marked with lime first
   - Students who have divided the group occupy their respective areas
   - Students hold 2 balls in hand
   - After hearing the cue from the teacher the students start throwing each other's law
   - If the ball in hand can be taken again
   - The game will stop if the ball stock in the cart is exhausted.
   - The game will start again if the ball has accumulated in the basket
   - Students self-count how many throws are hit by the opponent

Unauthorized pitch:

- Student throws forward to the gray field area
- Throws the head
- Conducting a toss outside the game area

Determination of winners: highest points

(Picture 2)

Game Throw tires

1. Number of participants: unlimited divided into 2 groups
2. Tools and materials: 4 pancal bike tires, chalk, marker, raffia strapAlokasi waktu : bebas
3. How to play:

- Students enter within the throwing area
- Each group appoints representatives to make a throw
- Student throws forward as far as possible
- Each student gets 2 chance of throwing

Unauthorized pitch:

- Students who throw their legs through the throwing area
- Ban tumbling
- The tires fall in the middle between 10 and 20 or 20 and 30 and so on

4. Determination of the winner: the highest score to be a winner

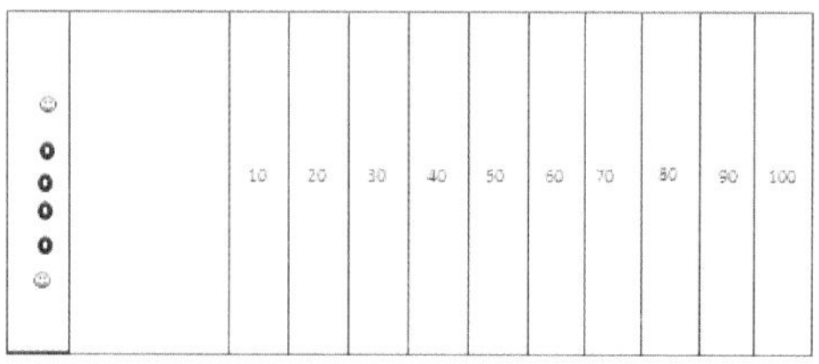

Game push the ball

1. Number of participants: not limited to sharing in 2 groups
2. Tools and materials: volleyball / football 2, plastic soccer ball 2, raffia strap
3. Time allocation: 30 seconds per student
4. How to play:

- Each group appoints representatives for encouragement
- Student stands in front of a volleyball / soccer ball in hanging
- When hearing the cue from the teacher immediately melakun movement push the ball by wearing a plastic ball in the hanging next to it
- Do it repeatedly until the time is finished

5. Unlawful encouragement

- Encourages to cross the line

6. Winner determination: highest score

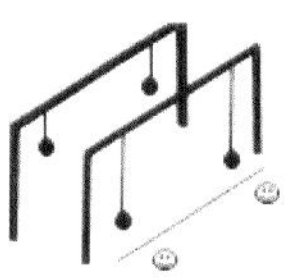

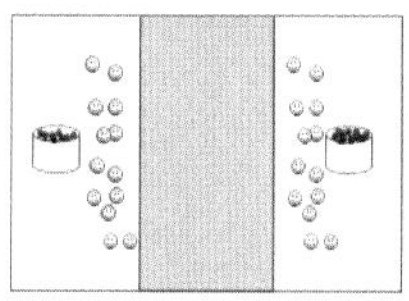

(Picture 2)

Permissions

All chapters in this book were first published in ACTIVE: JPESHR, by Universitas Negeri Semarang ; hereby published with permission under the Creative Commons Attribution License or equivalent. Every chapter published in this book has been scrutinized by our experts. Their significance has been extensively debated. The topics covered herein carry significant findings which will fuel the growth of the discipline. They may even be implemented as practical applications or may be referred to as a beginning point for another development.

The contributors of this book come from diverse backgrounds, making this book a truly international effort. This book will bring forth new frontiers with its revolutionizing research information and detailed analysis of the nascent developments around the world.

We would like to thank all the contributing authors for lending their expertise to make the book truly unique. They have played a crucial role in the development of this book. Without their invaluable contributions this book wouldn't have been possible. They have made vital efforts to compile up to date information on the varied aspects of this subject to make this book a valuable addition to the collection of many professionals and students.

This book was conceptualized with the vision of imparting up-to-date information and advanced data in this field. To ensure the same, a matchless editorial board was set up. Every individual on the board went through rigorous rounds of assessment to prove their worth. After which they invested a large part of their time researching and compiling the most relevant data for our readers.

The editorial board has been involved in producing this book since its inception. They have spent rigorous hours researching and exploring the diverse topics which have resulted in the successful publishing of this book. They have passed on their knowledge of decades through this book. To expedite this challenging task, the publisher supported the team at every step. A small team of assistant editors was also appointed to further simplify the editing procedure and attain best results for the readers.

Apart from the editorial board, the designing team has also invested a significant amount of their time in understanding the subject and creating the most relevant covers. They scrutinized every image to scout for the most suitable representation of the subject and create an appropriate cover for the book.

The publishing team has been an ardent support to the editorial, designing and production team. Their endless efforts to recruit the best for this project, has resulted in the accomplishment of this book. They are a veteran in the field of academics and their pool of knowledge is as vast as their experience in printing. Their expertise and guidance has proved useful at every step. Their uncompromising quality standards have made this book an exceptional effort. Their encouragement from time to time has been an inspiration for everyone.

The publisher and the editorial board hope that this book will prove to be a valuable piece of knowledge for researchers, students, practitioners and scholars across the globe.

List of Contributors

Eka Nandasari
SD N Larikan, Jl. Ds. Larikan-larikan, Kecamatan Doro Kabupaten Pekalongan, Indonesia, 51191

Agus Pujianto and Tri Nur Harsono
Jurusan Pendidikan Jasmani Kesehatan dan Rekreasi, Fakultas Ilmu Keolahragaan, Universitas Negeri Semarang, Indonesia

Muhamad Faozan, Imam Santosa and Mohamad Annas
Department of Health Physical Education and Recreation, Sport Science Faculty, Universitas Negeri Semarang, Indonesia

Agni Herarta Anindya Satria, Sugiyanto and Agus Kristiyanto
Prodi Ilmu Keolahragaan Program Pascasarjana,Universitas Sebelas Maret Surakarta, Indonesia

Suratmin, Gede Eka Budi Darmawan and I Putu Darmayasa
Department of Sport Coaching Education, FOK UNDIKSHA, Indonesia

Indriyanti, Tri Nur Harsono and Rumini
Department of Health Physical Education and Recreation, Sport Science Faculty, Universitas Negeri Semarang, Indonesia

Gestiawan Candra Pramulyarso and Imam Santosa CWW
Jurusan Pendidikan Jasmani Kesehatan dan Rekreasi, Fakultas Ilmu Keolahragaan, Universitas Negeri Semarang, Indonesia

Pandora Wahyu Herjanata
Department of Health physical education and recreation, Sport Science Faculty, Universitas Negeri Semarang, Indonesia

Lina Dewi Nurutami, Heny Setyawati and Agus Raharjo
Department of Health Physical Education and Recreation, Sport Science Faculty, Universitas Negeri Semarang, Indonesia

Farizha Irmawati, Erfitra Rezqi and Ika Oktaviana
Physical Education Program of Health and Recreation, IKIP Budi Utomo Malang, Indonesia

Moch Fahmi Abdulaziz, Harry Pramono, Anirotul Qoriah and Bagus Ginanjar MS
Jurusan Pendidikan Jasmani Kesehatan dan Rekreasi, Fakultas Ilmu Keolahragaan, Universitas Negeri Semarang

Farid Mouissi
APSSES Laboratory, Institute of Physical Education and Sports, University of Chlef, Algeria

Martin Hofmeister
Consumer Centre of the German Federal State of Bavaria, Department Food and Nutrition, Germany

Ketut Chandra Adinata Kusuma and I Kadek Happy Kardiawan
Department of Sport Coaching Education, Faculty of Sport and Health, Universitas Pendidikan Ganesha, Indonesia

Agung Wahyudi
Jurusan Pendidikan Jasmani Kesehatan dan Rekreasi, Fakultas Ilmu Keolahragaan, Universitas Negeri Semarang, Indonesia

Katsran Zalaff and M. Furqon Hidayatullah
Prodi Ilmu Keolahragaan Program Pascasarjana,Universitas Sebelas Maret Surakarta, Indonesia

Devi Fatma Nurlina and Supriyono
Department of Health Physical Education and Recreation, Sport Science Faculty, Universitas Negeri Semarang, Indonesia

Pramoda Wardana and Kiyatno
Prodi Ilmu Keolahragaan Program Pascasarjana, Universitas Sebelas Maret Surakarta, Indonesia

Isnaini Nurul Hidayah and Bambang Priyono
Department of Health Physical Education and Recreation, Sport Science Faculty, Universitas Negeri Semarang, Indonesia

Fraser Carson, Clara McCormack and Julia Walsh
Deakin University, Australia

Novri Gazali and Romi Cendra
Jurusan Pendidikan Jasmani Kesehatan dan Rekreasi, Fakultas Keguruan dan Ilmu Pendidikan Universitas Islam Riau, Indonesia

Ajib Nasir Hanifa, Agus Tomi and Oni Bagus Januarto
Universitas Negeri Malang, Indonesia

Ricky Wibowo, Eka Nugraha and Kuston Sultoni
Universitas Pendidikan Indonesia, Indonesia

Tri Rustiadi, Billy Castyana and Dwi Gansar Santi Wijayanti
Jurusan Pendidikan Jasmani Kesehatan dan Rekreasi, Fakultas Ilmu Keolahragaan, Universitas Negeri Semarang, Indonesia

Sri Febriyani
Jurusan Pendidikan Jasmani Kesehatan dan Rekreasi, Fakultas Ilmu Keolahragaan, Universitas Negeri Semarang, Indonesia

Cheng Yun-Wen
Department of Physical Education Master, National Kaohsiung Normal University, Taiwan

Muhammad Virga Gustifajar, Wasis D. Dwiyogo and Febrita Paulina H
Universitas Negeri Malang, Indonesia

Dhian Kusmiyanti, Agus Kristiyanto and Tri Aprilijanto Utomo
Program Studi Ilmu Keolahragaan, Program Pascasarjana Universitas Sebelas Maret, Surakarta Jawa Tengah, Indonesia

Hartini
Pendidikan Kepelatihan Olahraga, Fakultas Keguruan Dan Ilmu Pendidikan, Universitas Tunas Pembangunan, Surakarta, Jawa Tengah, Indonesia

Yogha Tri Pamungkas, Aris Mulyono and Uen Hartiwan
Department of Physical Education, Faculty of Sport Science, Universitas Negeri Semarang, Indonesia

Jasmani
Department of Sport Coaching Education, Faculty of Teacher Training and Education, Universitas Tunas Pembangunan, Indonesia

Angga Adi Prasetya, M E Winarno and Dona Sandy Yudasmara
Universitas Negeri Malang, Malang, Indonesia

Kartika Septianingrum and Sugiyanto
Postgraduate Program, Sebelas Maret University, Surakarta, Indonesia

Nuril Lolita Hudayhana
Departement of Sport Science, Surabaya State University, Surabaya, Indonesia

Dhevana Pradika Yanda Putra
Project Fellow, University of Muhammadiyah Semarang, Semarang, Indonesia

Abdurrachman and Mucshin Doewes
Program Pascasarjana, Universitas Sebelas Maret, Surakarta, Indonesia

Umar Nurzaman, Sulaiman and Agus Widodo Suripto
Jurusan Pendidikan Jasmani, Kesehatan dan Rekreasi Fakultas Ilmu Keolahragaan, Universitas Negeri Semarang, Semarang, Indonesia

Roas Irsyada and Uen Hartiwan
Jurusan Pendidikan Jasmani, Kesehatan dan Rekreasi Fakultas Ilmu Keolahragaan, Universitas Negeri Semarang, Semarang, Indonesia

Olufunmilola Leah Dominic, Chioma Esther Whoba, Adetayo Ebun Talabi, Surajudeen Tosho Bakinde, Sikiru Adewale Adeoye, Tajudeen Olarewaju Ibraheem and Iliasu Yakubu Seidina
Department of Human Kinetics Education, University of Ilorin, Nigeria

Moses Monday Omoniyi, Asamoah Richmond, Doku Abigail Oforiwaa, Afrifa Daniel, Asamoah-Mensah Anthony, Deku Prince De-Gualle and Tiguridaane Isaac Azo
Department of Sports and Exercise Science, Faculty of Allied Health Sciences, College of Health sciences, Kwame Nkrumah University of Science and Technology, Kumasi, Ghana

Ketut Chandra Adinata Kusuma and I Kadek Happy Kardiawan
Jurusan Pendidikan Kepelatihan Olahraga, Fakultas Olahraga dan Kesehatan, Universitas Pendidikan Ganesha,Indonesia

Barbara A. Masberg and Andrea Eklund
Department of Family and Consumer Sciences Central Washington University

Henri Gunawan Pratama, Khamim Hariyadi and Rohmat Febrianto
STKIP PGRI TRENGGALEK, Indonesia

Irwansyah and Guntur Firmansyah
Pendidikan Jasmani Kesehatan dan Rekreasi, Fakultas Pendidikan Ilmu Eksakta dan Keolahragaan IKIP Budi Utomo, Indonesia

Index

S

T

U

V